MEDICAL RADIOLOGY
Diagnostic Imaging

Editors:
A. L. Baert, Leuven
M. Knauth, Göttingen

Henrik S. Thomsen · Judith A. W. Webb (Eds.)

Contrast Media

Safety Issues and ESUR Guidelines

2nd Revised Edition

With Contributions by

P. Aspelin · M.-F. Bellin · G. Biondi-Zoccai · G. Heinz-Peer · J. Å. Jakobsen · M. Lotrionte
S. K. Morcos · R. Oyen · J. M. Raine · F. Stacul · D. I. Stenver · H. S. Thomsen
A. J. van der Molen · J. A. W. Webb

Foreword by

A. L. Baert

With 10 Figures, 5 in Color and 24 Tables

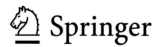 Springer

Henrik S. Thomsen, MD
Professor of Radiology
Consultant, Department of Diagnostic Radiology
Copenhagen University Hospital, Herlev
Director, Department of Diagnostic Sciences
Faculty of Health Sciences
University of Copenhagen
Herlev Ringvej 75
2730 Herlev
Denmark

Judith A.W. Webb, MD, FRCP, FRCR
Consultant (retired)
Department of Radiology
St. Bartholomew's Hospital
University of London
West Smithfield
London EC1A 7BE
UK

Medical Radiology · Diagnostic Imaging and Radiation Oncology
Series Editors:
A. L. Baert · L. W. Brady · H.-P. Heilmann · M. Knauth · M. Molls · C. Nieder

Continuation of Handbuch der medizinischen Radiologie
          Encyclopedia of Medical Radiology

ISBN: 978-3-540-72783-5   e-ISBN: 978-3-540-72784-2

DOI: 10.1007/978-3-540-72784-2

Medical Radiology · Diagnostic Imaging and Radiation Oncology ISSN 0942-5373

Library of Congress Control Number: 2008934596

Cover design: PublishingServices Teichmann, 69256 Mauer, Germany

Printed on acid-free paper

9 8 7 6 5 4 3 2 1

springer.com

Foreword

Two years only after the publication of the first edition of "Contrast media – Safety issues and ESUR guidelines" in our book series Medical Radiology in 2006, it appeared that a second edition was urgently needed.

The first edition was indeed an exceptional success with our readership and sold out rapidly, but moreover the safety of MR contrast media urgently required a reappraisal after the publication of a new and dramatic adverse reaction to some of the gadolinium-based agents: the so called NSF syndrome.

I am very much indebted to Professor Henrik S. Thomsen and his academic colleagues from the ESUR Contrast Medium Safety Committee for accepting the task to prepare a second edition of their remarkable book. Within a record short period of time they have been able to complete this fully revised new volume.

It offers to the readers a comprehensive overview of all problems related to the use of contrast media in modern radiology and of our latest knowledge and insights in the mechanisms of adverse reactions related to contrast media. It answers all questions that radiologists and referring physicians are confronted with in their daily practice when they consider the administration of these agents to their patients.

I congratulate the editors and all contributing authors for this exceptional work, which should again be considered as the standard text for reference and consultation on the highly important issue of safety of contrast media. I am convinced that this second edition will meet the expectations of the readers and that it will soon be available in many radiological offices.

Leuven   ALBERT L. BAERT

Preface to the 2nd Edition

A new edition of *Contrast Media: Safety Issues and ESUR Guidelines* has become necessary relatively soon after the first edition. Unusually for a book on contrast media (CM), the first edition sold out in 30 months. Since the first edition, nephrogenic systemic fibrosis, a serious adverse reaction after some of the gadolinium-based contrast agents, has been recognised, and this has necessitated a reappraisal of these agents.

This second, fully revised edition continues to provide a unique and invaluable source of information on the safety issues relating to CM. It contains a number of completely new chapters, for example, on gadolinium-based CM, meta-analyses in CM research, and various regulatory issues. Comprehensive consideration is given to the many different safety issues relating to iodine based, MR, barium, and ultrasound CM. There are chapters on both acute and delayed non-renal adverse reactions and on renal adverse reactions. All the questions that commonly arise in radiological practice are addressed, and the latest version of the well-known European Society of Urogenital Radiology guidelines on CM is included. We hope that all radiologists will find this book helpful in their everyday practice.

We are very grateful to our academic colleagues in the European Society of Urogenital Radiology Contrast Medium Safety Committee for their invaluable help. They deserve thanks for their continuing involvement in our many debates and discussions. We also thank Prof Albert L. Baert, as well as Ursula N. Davis and her colleagues at Springer Verlag, for their continuous support of this book.

Finally, Henrik thanks his wife, Pia, for endorsing this project again and again.

Herlev, Denmark
London, UK

Henrik S. Thomsen
Judith A. W. Webb

Preface to the 1st Edition

The European Society of Urogenital Radiology established its Contrast Media Safety Committee in 1994. Over the years it has consisted of between 12 and 14 members, the majority of whom are experts in the field of contrast media research. There is currently one member from the scientific section of each of the pharmaceutical companies producing contrast agents (Bracco, Italy; GE Healthcare Diagnostics, USA; Guerbet, France; Schering, Germany). Although the members of the committee have diverse views the Contrast Media Safety Committee works as one group for the good of patients. The committee benefits from the wealth of knowledge on contrast agents brought to it by the representatives of the pharmaceutical companies. However, the rules of the Contrast Media Safety Committee forbid any commercial promotion and the committee deals with all types of contrast agents based purely on objective analysis, sound scientific data, well documented clinical experience and clinical common sense. Disagreement within the committee is discussed rationally and without commercial influence. All contrast media are referred to by their generic names, except when the generic name is confusing (e.g. ultrasound contrast agents). After 11 years of work the committee has covered all the topics of clinical importance regarding the safe use of contrast media. The current book is mainly a collection of this work together with a few new chapters. The chapters have been prepared by the individual authors based on their original papers (see Appendix) when applicable and an up to date review of the literature. Some chapters are new and have never been published as papers by the committee. The chapters have not been circulated among or discussed by the members of the committee and have been edited by myself. In the appendix the latest version of the ESUR guidelines agreed at the meeting of the committee in Copenhagen, February 2005, is presented.

The ESUR guidelines have been well received by the radiological community. They are frequently cited in the literature. They have been incorporated into the protocols of many departments all over the world. They are also used by the health authorities in many countries as a reference for good radiological practice. Several of the guidelines have been translated into languages other than English, for example Spanish, Russian and Japanese.

I am sure the readers will agree that this book offers an invaluable, unique, practical and unparalleled resource dealing with safety issues related to radiographic, MR and ultrasound contrast media, and that it will ultimately benefit patients.

It has been a great honor for me to serve as chairman of this prestigious committee for 9 years. Special mention goes to the secretary of committee, Dr. Sameh Morcos, whose close cooperation has always been highly productive and inspirational. Without his energy and enthusiasm we would never have accomplished what we have. Also, the past and current members of the committee deserve sincere thanks for their continuing involvement and for the outstanding discussions at the annual committee meeting. Despite disagreements we have always reached a consensus. A special thank you goes to Dr. Judith Webb, who has not only participated actively in our work but has also ensured that our manuscripts were published in correct English. Dr. Webb has revised the English throughout this book and I am most grateful for her outstanding and continuous support. We also thank Professor Albert L. Baert, Editor-in-Chief of European Radiology and Editor-in-Chief of this book series, as well as Springer-Verlag for their immediate endorsement and support of the book.

Finally, I wish to thank my family, especially my wife Pia, for allowing me to invest so many hours of family time in this project.

Herlev, Denmark   HENRIK S. THOMSEN

Contents

General Issues

Classification and Terminology

PETER ASPELIN, MARIE-FRANCE BELLIN, JARL Å. JAKOBSEN, and JUDITH A. W. WEBB

CONTENTS

1.1
Introduction

Current radiological imaging uses either electro-magnetic radiation (X-rays or radiowaves) or ultra-sound. X-rays have a frequency and photon energy several powers higher than that of visible light and can penetrate the body. The radiation that emerges from the body is detected either by analogue radiological film or by a variety of digital media. The radiowaves used in magnetic resonance imaging have a frequency and photon energy several powers lower than that of visible light. The radiowaves cause deflection of protons in the body, which have aligned in the magnetic field in the scanner, and as the protons relax back to their resting position, they emit radiowaves, which are used to generate the image. Ultrasound imaging uses sound (pressure) waves several powers higher than audible sound, which are reflected back from tissue interfaces in the body to generate the image.

Contrast agents may be used with all of these imaging techniques to enhance the differences seen between the body tissues on the images. Contrast agents alter the response of the tissues to the applied electromagnetic or ultrasound energy by a variety of mechanisms. The ideal contrast agent would achieve a very high concentration in the tissues without producing any adverse effects. Unfortunately, so far this has not been possible and all contrast agents have adverse effects.

This chapter deals with the classification of contrast agents and the terminology used to describe them.

PETER ASPELIN
Department of Radiology, Karolinska University Hospital, 14186 Stockholm, Sweden
MARIE-FRANCE BELLIN
Department of Radiology,
University Paris-Sud 11, Paul Brousse Hospital,
AP-HP, 12–14 avenue. Paul Vaillant Couturier,
94804 Villejuif Cedex, France
JARL Å. JAKOBSEN
Department of Diagnostic Radiology, Rikshospitalet,
0027 Oslo, Norway
JUDITH A. W. WEBB
Department of Diagnostic Imaging, St. Bartholomew's Hospital, West Smithfield, London EC1A 7BE, UK

1.2
Radiographic Contrast Agents

Radiographic contrast media are divided into positive and negative contrast agents. The positive contrast media attenuate X-rays more than do the body soft tissues and can be divided into water-soluble iodine agents and non-water-soluble barium agents. Negative contrast media attenuate X-rays less than do the body soft tissues. No negative contrast agents are commercially available.

1.2.1
Iodine-Based Contrast Agents

Water-soluble iodine-based contrast agents that diffuse throughout the extracellular space are principally used during computed tomography (CT), angiography and other conventional radiography. They can also be administered directly into the body cavities, for example the gastrointestinal tract and the urinary tract.

All these contrast agents are based on a benzene ring to which three iodine atoms are attached. A monomer contains one tri-iodinated benzene ring and a dimer contains two tri-iodinated benzene rings.

Iodine-based contrast agents can be divided into two groups, ionic and nonionic, based on their water solubility. The water in the body is polarised unevenly with positive poles around the hydrogen atoms and negative poles around oxygen atoms. Ionic contrast agents are water soluble because they dissociate into negative and positive ions, which attract the negative and positive poles of the water molecules. Nonionic contrast agents do not dissociate and are rendered water soluble by their polar OH groups. Electrical poles in the contrast medium OH groups are attracted to the electrical poles in the water molecules.

The osmolality of contrast agents affects the incidence of side-effects, particularly above 800 mosm kg^{-1}. The early contrast media had very high osmolalities (1,500–2,000 mosm kg^{-1}) and subsequently agents of lower osmolality have been developed. Contrast agents may be divided into high-, low- and iso-osmolar agents. An indication of the osmolality of an agent is given by the contrast agent ratio, which is derived by dividing the number of iodine atoms in solution by the number of particles in solution:

$$\text{Contrast agent Ratio} = \frac{\text{Number of iodine atoms}}{\text{Number of particles in solution}}.$$

The higher osmolality agents have more particles per iodine atom and therefore have lower ratios. Thus the ionic monomers have a ratio of 1.5 (three iodine atoms per two particles in solution), the nonionic monomers and the ionic dimers have a ratio of 3 (three iodine atoms per particle in solution), and the nonionic dimers have a ratio of 6 (six iodine atoms per particle in solution) (Fig. 1.1). The nonionic dimers are iso-osmolar with blood (300 mosm kg^{-1}) at all concentrations.

Using these properties four different classes of iodine-based contrast agents may be defined:
1. Ionic monomeric contrast agents (high-osmolar contrast media, HOCM), for example amidotrizoate, iothalamate and ioxithalamate

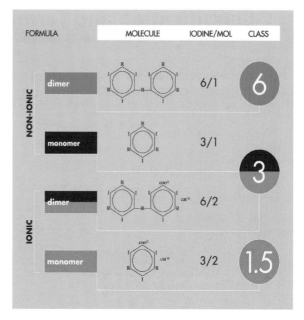

Fig. 1.1. Classification of iodine-based contrast agents

2. Ionic dimeric contrast agents (low-osmolar contrast media, LOCM), for example ioxaglate (Fig. 1.2)
3. Nonionic monomeric contrast agents (low-osmolar contrast media, LOCM), for example iohexol, iopentol, ioxilan, iomeprol, ioversol, iopromide, iobitridol and iopamidol (Fig. 1.2)
4. Nonionic dimeric contrast agents (iso-osmolar contrast media, IOCM), for example iotrolan, iodixanol (Fig. 1.2)

1.2.2
Barium Contrast Agents

Barium sulphate preparations used to visualise the gastrointestinal tract consist of a suspension of insoluble barium sulphate particles, which is not absorbed from the gut. Differences between the different commercially available agents are very minor and relate to the additives in the different barium sulphate preparations.

1.3

MR Contrast Agents

Magnetic resonance (MR) imaging contrast agents contain paramagnetic or superparamagnetic metal ions, which affect the MR signal properties of the

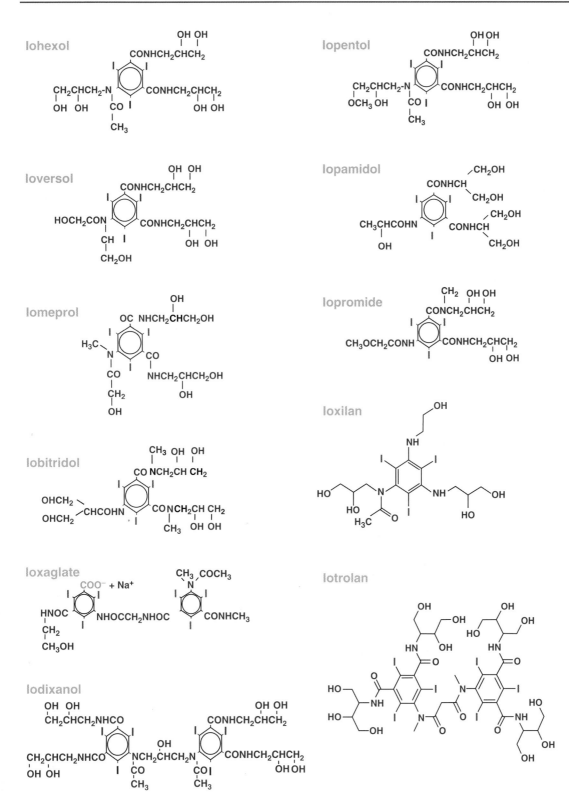

Fig. 1.2. Iodine-based contrast agents (nonionic monomers, ionic and nonionic dimers)

surrounding tissues. They are used to enhance contrast, to characterise lesions and to evaluate perfusion and flow-related abnormalities. They can also provide functional and morphological information.

1.3.1
Paramagnetic Contrast Agents

Paramagnetic contrast agents are mainly positive enhancers that reduce T1 and T2 relaxation times and increase signal intensity on T1 weighted MR images. In most paramagnetic agents, the active constituent is gadolinium, a paramagnetic metal in the lanthanide series, which has a high magnetic moment and a relatively slow electronic relaxation time. In two other paramagnetic agents, the active constituent is manganese, which has similar relaxivity properties to gadolinium, but in contrast to gadolinium is an ion that occurs naturally in the body. In all paramagnetic agents, which are used intravascularly, the active gadolinium or manganese is bound to a ligand in a chelate to minimise its toxicity.

1.3.1.1
Gadolinium Contrast Agents

Gadolinium contrast agents may be considered in two categories: non-specific extracellular gadolinium chelates and high relaxivity agents. The non-specific extracellular gadolinium chelates do not bind to protein and are excreted by the kidney only, while the high relaxivity agents show protein binding and are excreted to a varying extent through the bile as well as by the kidney.

Gadolinium agents are also classified by the chemical structure of the ligand to which the gadolinium is bound. The ligands are either linear or cyclic, and may be ionic, which have a charge in solution, or nonionic. The stability of gadolinium contrast agents depends on their kinetic, thermodynamic and conditional stability. Although these parameters do not directly relate to molecular structure, the contrast agents with cyclic ligands, in which gadolinium is caged in a preorganised cavity, are more stable than those with linear ligands.

Currently available gadolinium contrast agents may be classified as follows (Figs. 1.3, 1.4):
A. Non-specific extracellular gadolinium chelates
   1. Ionic, linear ligand, e.g. gadopentetate dimeglumine
   2. Nonionic, linear ligand, e.g. gadodiamide, gadoversetamide
   3. Ionic, cyclic ligand, e.g. gadoterate dimeglumine
   4. Nonionic, cyclic ligand, e.g. gadobutrol, gadoteridol
B. High relaxivity agents
   Ionic, linear ligand, e.g. gadobenate dimeglumine, gadofosveset trisodium and gadoxetate disodium.

Extracellular non-specific gadolinium contrast agents are given by bolus injection, and their biodistribution and pharmacokinetics are similar to those of iodine-based radiographic contrast agents. High relaxivity gadolinium contrast agents behave similarly to the extracellular non-specific agents immediately after intravascular injection. However, because of their protein binding and biliary excretion, their pharmacokinetics differ and the later liver uptake phase may be used for liver imaging. Of the available high relaxivity agents, gadobenate is mainly used as an extracellular agent, gadofosveset was specifically designed for MR angiography, and gadoxetate, which has the greatest biliary excretion, is mainly used for liver imaging.

1.3.1.2
Liver Specific Agents

As well as the high relaxivity gadolinium contrast agents described in Sect. 1.3.1.1, liver specific agents include two manganese compounds, the manganese chelate mangafodipir trisodium and manganese-chloride together with promoters for oral intake (CMC–001) (Fig. 1.5).

The gadolinium based agents and manganese are taken up to a varying degree by hepatocytes and excreted in the bile. Mangafodipir trisodium releases manganese ions by transmetallation with zinc, and these are bound by alpha 2 macroglobulin and transported to the liver. The manganese chloride preparation is given orally and reaches the liver via the portal system. Manganese has five unpaired electrons and is a powerful T1 relaxation agent. It has greater intracellular uptake than gadolinium and has three times greater T1 relaxivity in liver tissue.

1.3.2
Superparamagnetic Contrast Agents

Superparamagnetic contrast agents include superparamagnetic iron oxides (SPIOs) and ultra small

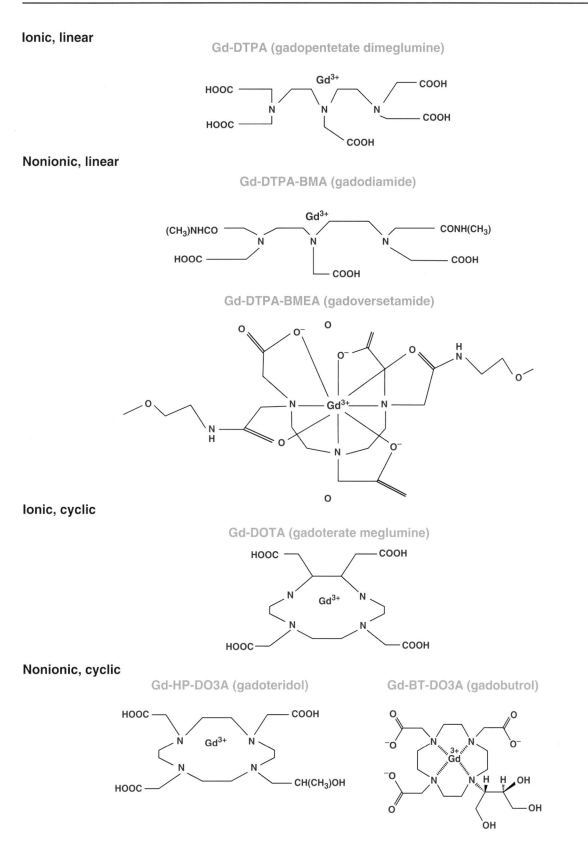

Fig. 1.3. Extracellular gadolinium-based contrast agents

Ionic, linear

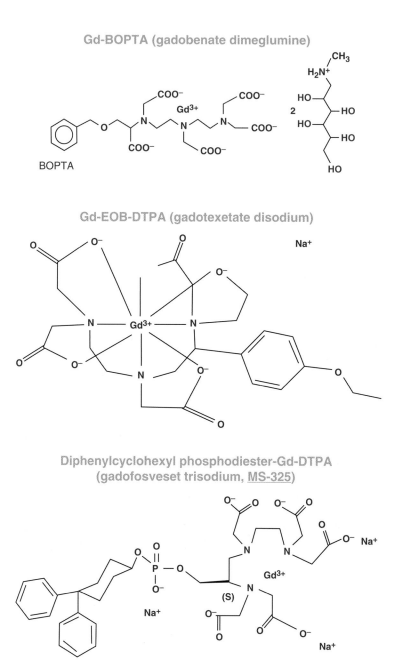

Fig. 1.4. High relaxivity gadolinium-based contrast agents

superparamagnetic iron oxides (USPIOs). Two preparations of SPIOs are available: ferumoxides and ferucarbotran. These particulate agents are composed of an iron oxide core, 3–5 nm in diameter, covered by low molecular weight dextran for ferumoxides and by carbodextran for ferucarbotran, which prevent uncontrolled aggregation of the magnetic crystals.

SPIOs and USPIOs are extremely effective T2 relaxation agents, which produce signal loss on T2 and T2*-weighted images. They also have a T1 effect, which is substantially less than their T2 effect.

In principle, smaller particles circulate longer in the blood space and may accumulate in the macrophages of the lymph nodes, liver and spleen, while large particles have a shorter half life and target the liver more specifically.

Ferumoxides amd ferucarbotran are approved for adult patients and liver imaging while USPIOs

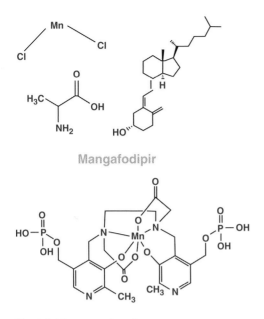

CMC-001

Mangafodipir

Fig. 1.5. Manganese-based contrast agents

are under investigation for MR lymphography. The surface structure of USPIOs gives them an extended circulation time and they also have the potential to be used as positive blood pool contrast agents.

After injection, SPIO and USPIO particles are metabolised into a soluble, non-superparamagnetic form of iron. Iron is incorporated into the body pool of iron (e.g. ferritin, hemosiderin and hemoglobin) within a few days.

1.4
Ultrasound Contrast Agents

Ultrasound contrast agents produce their effect by increased back-scattering of sound compared to that from blood, other fluids, and most tissues. On grey-scale images, microbubble contrast agents change grey and dark areas to a brighter tone when the contrast enters in fluid or blood. The spectral Doppler intensity is also increased, with a brighter spectral waveform displayed and a stronger sound heard. Using color Doppler technique, ultrasound contrast agents enhance the frequency or the power intensity, giving rise to stronger color encoding. The level of enhancement of the Doppler signals may be in the order of up to 30 dB.

Ultrasound contrast agents can be used to enhance Doppler signals from most main arteries and veins.

They may be useful for imaging solid organs, e.g. liver, kidney, breast, prostate and uterus. They can also be used to enhance cavities, e.g. bladder, ureters, Fallopian tubes and abscesses.

1.4.1
Classification

Ultrasound contrast agents can be divided into five different classes: (1) Nonencapsulated gas microbubbles (e.g. agitated or sonicated), (2) stabilised gas microbubbles (e.g. with sugar particles), (3) encapsulated gas microbubbles (e.g. by protein, liposomes or in polymers), (4) microparticle suspensions or emulsions [perfluorooctyl bromide (PFOB), phase-shift], and (5) gastrointestinal (for ingestion). Products from all classes are not commercially available.

Ultrasound contrast agents (USCA) can also be classified based on their pharmacokinetic properties and efficacy: (1) Non-transpulmonary USCAs, which do not pass the capillary bed of the lungs following a peripheral intravenous injection, show on B-mode only in the right ventricle and have a short duration effect, (2) transpulmonary blood pool USCAs with a short half-life (<5 min after an intravenous bolus injection), which produce low signals using harmonic imaging at low acoustic power, (3) transpulmonary blood pool USCAs with a longer half-life (>5 min after an intravenous bolus injection), which produce high signals using harmonic imaging at low acoustic power, (4) transpulmonary USCAs with a specific liver and spleen phase, which can be short- or long-lived. They lodge in the small vessels of the liver or spleen, or are taken up by either the reticuloendothelial system or by the hepatocytes.

Agents that are currently available commercially or are close to being available commercially are listed in Table 1.1.

Table 1.1. Some ultrasound contrast agents

Product name	Constituents
Definity™ (DMP 115)	Fluorocarbon gas in liposomes
SonoVue® (BR1)	Sulphur hexafluoride gas in polymer with phospholipid
Optison™ (FS069)	Octafluoropropane-filled albumin microspheres
Sonazoid™ (NC100100)	Perfluorinated gas-containing microbubbles
Levovist® (SHU 508A)	Galactose-based, palmitic acid stabilised air-bubbles

Requests for Imaging Using Contrast Agents: What Information Must be Provided

2

Sameh K. Morcos and Marie-France Bellin

CONTENTS

2.1
Introduction

There are potential risks associated with the administration of contrast agents and adverse reactions may occur. In addition, contrast agents may interact with some of the drugs and clinical tests used in the management of patients (Thomsen 2006; Morcos 2005a, b; Morcos and Thomsen 2001, Morcos et al. 2001, 2005). Although most serious reactions are observed after intravascular injection, adverse effects may also develop

Sameh K. Morcos
Department of Diagnostic Imaging, Northern General Hospital,
Sheffield Teaching Hospitals NHS Trust,
Sheffield S5 7AU, UK
Marie-France Bellin
Department of Radiology, University Paris-Sud 11,
Paul Brousse Hospital, AP-HP, 12–14 avenue.
Paul Vaillant Couturier, 94804 Villejuif Cedex, France

after oral or intra-cavitary administration because some of the contrast molecules may be absorbed into the circulation (Morcos 2005). Reactions to contrast agents can be divided into non-renal and renal adverse reactions. Non-renal reactions may be acute (developing within 1h of contrast agent administration) or delayed (developing after 1h but less than a week) (Morcos and Thomsen 2001). Some reactions, such as thyrotoxicosis and nephrogenic systemic fibrosis, may occur after 1 week and are termed very late reactions. Patients at high risk of these reactions should be identified before contrast administration to ensure that all necessary measures to reduce the risk are taken.

2.2
Iodine-Based Contrast Media

2.2.1
Risk Factors for Acute Non-Renal Adverse Reactions

There is a sixfold increase in incidence of severe reactions to both ionic and nonionic contrast agents in patients with a history of previous severe adverse reaction to contrast agents. Asthma is also an important risk factor with reported six- to tenfold increase in the risk of a severe reaction in such patients. Patients with a strong history of allergic reactions to different substances including those with a history of troublesome hay fever are also at risk (Morcos 2005a).

2.2.2
Risk Factors for Delayed Skin Reactions

A previous reaction to contrast medium is an important predisposing factor increasing the risk of reaction by a factor of 1.7–3.3. A history of drug or contact allergy is a further risk factor increasing the likelihood of a reaction by approximately a factor of two (Chap. 16). There is an increased incidence of delayed skin reactions to contrast agents in patients who have received nonionic dimers or interleukin-2 (IL-2) (Morcos et al. 2005; Webb et al. 2003).

2.2.3
Risk Factors for Contrast-Induced Nephropathy

Pre-existing renal impairment [serum creatinine > 130 μmol l^{-1} or preferably eGFR < 60 ml min^{-1} 1.73 m^{-2}] calculated according to the Modification of Diet in Renal Disease (MDRD) study equation (Bostom et al. 2002) is an important risk factor particularly if it is associated with diabetes mellitus. The degree of renal insufficiency is a major determinant of the severity of contrast-induced nephropathy (CIN) (Thomsen 2006). An eGFR of 30 ml min^{-1} 1.73 m^{-2} or less markedly increases the incidence and severity of CIN (Morcos et al. 1999; McCullough et al. 1997). Other risk factors include dehydration, congestive cardiac failure, concurrent use of nephrotoxic drugs such as nonsteroidal anti-inflammatory drugs (NSAID) and aminoglycosides, hypertension, hyperuricemia or proteinuria (Morcos et al. 1999; McCullough et al. 1997; Morcos 2004, 2005b).

Since pre-existing renal impairment is a crucial risk factor for CIN, it is important to know the renal function before contrast agents are given, as precautions must be taken in patients with renal insufficiency. Measurement of serum creatinine is used in many centers for this purpose, but has several limitations for accurate assessment of renal function (Morcos 2005b; Thomsen et al. 2005) and eGFR is a better test, when serum creatinine is abnormal, but it is not perfect as all equations overestimate renal function to various degrees.

2.2.4
Risk Associated with Concomitant Medications

Although contrast agents are not highly active pharmacologically, interaction with other drugs may occur with possible serious consequences to the patient (see Chaps. 11, 14). This is an important issue to be included in a questionnaire.

2.2.5
Patients with Thyroid Disease

Radiographic water-soluble iodine-based contrast media solutions contain small amounts of free iodide, which may cause thyrotoxic crisis in patients with Graves' disease or with multinodular goiter and thyroid autonomy, especially if they are elderly and living in areas of iodine-deficiency. Patients at risk of thyrotoxicosis should be closely monitored by endocrinologists after iodine-based contrast medium injection. Prophylaxis is generally not necessary but in high-risk patients, particularly those in areas of dietary iodine deficiency, prophylactic treatment may be given by an endocrinologist (see Chap. 18).

2.3
MRI Contrast Agents

MR contrast agents include extracellular and liver-specific agents. Patients at risk of adverse reactions to these agents are briefly discussed further.

2.3.1
Extracellular Gadolinium-Based Contrast Agents

Most adverse reactions to extracellular agents are mild and transient. Risk factors for acute reactions include a history of allergy, bronchial asthma or previous reaction to gadolinium-based contrast media (Niendorf et al. 1993; Shellock and Kanal 1999).

CIN is rare with doses not exceeding 0.3 mmol kg body weight^{-1} (Ergün et al. 2006; Thomsen 2004; Zhang et al. 2006; Briguori et al. 2006; Sam et al. 2003). However, patients with preexisting severe renal impairment may be at risk of CIN after administration of extracellular non-organ-specific gadolinium-based contrast media (Ergün et al. 2006). High doses of gadolinium agents used for X-ray procedures have a significant risk of inducing nephrotoxicity (Thomsen et al. 2002).

Nephrogenic systemic fibrosis has recently been reported in patients on dialysis or with a glomerular filtration below 30 ml min^{-1}, following administration of lower stability gadolinium-based contrast agents (Chap. 24).

2.3.2
Liver-Specific MR Contrast Agents

MR liver-specific contrast agents include superparamagnetic oxides, manganese contrast agents and hepatobiliary gadolinium chelates. The risk factors with these agents are summarized below.

Superparamagnetic iron oxides (SPIO). Back pain and flushing are the most frequently reported adverse reactions to these agents, but no risk factors have been identified (Ros et al. 1995). However, the administration of these agents in patients with known allergy or hypersensitivity to parenteral iron or dextran should be avoided and they should be used with caution in patients with hemosiderosis or hemochromatosis (Bellin et al. 2005).

Manganese-based contrast agents. Nausea, headache and pruritus may develop after infusion of the intravascular formulation, but no predisposing factors have been identified (Bellin et al. 2005).

Hepatobiliary gadolinium chelates. The most common adverse reactions include headache, nausea, and flushing (Bellin et al. 2005). Serious adverse reactions are rare. No risk factors have been identified for these reactions.

2.4

Discussion

It is vital that all the relevant information about the patient is readily available before contrast agent administration to minimize the potential risks and to take the necessary measures to prevent an adverse reaction. Of all the potential adverse reactions to contrast agents, those which are most likely to have serious sequelae are severe anaphylactoid reactions and CIN. It is proposed that the request for an imaging test requiring contrast agent administration should provide information about important risk factors for these complications. An awareness of the drug history is also important as there is the possibility of interaction between contrast agents and other drugs. In addition, patients with thyroid disease, particularly elderly patients living in regions with iodine deficiency, can be adversely affected by contrast media. Information about risk factors should be available before the appointment for a contrast agent

enhanced examination to plan prophylactic measures or to advise an alternative imaging technique not requiring contrast agent administration. Some of the prophylactic measures such as hydration or steroid prophylaxis require time to produce the desired pharmacological effect. In emergency situations the radiologist should try to obtain as many of the questionnaire answers as possible before contrast agent administration and make a judgment of benefit against risk depending on the clinical problem under investigation.

Demanding an extensive list of information with the request is not practical and may not receive the cooperation of referring clinicians. Thus, it is important to focus the questionnaire on important risk factors for serious complications that are most likely to be encountered in clinical practice. The ESUR contrast agent questionnaire should be considered as a supplement to the standard referral for imaging examinations. It offers a practical approach for identifying patients at high risk of contrast agent reactions without omitting important risk factors or being excessively demanding to use routinely. The completed contrast agent questionnaire should be sent with the request to the Imaging Department for further action. The ESUR questionnaire can be found in Chap. 29.

References

Bellin MF, Webb JAW, van der Molen A, Thomsen HS, Morcos SK, Members of Contrast Media Safety Committee of European Society of Urogenital Radiology (ESUR) (2005). Safety of MR liver specific contrast media. Eur Radiol 15:1607–1614

Bostom AG, Kronenberg F, Ritz E (2002) Predictive performance of renal function equations for patients with chronic kidney disease and normal serum creatinine levels. J Am Soc Nephrol 13:2140–2144

Briguori C, Colombo A, Airoldi F et al. (2006) Gadolinium-based contrast agent and nephrotoxicity in patients undergoing coronary artery procedures. Catheter Cardiovasc Interv 67:175–180

Ergün I, Keven K, Uruç I et al. (2006) The safety of gadolinium in patients with stage 3 and 4 renal failure. Nephrol Dial Transplant 21:697–700

McCullough PA, Wolyn R, Rocher LL et al. (1997) Acute renal failure after coronary intervention: incidence, risk factors and relationship to mortality. Am J Med 103:368–375

Morcos SK (2004) Prevention of contrast media nephrotoxicity – the story so far. Clin Radiol 59:381–389

Morcos SK (2005a) Acute serious and fatal reactions to contrast media: our current understanding. Br J Radiol 78:686–693

Morcos SK (2005b) Prevention of contrast media-induced nephrotoxicity after angiographic procedures. J Vasc Interv Radiol 16:13–23

Morcos SK, Thomsen HS (2001) Adverse reactions to iodinated contrast media. Eur Radiol 11:1267–1275

Morcos SK, Thomsen HS, Webb JAW and members of Contrast Media Safety Committee of the European Society of Urogenital Radiology (ESUR) (1999) Contrast media induced nephrotoxicity: a consensus report. Eur Radiol 9:1602–1613

Morcos SK, Thomsen HS, Webb JAW, Contrast Media Safety Committee of the European Society of Urogenital Radiology (2001) Prevention of generalized reactions to contrast media: a consensus report and guidelines. Eur Radiol 11:1720–1728

Morcos SK, Thomsen HS, Exley CM, Members of Contrast Media Safety Committee of European Society of Urogenital Radiology (ESUR) (2005) Contrast media: interaction with other drugs and clinical tests. Eur Radiol 15:1463–1468

Niendorf HP, Alhassan A, Haustein J, Clauss W, Cornelius I (1993) Safety and risk of gadolinium–DTPA: extended clinical experience after more than 5 000 000 applications. Adv MRI Contrast 2:12–19

Ros PR, Freeny PC, Harms SE, Seltzer SE et al. (1995). Hepatic MR imaging with ferumoxides: a multicenter clinical trial of the safety and efficacy in the detection of focal hepatic lesions. Radiology 196:481–488

Sam AD, Morash MD, Collins J et al. (2003) Safety of gadolinium contrast angiography in patients with chronic renal insufficiency. J Vasc Surg 38:313–318

Shellock FG, Kanal E (1999) Safety of magnetic resonance imaging contrast agents. J Magn Reson Imaging 10: 477–484

Thomsen HS (2004) Gadolinium-based contrast media may be nephrotoxic even at approved doses. Eur Radiol 14: 1654–1656

Thomsen HS (ed) (2006) Contrast media: safety issues and ESUR guidelines. Springer, Heidelberg

Thomsen HS, Almén T, Morcos SK, Members of Contrast Media Safety Committee of European Society of Urogenital Radiology (2002) Gadolinium-containing contrast media for radiographic examinations: a position paper. Eur Radiol 12:2600–2605

Thomsen HS, Morcos SK, Members of Contrast Media Safety Committee of European Society of Urogenital Radiology (ESUR) (2005) In which patients should serum-creatinine be measured before contrast medium administration? Eur Radiol 15:749–754

Webb JAW, Stacul F, Thomsen HS, Morcos SK, members of the Contrast Media Safety Committee of the European Society of Urogenital Radiology (ESUR) (2003) Late adverse reactions to intravascular iodinated contrast media. Eur Radiol 13:181–184

Zhang HL, Ersoy H, Prince MR (2006) Effects of gadopentetate dimeglumine and gadodiamide on serum calcium, magnesium, and creatinine measurements. JMRI 23:383–387

Off-Label Use of Medicines: Legal Aspects

3

JUNE M. RAINE

CONTENTS

3.1
Introduction

In Europe, subject to certain exemptions explained later, no medicine can be marketed for human use without a Marketing Authorisation granted either by a Member State competent authority or by the European Commission. The regulatory system exists to protect patients by ensuring that marketed medicines meet acceptable standards of safety, quality and efficacy in their indications. Nonetheless, for a range of reasons use of medicines outside their authorised indications, commonly known as off-label use, and use of unlicensed medicines (i.e. medicines without a marketing authorisation) are

J. M. RAINE
Medicines and Healthcare Products Regulatory Agency,
Market Towers, 1 Nine Elms Lane, London, SW8 5NQ, UK

common. This chapter outlines the definition of a medicine and the current regulatory framework; reviews the legal position of prescribers of off-label use and the use of unlicensed medicines; considers special populations and therapeutic areas where off-label use or the use of unlicensed medicines is common; and provides some general guidance for prescribers considering off-label use or the use of unlicensed medicines.

3.2
Definition of a Medicine

As diagnostic agents, contrast media fall within the definition of a medicine in European law, since the definition includes

'Any substance or combination of substances which may be used in or administered to human beings ... with a view to ... making a medical diagnosis'.

The legislation also encompasses radiopharmaceuticals:

'Any medicinal product which, when ready for use, contains one or more radionuclides (radioactive isotopes) included for a medicinal purpose'.

Marketing authorisation is required for radionuclide generators, kits, radionuclide precursor radiopharmaceuticals and industrially prepared radiopharmaceuticals. A marketing authorisation is not required for a radiopharmaceutical prepared at the time of use by a person or by an authorised establishment, according to national legislation, to use such medicinal products in an approved health care establishment exclusively from authorised radionuclide generators, kits or radionuclide precursors in accordance with the manufacturer's instructions.

European medicine legislation does not apply to the following:

- Medicines prepared in a pharmacy in accordance with a medical prescription for an individual patient (the 'magistral formula')
- Medicines prepared in a pharmacy in accordance with the prescriptions of a pharmacopoeia and intended to be supplied directly to the patients served by the pharmacy (the 'officinal formula')
- Medicines for research and development trials [covered by the Directive 2001/20/EC on good clinical practice in the conduct of clinical trials for human use ('the Clinical Trials Directive')]
- Intermediate products intended for further processing by an authorised manufacturer
- Any radionuclides in the form of sealed sources

3.3

The European Regulatory System

The European regulatory system governing the marketing of medicines for human use is set out in Directive 2001/83/EC as amended, Regulation (EC) No.726/2004 and associated legislation. The regulation lays down community procedures for the authorisation, supervision and pharmacovigilance of medicines, establishes a European Medicines Agency and sets up a scientific committee attached to the Agency, the Committee for Human Medicinal Products. It makes provision for medicines to be approved by the European Commission via centralised authorisations valid in all member states.

The centralised procedure must be used for certain specified categories of medicines and can also be used for medicines that contain a new active substance or that constitute a significant therapeutic, scientific or technical innovation. It is therefore unsurprising that a number of new diagnostic imaging agents have been authorised by the centralised route. The Directive sets in place decentralised and mutual recognition systems, enabling authorisations to be granted nationally by Member States. For the foreseeable future, depending on the route by which a medicine has been authorised, differences may exist in Europe between member states' authorisations for the same product and in availability of medicines. The result is that use may be within an authorisation in one country and off-label in another.

The terms in which a marketing authorisation is granted are specified in the Summary of Product Characteristics (SPC), with which all advertising must comply. The SPC contains detailed provisions covering indications, recommended dosage, contra-indications, special warnings and precautions, and adverse effects associated with the medicine. Copies of SPCs are available from the marketing authorisation holder, from the European Medicines Agency, from some Member State competent authorities and via the Electronic Medicines Compendium on www.medicines.org.uk. The SPC also forms the basis for the Patient Information Leaflet (PIL), which accompanies the medicine and is written in terms that are understandable by patients. Clearly, a medicine that is unlicensed will not have an SPC or PIL. Marketing authorisation holders are required to keep their authorisations up to date as new information accrues in clinical use, and there is naturally a particular focus on safety data. New evidence on efficacy may not be so readily identified and manufacturers may legitimately decline to market a medicine for a purpose they do not wish to support.

3.4

Definition of Off-Label Use

The term "off-label use" applies to prescribing or administration outside any of the terms of the marketing authorisation, generally in relation to indications, dosage, or contra-indications. The expression relates to a term used in the US authorisation process: the Food and Drug Administration (FDA) approves product labelling. A medicine that is prescribed off-label will be accompanied by information that may not be consistent with its off-label use, creating the potential for concern or confusion on the part of the patient, parent or carer.

In the light of the regulatory framework, there are a number of situations where off-label use or the use of unlicensed medicines occurs:

- Products for which a marketing authorisation application or variation has yet to be made. These include drugs in development and undergoing clinical trials.
- Medicines for which a marketing authorisation application or variation has been refused.
- Medicines that no longer have a relevant marketing authorisation because it has been suspended, revoked, not renewed or compulsorily varied.
- Products prepared in formulations specially adapted to special populations such as lower

strengths for children or liquids for the elderly or without particular excipients for patients allergic to them.

The use of unlicensed medicines in clinical trials is subject to the provisions of the Clinical Trials Directive and is not dealt with in this chapter.

3.5

Special Populations and Special Therapeutic Areas

Off-label prescribing of medicines, and the prescribing of unlicensed medicines, is common in the areas of oncology, obstetrics, and infectious disease in particular in HIV/AIDS, and is particularly common in the paediatric population. Hospital-based studies have shown that many drugs used in children are either not licensed or are prescribed off-label. On general paediatric surgical and medical wards 36% of children received at least one drug that was unlicensed or off-label during their in-patient stay. In paediatric intensive care this figure was 70% and in neonatal intensive care it was 90%. A study of children's wards in five European countries found that almost half of all prescriptions were either unlicensed or off label. This is consistent with the UK licensing position on contrast media – of around 90 licensed products, about 50% are indicated in children.

This situation has resulted from practical, ethical and commercial considerations relating to conducting clinical trials in children. There are difficulties in developing formulations appropriate for children, and funding for research into the paediatric use of established medicines has been lacking. Following initiatives taken by the FDA in 1997 and 1999 to create incentives and obligations to conduct trials in children, the position is changing. Drawing on the experience of the US legislation, the European Commission subsequently published its own proposals, and in January 2007, a new Paediatric Regulation ((EC) No. 1901/2006) came into force, which established a system of incentives and requirements to improve the availability of licensed medicines for children. Importantly, the European Regulation contains provisions for research funding, improved information on the use of medicines in children and publication of information from clinical trials in children, by the end of 2009.

3.6

Legal Position of the Prescriber

The regulatory system aims to control the activities of pharmaceutical companies manufacturing, selling or supplying medicines. It is not intended to impact on the practice of medicine. European legislation does not require member states to prohibit the prescription or administration of medicines outside their authorised indications. Medicines prescribed outside the terms of the marketing authorisation may be dispensed by pharmacists and administered by nurses or midwives. In addition, the legislation contains a specific exemption, which enables Member States to permit the supply of unlicensed medicines for individual patients at the order of their doctor – Article 5 of Directive 2001/83/EC provides that 'a Member State may, in accordance with the legislation in force and to fulfil special needs, exclude from the provisions of this Directive medicinal products supplied in response to a bona fide unsolicited order, formulated in accordance with the specifications of an authorised health-care professional and for use by an individual patient under his direct personal responsibility'. This provision is the basis for what is referred to as the 'specials' regime. The exemption helps preserve the clinical freedom to act in what is judged to be in the best interests of the individual patient.

The way in which European legislation is framed means that doctors can

- Prescribe medicines off-label
- Prescribe unlicensed products for individual patients, either under the specials regime (i.e. when no suitable licensed alternative is available) or where they are specially prepared in a pharmacy
- Supply another doctor with an unlicensed medicine, in accordance with the specials regime
- Use unlicensed medicines in clinical trials
- Use or advise the use of licensed medicines for indications or in doses or by routes of administration outside the recommendations given in the licence (i.e. off-label)
- Subject to the points made below, prescribe or recommend the use of a medicine contrary to any warnings or precautions given in the marketing authorisation

While European legislation and the regulatory system permits the off-label use or, in certain circumstances, the use of unlicensed medicines, consideration also needs to be given to potential civil liability of the prescriber, in particular for negligence, in the event that such use results in an injury to a patient.

Even in relation to an unlicensed product, manufacturers retain a responsibility for the efficacy and safety of their product under Directive 85/374/EEC on the liability for defective products (in the UK, see the Consumer Protection Act 1987), subject to the product being stored and administered correctly. A manufacturer is, however, unlikely to be liable if injury results not from an inherent defect in the product or its accompanying information, but from the decision of the doctor to use the product off-label or to use an unlicensed product for a particular patient.

The law relating to medical negligence differs in different Member States, but generally provides for the imposition of liability on individual prescribers in certain circumstances. In the UK, a doctor owes a duty of care to his individual patients; if he breaches that duty by failing to take reasonable care and a patient is injured as a result, he will be liable for negligence. A doctor will generally not be considered negligent if his actions would be accepted as proper by a responsible body of medical professional opinion. The courts will not, however, consider a body of opinion as responsible if that opinion is not capable of withstanding logical analysis.

A doctor is also responsible for obtaining the consent of the patient to the treatment in question. Failure to obtain fully informed consent may amount to negligence.

3.7

Guidance for Prescribers

The responsibility for prescribing any medicine falls on the prescribing physician or health care professional. If the prescription is for an unlicensed medicine or for off-label use, these responsibilities are enhanced.

First, when prescribing an unlicensed medicine or a medicine for off-label use, the prescriber is responsible for determining whether it is appropriate to use the medicine as proposed for the individual patient. Where the proposed use is not covered by the terms of a marketing authorisation, the prescriber should consider the safety and efficacy of the product in relation to the proposed use. The prescriber needs to be satisfied that there is sufficient evidence and/or experience of using the medicine to demonstrate its safety and efficacy. The prescriber should consider

any relevant published literature, clinical guidance or clinical trial data made available by regulatory authorities or companies themselves. Prescribers can also rely on information and guidance from a responsible body of medical opinion. In the area of paediatrics, for example the UK benefits from the availability of the British National Formulary for Children, which itself was based on the publication 'Medicines for Children' produced by the Royal College of Paediatrics and Child Health. Other examples of specific therapeutic guidance are available.

In relation to unlicensed medicines, other than a medicine prepared in a pharmacy in accordance with a prescription, the doctor must also be satisfied that an alternative licensed medicine would not meet the patient's needs.

The second responsibility of prescribers undertaking off-label prescribing or the prescribing of unlicensed medicines is to ensure that the patient, parent or carer is adequately informed about the risks and benefits of the medicine, in the absence of authorised product information. It has been recommended that, when obtaining consent to treatment, the doctor should tell the patient of the drug's licence status, and that for an unlicensed medicine its effects will be less well known and understood than those of a licensed product. The provision of information by the prescriber is particularly important in relation to off-label use, where the patient information leaflet may provide conflicting information or information not relevant to such use, and in relation to unlicensed medicines, where no such leaflet is available. In relation to off-label use, the prescriber should have access to the up-to-date Summary of Product Characteristics to give appropriate information and advice.

Providing a full verbal or written explanation to the patient and recording that in writing helps ensure that the patient understands the risks involved and gives genuine and informed consent. This also reduces the risk of liability on the part of the prescriber in the event of injury to the patient.

Third, prescribers have a professional responsibility for monitoring the safety of medicines and for submission of reports of any suspected adverse drug reactions to the competent authority of the Member State. This applies to unlicensed medicines no less than authorised products. Some Member States have introduced a legal requirement requiring health professionals to report suspected adverse drug reactions, but this does not appear to have resulted in higher reporting rates.

3.8

Conclusion

The use of medicines according to the terms of the marketing authorisation is supported by evidence of safety, quality and efficacy, which has satisfied regulatory authorities of Member States or the European Commission. It is generally understood and accepted that there are clinical situations where off-label use or the use of unlicensed medicines may be judged by the prescriber to be in the patient's best interests, on the basis of the evidence available, indicating a likely favourable benefit:risk balance. In such cases, the onus is on the prescriber to be familiar with the available evidence of risk and benefit, to make appropriate information available to the patient, parent or carer, and to monitor safety in use. If appropriate care is taken, information provided and decisions related to off-label use or use of unlicensed medicines recorded, the risk of a prescriber being found liable for any mishap should be minimised.

Pharmacovigilance: When to Report Adverse Reactions

Doris I. Stenver

4.1

Introduction

Effective drug safety surveillance – pharmacovigilance – is of the utmost importance for patients. A surveillance system should be in place for all medicinal products, including contrast agents. The main objectives of pharmacovigilance are the early *detection* of new adverse drug reactions, risk *assessment*, risk *minimization*, and risk *communication*.

Health care professionals play a key role in safety surveillance, as they are front line observers when serious and unexpected adverse effects (Table 4.1) occur. They are under an obligation to report their observations and suspicions to the regulatory authorities, which can then react in an appropriate and timely manner. The responsibility of the health care professionals starts before administration of any medicinal product to patients – whether for therapeutic, preventive, or diagnostic purposes – when they should always make a careful risk/benefit assessment.

Doris I. Stenver
Danish Medicines Agency
Member of the CHMP Pharmacovigilance Working Party,
Axel Heides gade 1, DK-2300 København S, Denmark

It is important to be aware that drug safety surveillance is necessary for the entire life cycle of drugs, beginning in the premarketing phase and continuing throughout the postmarketing period. The recently identified condition of *nephrogenic systemic fibrosis* associated with the administration of gadolinium-based MR contrast agents to patients with renal impairment underlines this fact (STENVER 2008). Occasionally, it is necessary to monitor safety after marketing has been discontinued, for example, in the case of suspected late-onset adverse events, or to gather information on the outcome of observed events.

During the premarketing phase, information on risk is provided from the various preclinical and clinical studies. After market authorization, information on risk is collected from several sources, mainly through the spontaneous reporting system and from postmarketing safety studies.

4.2

The Adverse Drug Reaction Reporting System

For four decades the system for adverse drug reaction reporting has been a cornerstone and mainstay of drug safety surveillance.

The thalidomide tragedy in the 1960s (LENZ 1966) lead to the establishment in many countries of national public institutions responsible for collecting, registering, and assessing adverse drug reaction reports (FINNEY 1965; DUKES 1985). Since then, the field of pharmacovigilance has undergone significant development, and is today primarily governed by internationally agreed legislative rules (DIRECTIVE 2001).

The *key stakeholders* in the spontaneous reporting system are health care professionals, national and

Table 4.1. Definitions

Adverse reaction: A response to a medicinal product which is noxious and unintended and which occurs at doses normally used in man for the prophylaxis, diagnosis, or therapy of disease or for the restoration, correction, or modification of physiological function

Unexpected adverse reaction: an adverse reaction, the nature, severity, or outcome of which is not consistent with the summary of product characteristics

international authorities, and marketing authorization holders.

Health care professionals are responsible for reporting suspected adverse reactions to the authorities[1]. In some countries, reporting of adverse drug reactions by health care professionals is voluntary and in other countries either mandatory or a mixture of mandatory and voluntary. In Denmark, for example, reporting is mandatory during the first 2 years of marketing, during which period health care professionals should report *all* suspected adverse drug reactions they observe. Following the first 2-year period, health care professionals in Denmark are obliged to report all suspected or serious unexpected adverse reactions they observe for the entire marketing period.

The authorities are responsible not only for registration of the reports in a national database, but also for forwarding the reports to the marketing authorization holder responsible for putting the product on the market. Once they have received adverse drug reaction reports from health care professionals, the authorities are also obliged to forward the reports to the Eudravigilance database established at the European drug regulatory authority, EMEA, and to the WHO. All adverse drug reactions classified as serious should be exchanged between the authorities and the marketing authorisation holders (and vice versa) within 15 days of receipt. The reports are also submitted to the WHO database. Thus *through the reporting system all the observations made by health care professionals at a national level are in effect provided to a large international community.*

The *assessment* is undertaken by the authorities and the marketing authorization holders in collabo-

ration. The assessment is made on the basis of individual case reports when they are received, and also after individual reports have been included in the periodic safety update reports, which marketing authorization holders are obliged to submit to the authorities at intervals after marketing has started.

Every assessment concludes with a decision about whether new safety data have been discovered, and – if this is the case – whether the safety profile of the product has in fact changed. The need to revise the labeling (Summary of Product Characteristics, Package Insert Leaflet) by introducing, for example, new contraindications, warnings, or precautionary measures or by adding new adverse drug reactions has to be considered. Whether further risk minimization measures, for example, a request for further studies or creation of registries is required, and whether information should be provided to health care professionals and the public also need to be considered.

4.3
When Should Adverse Reactions be Reported?

Ideally health care professionals should report all suspected serious adverse drug reactions to the authorities, even though the adverse reaction may be known and appears on the package insert leaflet. In addition, health care professionals should consider reporting known non-serious reactions, because the perceived frequency of these based on clinical trials may in fact differ from that observed in the post-marketing setting.

It is well recognized that adverse drug reactions are under-reported all over the world. The many reasons for under-reporting of adverse drug reactions include insufficient time to complete reporting forms, lack of knowledge of the impact of reporting, and the fact that the patient's symptoms may not be recognized by health professionals to be drug-related.

The recently discovered association of the severe, disabling, and occasionally fatal condition nephrogenic systemic fibrosis (NSF) with the use of gadolinium-based MR contrast agents in patients with renal impairment illustrates the challenges of drug safety surveillance. It is noteworthy that gadolinium-based contrast agents had been used for more than a decade in a huge number of patients, and that the condition of *nephrogenic systemic fibrosis* had been described in the

---

[1] In recent years patient reporting (adverse drug reaction reports received directly from consumers/citizens) has become accepted by several European authorities, and it is foreseen that the legislative basis for patient or consumer reporting will be introduced by the upcoming revision of the European Union (EU) legislation.

literature for some years before GROBNER in 2006 finally realized that NSF and gadolinium could be linked.

It is also noteworthy that many health care professionals seemed to be reluctant to report new suspected cases of NSF to the national regulatory authorities and instead preferred to publish small case series in scientific journals. This led to considerable delay in the collection of sufficient data for the necessary regulatory actions to be taken to prevent further cases and to protect patients.

In addition, the adverse drug reaction reports have facilitated an increased understanding of the risk profile across the whole class of gadolinium agents. This meant that it was possible to introduce risk minimization measures to the benefit of all patients who receive gadolinium-based MR contrast media.

References

Directive 2001/83/EC, Pharmacovigilance for medicinal products for human use, vol. 9A. Regulation (EC) No. 726/2004 (http://ec.europa.eu/enterprise/pharmaceuticals/eudralex/)

Dukes G (1985) The effects of drug regulation. A survey based on European studies of drug regulation. MTP Press, Falcon House, Lancaster, England

Finney DJ (1965) The design and logic of a monitor of drug use. J Chronic Dis 18:77–98

Grobner T (2006) Gadolinium – a specific trigger for the development of nephrogenic fibrosing dermatopathy and nephrogenic systemic fibrosis? Nephrol Dial Transplant 21:1104–1108

Lenz W (1966) Malformations caused by drugs in pregnancy. Am J Dis Child 112:99–106

Stenver DI (2008) Pharmacovigilance: What to do if you see an adverse reaction and the consequences. Eur J Radiol 66:184–186

What is Required in Order to Get the Authorities to Approve a New Contrast Agent?

Doris I. Stenver

CONTENTS

5.1
Introduction

The evaluation of diagnostic agents is governed by the same regulatory rules and principles as those for other medicinal products. The requirements for applications for Marketing Authorization for medicinal products in the EU, including all contrast agents, are provided in Directive 2001/83/EC as amended.

Several guidance documents have been developed to further amplify the requests laid down in the legislation.

The most important guidelines which give advice on *clinical* evaluation are the following:

Doris I. Stenver
Danish Medicines Agency
Member of the CHMP Pharmacovigilance Working Party, 1 Axel Heides Gade, DK-2300 Copenhagen S, Denmark

- Guideline on clinical evaluation of diagnostic agents (Emea 2008)
- Good clinical practice (International Conference for Harmonization, ICH, topic E6)
- Statistical principles for clinical trials (ICH topic E9)
- Choice of control group (ICH topic E10)
- Structure and content of clinical study reports (ICH topic E3)

This chapter summarizes the Guideline on Clinical Evaluation of Diagnostic Agents (Emea 2008), which outlines the principles for the clinical evaluation of diagnostic agents intended for in vivo administration.

The European Public Assessment Reports for the two latest approved gadolinium-containing MR contrast agents, gadofosveset trisodium (Vasovist®) and gadoversetamide (Optimark®), will be used to illustrate the nonclinical and clinical parts of the process of application for approval.

5.2
General Principles of Evaluation

The principles used for the evaluation of medicinal products with respect to quality, pharmacology, toxicology, pharmacokinetics, and safety also apply to diagnostic agents. However, since contrast agents are used to diagnose and monitor diseases or conditions and not for treatment, the clinical development programs have to be adapted accordingly.

In general, approval of a contrast agent is usually based on the clinical indications for its use rather than the general properties of a specific molecule. However, the general properties should be described in the application.

In practice, the requirements for authorization for completely *new* contrast agents may differ from those for contrast agents *similar to* contrast agents that have already been approved. Examples of the latter would be iodinated monomers or nontissue-specific extracellular gadolinium chelates which share several similarities with an already approved contrast agent (such as chemical structure/class, pharmacokinetic profile, dose and dosing regimen of the active moiety), but frequently differ in the chemical structure of the carrier molecule. For such compounds, so-called noninferiority comparative trials against a similar already approved agent are recommended. The aim is to show similar technical and diagnostic performances (sensitivity and specificity) as well as similar or better safety profile for the same patient population or indication. This relatively limited evidence for assessing the clinical benefit of these products is based on the claim(s) for the same indication that has already been granted to the similar approved contrast agent (the comparator). If the aim is to show superiority of the new contrast agent, this limited evidence may not be sufficient and, in addition to better technical and diagnostic performance, the impact on diagnostic thinking and patient management (see below) may need to be shown or at least discussed in the submission. However, if the impact of the diagnosis provided by the comparator contrast agent that has already been approved is widely accepted, better technical and diagnostic performance may be sufficient to support a claim of superiority.

If use for a new indication not approved for the similar contrast agent is claimed, the requirements for approval are identical to those required for a new product. It is then necessary to show adequate technical and diagnostic performance in relation to a *standard of truth* (e.g., the histopathological diagnosis). In addition, when appropriate, technical and diagnostic performance should be compared to an established contrast agent in the clinical context in which the new agent is to be used.

Quality Aspects

Chemical, pharmaceutical, and biological aspects of the contrast agent should be presented in detail in the application.

A wide range of information about the *active substance* of the contrast agent should be provided, such as the composition and molecular structure and the administration form and dosage.

The stepwise manufacturing process should be adequately described, for example, the chemical synthesis, purification steps, etc. Specifications for starting materials, reagents, catalysts, and solvents should be provided. Information on how the structure has been elucidated (e.g., elemental analysis, infrared spectroscopy, ultraviolet spectroscopy, optical rotation, mass spectrometry) should be given, together with data on how physico-chemical parameters (e.g., polymorphism, solubility, particle size) have been analyzed.

The active substance specification should include data on appearance, identification tests, purity control, and stability.

Also for the *medicinal product*, the manufacturing process, product specification, and stability data should be provided.

Nonclinical Evaluation

The nonclinical data comprises data on pharmacology, pharmacokinetics, and toxicology and studies should be performed in accordance with Good Laboratory Practice (GLP) requirements.

For example, when considering the pharmacological characteristics of magnetic resonance agents, the degree of albumin binding and the ability to alter proton relaxation times in vitro and in vivo are of the utmost importance. Depending on the claimed indication(s), other aspects such as renal contrast enhancement, imaging performance in cerebral metastatic disease, and permeability of the blood brain barrier should be documented. Comparisons between contrast agents with similar structure may facilitate the evaluation. As an example, in vitro and in vivo investigations of primary as well as secondary pharmacodynamics were performed for the recently approved contrast agent gadoversetamide in comparison with gadopentetate dimeglumine.

In vitro and in vivo safety pharmacology studies should provide data on the effect on vital organ functions, such as convulsive threshold and risk of QT-prolongation.

Ideally, the potential for pharmacodynamic drug interactions should also be investigated. For example, for gadofosveset trisodium, a series of drug interaction studies were performed to assess the ability to displace frequently used drugs, such as digoxin and warfarin, from their binding sites on human serum albumin. In addition, the potential effect of commonly used drugs on MRI efficacy was examined. For gadoversetamide, no studies on pharmacodynamic drug interactions were available before the marketing authorization was issued.

The pharmacokinetic data set should include data on absorption, biodistribution or bioavailability, metabolism, and excretion. The pharmacokinetic testing is typically performed in two or more of the species used for toxicology testing (rat, rabbit, dog, monkey) and using the administration route intended for use in man.

The toxicology test program should as a minimum include *single dose* toxicity, *repeat dose* toxicity, *geno*toxicity, *carcino*genicity, and *reproduction* toxicity.

Finally, potential *eco*toxic and environmental risks should be assessed.

5.5
Clinical Evaluation

5.5.1
Good Clinical Practice (GCP) and Ethics

The clinical trials used to support the marketing authorization application should be designed, conducted, recorded, and reported in compliance with the GCP principles as laid down in regulations and guidelines. In addition, all studies should be conducted in accordance with the Declaration of Helsinki.

5.5.2
Fundamental Requirements

The guideline on clinical evaluation of diagnostic agents (Emea 2008) states that in order to establish an indication for a contrast agent, it is necessary to demonstrate its benefit by assessing its technical performance (including procedural convenience), diagnostic performance, impact on diagnostic thinking, patient management, clinical outcome, and safety. In addition, a *clinical* pharmacology study program should be performed to provide data on safety, tolerance, pharmacokinetics, and pharmacodynamic dose-related effects.

It is necessary to assess technical performance, for example, from image quality, but this on its own is not enough to show the clinical benefit of a new contrast agent and cannot be the sole basis for approval.

The diagnostic performance consists of the sensitivity and specificity of a test. The trade-off between sensitivity and specificity requires careful analysis in relation to the intended applications and the implications for patient care. The impact of disease prevalence should also be taken into consideration.

The impact on diagnostic thinking refers to the impact of a test result on posttest vs. pretest probability of a correct diagnosis in a well-defined clinical context, which includes patient characteristics and other diagnostic procedures. Positive as well as negative predictive values are important parameters that influence the impact of use of the contrast agent on diagnostic thinking in a given patient.

A description and quantification of the impact of the diagnostic information obtained on the management of a patient and of the clinical outcome are generally obtained through an appropriate questionnaire. An assessment of the potential benefits and risks arising from the impact on therapeutic decisions should be made. In particular, the consequences of an incorrect diagnosis (false positive or false negative) must be considered.

For each claim, the contrast agent may be used alone or in combination with other diagnostic procedures necessary for the indication claimed. This should always be specified in the study protocol. If several indications or claims are planned for one imaging agent, it may be considered necessary to perform separate clinical trials.

5.5.3
Methodological Considerations

The protocol should describe the trial objectives or claim, the contrast agents and methods investigated (including the investigational agent, absolute or surrogate standard of truth, comparator, and other clinical assessments and procedures), testing procedures, trial population, sample size calculation, endpoint justification, blinding, randomization, statistical considerations, and principles for data presentation.

Relevant data on the diagnostic performance of the contrast agent obtained from earlier phases of its clinical development (phase II studies) should be used to design subsequent confirmatory trials.

Special attention should be given to the trade-off between sensitivity and specificity, taking the intended clinical use into consideration, and to the justification of power calculations and acceptance limits in relation to clinical relevance. It is particularly important to design the trials in relation to the intended clinical use of the contrast agent. For example, different trials will be required if the contrast agent under investigation will be used to provide additional information when insufficient diagnostic information is obtained from established tests or if it will be used as an alternative to established standard tests.

Comparative studies are required if the investigational contrast agent is being developed both as an alternative and as an improvement over existing contrast agents. An appropriate comparator agent would be one which is widely accepted in the EU for the claimed indication and reflects current good medical practice. The choice of comparator must be justified and the corresponding procedures clearly described. The comparison should include evaluation of both efficacy and safety data.

For contrast agents, the unenhanced procedure may serve as an appropriate comparator for evaluating the added value of the contrast agent. However, comparison with a marketed comparator contrast agent is ideal.

Two recent marketing authorization applications illustrate this process. For gadoversetamide (Optimark®), the four submitted pivotal studies shared the same design, and were multicenter, randomized, double-blind, noninferiority studies to evaluate the safety, tolerance, and efficacy of gadoversetamide compared to gadopentetate dimeglumine in CNS or liver lesions. For gadofosveset trisodium (Vasovist®), no head to head comparisons with currently available MRA contrast agents were carried out, because no extracellular agent had European-wide approval for MRA during the development of gadofosveset trisodium.

5.5.4
Strategy and Design of Clinical Trials

In phase I studies, the aim is to obtain pharmacokinetic and first human safety data assessments with single mass dose and increasing mass doses of the diagnostic agent. Phase I trials may be done in healthy volunteers or in patients.

In phase II studies, the aim is to determine the mass dose or dosing regimen in patients to be used in the phase III studies, and to provide preliminary evidence of efficacy and safety, as well as to optimize the technique and timing of, for example, image acquisition. In addition, phase II studies are important for developing methods or criteria by which images or test results can be evaluated.

For gadofosveset trisodium, seven clinical phase I/II pharmacological studies were performed in healthy volunteers, in patients with renal or hepatic impairment, or in patients with vascular disease. For gadoversetamide, five phase I and one phase II study were performed in healthy volunteers and patients with various CNS or liver pathologies as well as a variety of renal and hepatic dysfunction.

Phase III studies are large-scale trials that aim to establish the efficacy of the contrast agent in a well-defined target patient population. The primary efficacy variable should be clinically relevant and evaluable or measurable in all patients. Multiple primary endpoints should be avoided. When approval for multiple indications is requested, studies must be done in different clinical settings, each corresponding to the particular claim and intended use.

The clinical phase III study program for gadofosveset trisodium consisted mainly of four studies performed in different vascular territories, and enrolled from 136 to 268 patients in each study. The clinical phase III study program for gadoversetamide comprised two pivotal CNS studies and two pivotal liver studies, and enrolled from 198 up to 208 patients in each study.

5.5.5
Clinical Safety

A serious safety concern may prevent marketing authorization if there are alternative and safer diagnostic methods. Marketing authorization will always be based on the benefit/risk ratio of the new contrast agent. In some cases a contrast agent will have to show a positive impact on diagnostic thinking and patient management to support a marketing authorization claim.

Clinical safety assessments of contrast agents should be designed based on their characteristics and intended use(s) and on the results of other relevant clinical studies. Not only short term but also long-term safety data should be provided. As well as risk(s) related to the agent itself (e.g., immunogenicity, allergic reactions), risks related to the potential for incorrect diagnosis following its use should be taken into consideration.

References

EMEA.Doc. Ref. CHMP/EWP/1119/98/Rev 1. A draft dated 26 June 2008 was released for consultation in June 2008. End of consultation is 31 December 2008 http://www.emea.europa.eu/pdfs/human/ewp/111998enrev1.pdf

ICH http://www.ich.org/cache/compo/276-254-1.html
Vasovist http://www.emea.europa.eu/humandocs/PDFs/EPAR/vasovist/060105en6.pdf
Optimark http://www.emea.europa.eu/humandocs/PDFs/EPAR/optimark/H-745-en6.pdf

A Critical Review of Meta-Analysis of Adverse Events After Contrast Agents

6

Giuseppe Biondi-Zoccai and Marzia Lotrionte

CONTENTS

Giuseppe Biondi-Zoccai
Meta-analysis and Evidence-based medicine Training in Cardiology (METCARDIO), via Aurelia Levante 5, Ospedaletti 18014, Italy
Marzia Lotrionte
Cardiology and Cardiac Rehabilitation Unit, Catholic University, Largo A. Gemelli 8, Rome 00136, Italy

Introduction

'If I have seen further it is by standing on the shoulders of giants' *Isaac Newton*

'The great advances in science usually result from new tools rather than from new doctrines' *Freeman Dyson*

'I like to think of the meta-analytic process as similar to being in a helicopter. On the ground individual trees are visible with high resolution. This resolution diminishes as the helicopter rises, and in its place we begin to see patterns not visible from the ground' *Ingram Olkin*

Systematic reviews and meta-analyses are achieving ever increasing success among researchers and practitioners, because of the immediate appeal of a single piece of literature which can apparently summarize diverse data on a particular topic (Table 6.1 and Fig. 6.1) (Egger et al. 2001; Biondi-Zoccai et al. 2003).

However, despite their major strengths, systematic reviews and meta-analyses may, like any other analytical research tool, have significant weaknesses, especially when applied to a challenging topic such as adverse events after contrast agents. Nonetheless, adverse reactions following administration of contrast media are an ideal subject for systematic review because of their diversity and low incidence rates (Fig. 6.2).

The aim of this chapter is to provide a concise but sound framework to assist the critical reading of systematic reviews and meta-analyses, with particular focus on adverse events after contrast agents.

Table 6.1. Developmental milestones of systematic review and meta-analysis

Year	Individuals	Milestone
1904	Karl Pearson (UK)	Correlation between inoculation of vaccine for typhoid fever and mortality across apparently conflicting studies
1931	Leonard Tippet (UK)	Comparison of differences between and within the effects of farming techniques on agricultural yield adjusting for sample size across several studies
1937	William Cochran (UK)	Combination of effect sizes across different studies of medical treatments
1970s	Robert Rosenthal, Gene Glass (USA); Archie Cochrane (UK)	Combination of effect sizes across different studies of, respectively, educational/psychological and clinical treatments
1980s	The global scientific community	Exponential development and use of meta-analytic methods; birth of The Cochrane Collaboration

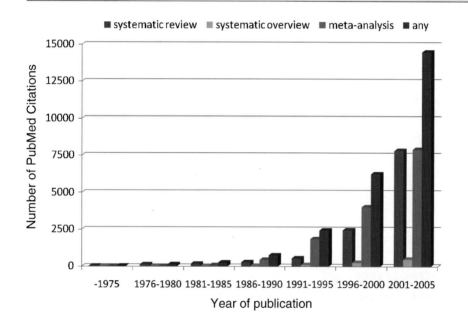

Fig. 6.1. Histogram showing the ongoing exponential increase in published systematic reviews, systematic overviews and meta-analyses. Based on a PubMed search performed on 30 September 2006 with the following strategy: ('2001' [PDAT]: '2005' [PDAT]) AND ('systematic' [title/abstract] AND 'review' [title/abstract]) OR ('systematic' [title/abstract] AND 'overview' [title/abstract]) OR ('meta-analysis' [title/abstract] OR 'meta-analyses' [title/abstract])

Greater flexibility – Lower validity

Qualitative reviews — Case reports and series

Systematic reviews — Observational studies

Meta-analyses from individual studies — Observational controlled studies

Randomized controlled trials

Meta-analyses from individual patient data — Multicenter randomized controlled trials

Lower flexibility – Greater validity

Fig. 6.2. Parallel hierarchy of scientific studies in clinical research. This figure does not establish reviews as strictly original research. However, it makes the case that meta-analysis, especially if it is based on individual patient data, can challenge the relevance and validity of even the most rigorous and comprehensive randomized trials

6.2
Basic Concepts of Systematic Reviews and Meta-Analyses

6.2.1
Definitions

A *systematic review* provides a point of view on a specific clinical problem, be it therapeutic, diagnostic or prognostic (Egger et al. 2001; Biondi-Zoccai et al. 2004). The term *systematic* means that all the steps underlying the reviewing process are explicitly and clearly defined, and so may be reproduced independently by other researchers. Thus, a formal set of methods is applied to study search (i.e. to the extensive search of the literature for primary/original studies), study selection, study appraisal, data abstraction and, when appropriate, data pooling using statistical methods. The term *meta-analysis* is used to describe a statistical method that combines results from several different primary studies to provide more precise and valid results. Thus, not all systematic reviews include a meta-analysis, as not all topics are suitable for sound and robust pooling of data. In addition, meta-analysis can be conducted outside the realm of a systematic review, without extensive and thorough literature searches, but then the results of the meta-analysis are

best viewed as only generating a hypothesis. This is mainly because meta-analyses outside the framework of a systematic review have a major risk of selection bias, for example small study bias or publication bias.

Additional definitions and pertinent examples useful for readers and writers of systematic reviews and meta-analyses are provided in Table 6.2.

6.2.2
Strengths

Systematic reviews have several unique strengths, especially if they include pooling of quantitative data by meta-analysis (Egger et al. 2001; Biondi-Zoccai et al. 2004). Specifically, they use systematic literature searches and so allow the whole body of evidence about a particular clinical question to be retrieved. Their standardized methods for search, appraisal and selection of primary studies allow reproducibility and objectivity. Thorough evaluation for internal validity and risk of bias in the individual primary studies clearly identifies the limitations of these studies. Often, the greatest strength of systematic reviews is their ability to pinpoint weaknesses and fallacies in apparently sound primary studies (Lau et al. 1998).

Quantitative synthesis by means of meta-analysis also substantially increases statistical power and provides narrower confidence intervals for statistical

Table 6.2. Brief glossary pertinent to systematic reviews and meta-analyses

Term	Characteristics
Review	A point of view on a given subject, which quotes different primary authors or studies
Overview	As above
Qualitative review	A review that avoids a systematic approach
Systematic review	A review that deliberately uses and reports a systematic approach to study search, selection, abstraction, appraisal and pooling
Quantitative review	A review that deliberately uses and reports quantitative methods to appraise or synthesize data
Meta-analysis	A study (not necessarily a review) which uses specific statistical methods for pooling data from separate datasets
Meta-regression	A study (not necessarily a review) that uses specific statistical methods for exploring interactions between dependent and independent variables (moderators) from a meta-analysis dataset
Individual patient data meta-analysis	A study (not necessarily a review) that uses specific statistical methods for pooling data from separate datasets using individual patient data
Overview of reviews	Deliberately uses a systematic approach to review search, selection, abstraction, appraisal and pooling

inferences. Assessing the effect of an intervention (an exposure or a diagnostic test) in many different settings and at many different times gives estimates and inferences of much greater external validity.

The huge sample sizes often achieved by systematic reviews may even provide the opportunity for testing post-hoc hypotheses or for exploring the effects in selected subgroups (THOMPSON and HIGGINS 2002). Clinical and statistical variability (i.e. heterogeneity and inconsistency) may be exploited by advanced statistical methods such as meta-regression, with the possibility of testing novel and hitherto untried hypotheses (BIONDI-ZOCCAI et al. 2005). Finally, meta-regression methods can even be used to perform adjusted indirect comparisons or network meta-analyses (BUCHER et al. 1997).

6.2.3
Limitations

There are also substantial drawbacks to systematic reviews and meta-analyses (EGGER et al. 2001). Since the first criticisms that they were 'an exercise in mega-silliness' and inappropriately 'mixing apples and oranges' (GLASS 1976), there has been ongoing debate about the correct approach to choose. Meta-analytic pooling should be used when there is statistical homogeneity and consistency but is not suitable when there is severe statistical heterogeneity [as testified by p values <0.10 at χ^2 test] or significant statistical inconsistency [as testified by I^2 values >50%]) (HIGGINS et al. 2003).

While Canadian authors have suggested that systematic reviews and meta-analyses from homogenous randomized controlled trials represent the apex of the evidence-based medicine pyramid (GUYATT et al. 2002), others have maintained that very large and simple randomized clinical trials offer several major advantages, and should always be preferred, when available, to systematic reviews (CAPPELLERI et al. 1996).

It is also all too common to retrieve only a few studies on a given clinical topic from the literature, or to find studies of such low quality that including or even discussing them in the setting of a systematic review may be misleading. This drawback is particularly associated with small study bias, which is a major threat to the validity of meta-analysis (EGGER et al. 2001). Especially when datasets are large, small primary studies are more likely to be reported, published and quoted if their results are significant. Conversely, small non-significant studies often fail to reach

publication or dissemination, and thus may be very easily missed, even after thorough literature searches. Combining results from these 'biased' small studies with those of larger studies, which are usually published even if negative or non-significant, may inappropriately deviate summary effect estimates away from the true value. Unfortunately, although several graphical and analytical tests are available (PETERS et al. 2006), small study bias, which also encompasses publication bias, is potentially always present in a systematic review and must not be forgotten.

Another common criticism is that systematic reviews and meta-analyses are not original research. The reader can form an independent opinion on this issue. Nonetheless, the main parameter for judging a systematic review should be its novelty and usefulness to the reader, not whether it represents original or secondary research (BIONDI-ZOCCAI et al. 2003).

Finally, a burning issue is whether results from large systematic reviews and meta-analyses can ever be applied to the single individual under our care. There is no universal answer to this question, and judgment always needs to be used about applying meta-analysis results to a particular patient. However, like the advocates of evidence-based medicine, we believe that all patients are likely to benefit similarly from a specific treatment or diagnostic strategy unless proven otherwise, for example by a significant test for statistical interaction (GUYATT et al. 2002).

6.2.4
Systematic Reviews and Meta-Analyses: How to do it Yourself

Even those who do not have to undertake a systematic review can obtain a helpful insight into this method of clinical research by understanding the key steps involved in the design, conduct and interpretation of a systematic review (BIONDI-ZOCCAI et al. 2004).

Briefly, a systematic review should always stem from a specific clinical question (Fig. 6.3). Even if the experienced reviewer can probably guess the answer to this question (i.e. the hypothetical solution), the goal of the systematic review is to confirm or disprove the hypothesis in a formal and structured way. With this goal in mind, the review should be designed as prospectively and in as much detail as possible, to avoid conscious or unconscious manipulation of the methods or data.

The next important steps define the boundaries of the review. Specifically, the reviewer needs to spell out the population of interest, the intervention or exposure

1. Definition of question and hypothetical solution
2. Prospective design of the systematic review
3. Problem formulation (Population, Intervention or exposure, Comparison, Outcome [PICO])
4. Data search
5. Data abstraction and appraisal
6. Data analysis ± quantitative synthesis (ie meta-analysis)
7. Results interpretation and dissemination

FEED-BACK ON HYPOTHESIS

Fig. 6.3. Simplified algorithm for the design and conduct of systematic reviews in clinical research. This scheme may appear quite rigid, but the systematic review process in fact requires repeat piloting of several steps of the reviewing process to adjust it to the limitations inherent in the primary literature, for example the lack of high-quality studies focusing on a given topic

to be appraised, the comparison(s) or comparator(s) and the outcome(s). The acronym PICO is often used to remember this approach. As an example, we might wish to conduct a systematic review of diabetics with critical limb ischemia undergoing digital subtraction angiography (P), with the intervention of interest being the administration of isosmolar contrast agents (I), the comparators being low-osmolar contrast agents (C) and the outcomes defined as risk of death or permanent hemodialysis within 30 days of the procedure (O).

After these preliminary steps, the actual review begins with a thorough and extensive search, encompassing several databases (not only MEDLINE/PubMed!) with the help of library personnel experienced in literature searches. When a list of potentially relevant citations has been retrieved, these should be assessed and then included or excluded based on criteria which stem directly from the PICO method of defining the clinical question. The study appraisal also includes a formal evaluation of study validity and of the risk of bias of the primary studies. Data abstraction is generally performed by at least two independent reviewers with any differences of opinion resolved by consensus, and provides the quantitative data which will eventually be pooled by meta-analysis (HIGGINS and GREEN 2008).

Provided that the studies are relatively homogeneous and consistent, meta-analytic methods are employed to combine effect estimates from single studies into a unique summary effect estimate, with corresponding *p* values for effect and confidence intervals.

The last step requires interpretation and dissemination of the results, possibly through publication in

a peer-reviewed journal. In many cases the results may lead the reviewer to go back to the original research question and, very often, to revise his/her working hypothesis.

6.3
Appraising Primary Studies, Systematic Reviews and Meta-Analyses

Appraisal of primary research studies as well as systematic reviews and meta-analyses should be based on their internal validity and, provided this is reasonably adequate, on their results and external validity (GUYATT et al. 2002). While interpretation of the results and the external validity of any research project is highly subjective and best left open to the individual judgment of the reader or decision-maker, internal validity can be appraised in a very structured and validated way.

Recent guidance on the appraisal of the risk of bias in primary research studies within the context of a systematic review has been provided by The Cochrane Collaboration, and includes separate assessment of the risk of selection, performance, attrition and adjudication bias, as clearly spelled out in Table 6.3 (HIGGINS and GREEN 2008). Other valid and complementary approaches, devised for specific study designs, have been proposed by advocates of evidence-based medicine methods (GUYATT et al. 2002).

The quality of a systematic review and meta-analysis also depends on a number of factors, including, obviously, the quality of the primary pooled studies. Nonetheless, the quality of report, for example the compliance with current guidelines on drafting and reporting of a meta-analysis by the Quality of Reporting of Meta-analyses [QUOROM] statement, should clearly be characterized by internal validity (MOHER et al. 1999; BIONDI-ZOCCAI et al. 2006). This can be low even in well reported reviews, but it is usually difficult to consider a poorly reported systematic review and meta-analysis to be of great value. The appraisal of the internal validity of a review is quite complex and based on several assumptions, including study search and appraisal, methods for data pooling and approaches to interpretation of study findings. However, useful guidance was provided by Oxman and Guyatt with their well validated method (Table 6.4).

Table 6.3. Risk of bias assessment tool recommended by The Cochrane Collaboration for the appraisal of primary studies

Question	Answers	Meaning
Adequate sequence generation?	Yes, no, or uncertain	Was the allocation sequence generated appropriately (e.g. computer or table of random numbers)?
Allocation concealment used?	Yes, no, or uncertain	Were physicians unaware of allocation code up to actual patient enrolment?
Blinding?	Yes, no, or uncertain	Were patients, caregivers, outcome assessors, ancillary personnel, and/or statisticians unaware of actual treatment?
Concurrent therapies similar?	Yes, no, or uncertain	Were concurrent medical and non-medical treatments similar in the groups under comparison?
Incomplete outcome data addressed?	Yes, no, or uncertain	Were all data analyzed, minimizing the impact of losses to follow-up?
Uniform and explicit outcome definitions?	Yes, no, or uncertain	Were definitions clearly spelled out and employed consistently to adjudicate events or outcomes?
Free of selective outcome reporting?	Yes, no, or uncertain	Were all relevant outcomes thoroughly reported?
Free of other bias?	Yes, no, or uncertain	Was the risk of any other bias low?
Overall risk of bias?	High, moderate, or low	What is the comprehensive assessment of the risk of bias of the study?

Table 6.4. Oxman and Guyatt index for the appraisal of reviews (EGGER et al. 2001)[a]

Question	Details
1	Were the search methods used to find evidence stated?
2	Was the search for evidence reasonably comprehensive?
3	Were the criteria for deciding which studies to include in the overview reported?
4	Was bias in the selection of studies avoided?
5	Were the criteria used for assessing the validity of the included studies reported?
6	Was the validity of all studies referred to in the text assessed using appropriate criteria
7	Were the methods used to combine the findings of the relevant studies reported
8	Were the findings of the relevant studies combined appropriately relative to the primary question the overview addresses?
9	Were the conclusions made by the author(s) supported by the data and/or analysis reported in the overview?
10	This question summarizes the previous ones and, specifically, asks to rate the scientific quality of the review from 1 (being extensively flawed) to 3 (carrying major flaws) to 5 (carrying minor flaws) to 7 (minimally flawed)

[a] The Oxman and Guyatt index evaluates the internal validity of a review on nine separate questions for which three distinct answers are eligible ('yes', 'partially/cannot tell', 'no'). The developers of the index specify that if the 'partially/cannot tell' answer is used one or more times in questions 2, 4, 6 or 8, a review is likely to have minor flaws at best and is difficult to rule out major flaws (i.e. a score ≤4). If the 'no' option is used on question 2, 4, 6 or 8, the review is likely to have major flaws (i.e. a score ≤3)

More recently, other investigators have suggested other tools for the appraisal of systematic reviews, such as the A Measurement Tool to Assess Systematic Reviews (AMSTAR), which, however, awaits further validation (SHEA et al. 2007).

6.4
Focus on Adverse
Events After Contrast Agents

While several limitations apply to systematic reviews and meta-analyses in general (EGGER et al. 2001), a number of drawbacks and potential threats to validity are specifically relevant to research on adverse reactions to contrast agents. These include analytical issues associated with low event rates and the resultant risk of alpha and beta errors, the common reliance on surrogate (thus softer) end-points, the impact of small study/publication bias and the possibility that funding or conflicts of interest will affect the analysis. We will provide a detailed description of these threats to validity, with some specific examples relevant to the contrast agent literature.

6.4.1
Analytical Challenges
Caused by Low Event Rates

Adverse reactions to contrast agents are relatively uncommon, so low event rates are often found in primary research studies, unless they are extensively powered, for example by enrolling more than 1,000 patients or by selectively recruiting very high-risk subjects. This fact may lead to null counts in one or more of the groups undergoing comparison in a controlled trial, and so producing severe difficulties for the analysis. Most statistical methods used for meta-analytic pooling require that at least one event has occurred in each study group. When this is not the case in one or more of the groups under comparison, bias may be introduced because of the common practice of adding 0.25 or 0.50 to each group without events (GOLDER et al. 2006).

In addition, when no event has occurred in any group, no comparison can be performed and data from such an underpowered study cannot be pooled for meta-analysis, as variance of the effect estimate approaches ∞.

6.4.2
Risk of Alpha Error

Alpha error is defined as the risk of incorrectly dismissing a null hypothesis, despite it being true. Even when all groups being compared in a particular study have one or more adverse events, the risk of biased estimates and alpha error may be present (EGGER et al. 2001). Minor differences in few and rare events may give nominally significant results (e.g., $p = 0.048$), which, however, may not be reliable. In such cases, we recommend reliance on the combined appraisal of p values and 95% confidence intervals, or even pushing for 99% confidence intervals. In other cases, a useful rule of thumb is only to trust meta-analyses reporting on at least 100 pooled events per group under comparison.

6.4.3
Risk of Beta Error

The beta error is the risk of erroneously accepting a null hypothesis despite it being false. This error is also common in systematic reviews and meta-analyses, especially when they include few studies with low event counts. This lack of statistical power (defined actually as 1-beta) is even more common with meta-regression analyses, which are usually underpowered because of the few studies included and because of regression to the mean phenomena (THOMPSON and HIGGINS 2002).

6.4.4
Reliance on Surrogate End-points

Surrogates may help the design of clinical research by increasing statistical power and by providing an insight into more than one clinical outcome. However, choosing the example of contrast-induced nephropathy (CIN), surrogates such as a greater than 25% increase in serum creatinine from baseline values may be less clinically relevant than hard clinical end-points, such as death or the permanent need for hemodialysis (GUYATT et al. 2002). Usually, only surrogates that have a direct impact on patient well being and are clearly and independently associated with hard clinical end-points should be accepted for the design of clinical research studies.

A study with significant results for surrogate end-points but not for hard end-points should be considered as generating a hypothesis or, at best, underpowered.

6.4.5
Small Study and Publication Bias

Small study bias is always a potential threat to the results of a systematic review, because this problem affects all clinical topics and research study designs (BIONDI-ZOCCAI et al. 2008). While this type of bias may have less impact in studies focusing on recent and well financed drugs or devices (e.g. fenoldopam), in other examples of cheaper interventions, publication bias may profoundly undermine the results of a systematic review. This applies particularly to the research evidence, which has now accumulated on acetylcysteine for the prevention of CIN (BIONDI-ZOCCAI et al. 2006), but also to other commonly prescribed agents such as contrast media.

6.4.6
Conflicts of Interest and Funding Issues

Another major threat to the validity of a systematic review, as to any other research project, depends on conflicts of interest and how studies are funded. It is well known that reviewers with underlying financial conflicts of interest are more likely to draw conclusions that favor an intervention, which benefits the source of any financial gain (BARNES and BERO 1998). Most studies performed on contrast agents are undertaken by investigators with either overt or probable conflicts of interest (ASPELIN et al. 2003; SOLOMON et al. 2007). Whether these facts should just lead to more critical reading of their work or should stimulate a comprehensive reevaluation of their whole research project is best left to the reader's discretion. It also depends on the overall internal validity of the study, for example the blinding of patients, physicians, adjudicators and analysts.

6.5
Conclusions and Future Perspectives

Systematic reviews and meta-analyses are powerful methods to assess the clinical effects of interventions in healthcare. They may prove particularly helpful in assessing the risk of contrast associated adverse events in terms of effect estimates for different contrast agents. More collaborative research effort is, however, needed to set up international research groups able to design, conduct and disseminate individual patient data meta-analyses, which can combine results from individual clinical trials in an unbiased and rigorous way (ANTITHROMBOTIC TRIALISTS' COLLABORATION 2002).

References

Antithrombotic Trialists' Collaboration (2002) Collaborative meta-analysis of randomised trials of antiplatelet therapy for prevention of death, myocardial infarction, and stroke in high risk patients. BMJ 324:71–86

Aspelin P, Aubry P, Fransson SG, Strasser R, Willenbrock R, Berg KJ (2003) Nephrotoxic effects in high-risk patients undergoing angiography. N Engl J Med 348:491–499

Barnes DE, Bero LA (1998) Why review articles on the health effects of passive smoking reach different conclusions. JAMA 297:1566–1570

Biondi-Zoccai GG, Abbate A, Agostoni P, Testa L, Burzotta F, Lotrionte M, Trani C, Biasucci LM (2005) Long-term benefits of an early invasive management in acute coronary syndromes depend on intracoronary stenting and aggressive antiplatelet treatment: a metaregression. Am Heart J 149:504–511

Biondi-Zoccai GG, Agostoni P, Abbate A (2003). Parallel hierarchy of scientific studies in cardiovascular medicine. Ital Heart J 4:819–820

Biondi-Zoccai GG, Lotrionte M, Abbate A, Testa L, Remigi E, Burzotta F, Valgimigli M, Romagnoli E, Crea F, Agostoni P (2006) Compliance with QUOROM and quality of reporting of overlapping meta-analyses on the role of acetylcysteine in the prevention of contrast associated nephropathy: case study. BMJ 332:202–209

Biondi-Zoccai GG, Lotrionte M, Anselmino M, Moretti C, Agostoni P, Testa L, Abbate A, Cosgrave J, Laudito A, Trevi GP, Sheiban I (2008). Systematic review and meta-analysis of randomized clinical trials appraising the impact of cilostazol after percutaneous coronary intervention. Am Heart J 155:1081–1089

Biondi-Zoccai GG, Testa L, Agostoni P (2004) A practical algorithm for systematic reviews in cardiovascular medicine. Ital Heart J 5:486–487

Bucher HC, Guyatt GH, Griffith LE, Walter SD (1997) The results of direct and indirect treatment comparisons in meta-analysis of randomized controlled trials. J Clin Epidemiol 50:683–689

Cappelleri JC, Ioannidis JP, Schmid CH, de Ferranti SD, Aubert M, Chalmers TC, Lau J (1996) Large trials vs meta-analysis of smaller trials: how do their results compare? JAMA 276:1332–1338

Egger M, Smith GD, Altman DG (2001) Systematic reviews in health care: meta-analysis in context, 2nd edn. BMJ Publishing Group, London

Glass G (1976) Primary, secondary and meta-analysis of research. Educ Res 5:3–8

Golder S, Loke Y, McIntosh HM (2006) Room for improvement? A survey of the methods used in systematic reviews of adverse effects. BMC Med Res Methodol 6:3

Guyatt G, Rennie D, Meade M, Cook D (2002) Users' guides to the medical literature. A manual for evidence-based clinical practice. AMA, Chicago

Higgins JP, Thompson SG, Deeks JJ, Altman DG (2003) Measuring inconsistency in meta-analyses. BMJ 327:557–560

Higgins JPT, Green S (2008) Cochrane handbook for systematic reviews of interventions. The Cochrane Collaboration, Oxford

Lau J, Ioannidis JP, Schmid CH (1998) Summing up evidence: one answer is not always enough. Lancet 351:123–127

Moher D, Cook DJ, Eastwood S, Olkin I, Rennie D, Stroup DF (1999) Improving the quality of reports of meta-analyses of randomised controlled trials: the QUORUM statement. Lancet 354:1896–1900

Peters JL, Sutton AJ, Jones DR, Abrams KR, Rushton L (2006) Comparison of two methods to detect publication bias in meta-analysis. JAMA 295:676–680

Shea BJ, Bouter LM, Peterson J, Boers M, Andersson N, Ortiz Z, Ramsay T, Bai A, Shukla VK, Grimshaw JM (2007) External validation of a measurement tool to assess systematic reviews (AMSTAR). PLoS ONE 2(12):e1350

Solomon RJ, Natarajan MK, Doucet S, Sharma SK, Staniloae CS, Katholi RE, Gelormini JL, Labinaz M, Moreyra AE (2007) Cardiac Angiography in Renally Impaired Patients (CARE) study: a randomized double-blind trial of contrast-induced nephropathy in patients with chronic kidney disease. Circulation 115:3189–3196

Thompson SG, Higgins JP (2002) How should meta-regression analyses be undertaken and interpreted? Stat Med 21:1559–1573

Iodinated and Gadolinium Contrast Media

General Adverse Reactions

Prevention of Acute Reactions

7

JUDITH A. W. WEBB

CONTENTS

JUDITH A.W. WEBB
Department of Diagnostic Radiology, St Bartholomew's
Hospital, West Smithfield, London EC1A 7BE, UK

7.1
Introduction

Acute idiosyncratic systemic reactions (also described as allergy-like or anaphylactoid) are defined as unpredictable reactions that occur within 1 h of contrast medium administration, and are unrelated to the amount of contrast medium above a certain level. This definition aims to distinguish them from chemotoxic reactions, which are dose-related and dependent on the physico-chemical properties of the contrast medium. However, in clinical practice, some reactions such as cardiovascular collapse may be difficult to characterise definitely into one or the other group.

Most of this chapter is concerned with acute idiosyncratic reactions to iodinated contrast media, particularly the factors predisposing to these reactions and the measures that may be taken to prevent them. At the end of the chapter, acute reactions to gadolinium contrast media are also discussed (see also Chap. 23).

7.2
Iodinated Contrast Media

7.2.1
Types and Timing of Acute Reactions

Many patients who are given intravascular iodinated contrast media experience some subjective sensations such as warmth, flushing, and altered taste. These common effects usually last for a few minutes and are not of clinical significance.

In radiological literature, acute idiosyncratic reactions have been classified as mild or minor, moderate, or severe (BUSH and SWANSON 1991). Mild or minor reactions usually do not need treatment and include nausea, mild vomiting, urticaria, and itching. Moderate reactions include more severe vomiting, marked urticaria, bronchospasm, facial or laryngeal oedema, and vasovagal reactions. Severe reactions include hypotensive shock, pulmonary oedema, respiratory arrest, cardiac arrest, and convulsions. While this type of classification is widely used in clinical practice, it has been suggested that Ring and Messmer's four-grade classification of anaphylactic reactions would provide more detailed and reproducible documentation of acute reactions (IDEE et al. 2005).

Most acute reactions occur early after contrast medium administration. In KATAYAMA et al's (1990) study of over 330,000 patients, over 70% of reactions to both ionic and nonionic contrast media occurred in the first 5 min. In all 44 patients who died after intravascular contrast medium (reviewed by SHEHADI (1985)), the acute reaction to contrast medium started within 15 min of administration.

The general incidence of anaphylactic reactions is increasing (RESUSCITATION COUNCIL (UK) 2008). It is not known whether this is also the case for anaphylactoid reactions to contrast media.

7.2.2
Mechanisms of Acute Reactions

The mechanisms by which acute adverse reactions to iodinated contrast media occur are still unclear (IDEE et al. 2005; MORCOS 2005; DEWACHTER et al. 2006) and this makes prevention of reactions more difficult.

True allergic hypersensitivity appears to account for at least some severe acute reactions. LAROCHE et al. (1998) showed immediate marked rises in plasma histamine and tryptase levels in patients who had severe acute reactions, with the levels being proportional to the severity of the reaction. The timing and size of the increases were similar to those observed in known allergic hypersensitivity reactions, which suggested that immediate mast cell degranulation had occurred. Contrast-medium-specific IgE levels were higher in severe reactors than controls (LAROCHE et al. 1998). In some severe reactors, skin testing with contrast medium was positive (LAROCHE et al. 1998; DEWACHTER et al. 2006). Some cross-reactivity between contrast media has been shown in reactors, and in some patients non-cross-reacting contrast media were subsequently administered without problems (DEWACHTER et al. 2006).

How iodinated contrast media act as antigens remains a problem, as they bind poorly to protein (LASSER et al. 1962). One suggestion, based largely on in vitro experiments, is that contrast media act as "pseudoantigens" that attach to the fixed Fc site on the IgE molecule rather than the variable Fab site of specific antigen binding (LASSER 2004). Lasser has proposed that in low concentrations contrast media cause binding of adjacent IgE molecules leading to mast cell activation, and that, in higher concentrations, contrast media inhibit IgE binding because the aggregation of contrast medium molecules causes steric hindrance (LASSER 2004). Others have not been able to show the aggregation of contrast medium molecules, considered necessary for this effect (SONTUM et al. 1998).

When mast cells are activated, heparin is also released and can activate the contact system with the release of bradykinin (LASSER 1987, 2004). In addition, other mediators, such as prostaglandins, leucotrienes, and cytokines, are likely to be involved (DEWACHTER et al. 2006).

Complement levels in the blood decrease after contrast medium, both in control subjects and reactors, with the decreases being greater in the reactors (ELOY et al. 1991). Although contrast media may be able to activate the complement system, it is considered unlikely that this mechanism is responsible for acute reactions (DEWACHTER et al. 2006).

The immediate non-allergic effects of contrast media could be caused by direct chemotoxicity. They could also relate to the non-specific release of small amounts of histamine from mast cells and/or basophils, which occurs in up to 80% of patients in the minutes immediately after contrast medium (ELOY et al. 1991; RODRIGUEZ et al. 2001; DEWACHTER et al. 2006). This effect relates to the nature of the contrast medium molecule as well as the dose and osmolality of the contrast agent.

7.2.3
Risk Factors for Acute Idiosyncratic Reactions

7.2.3.1
Type of Contrast Agent

With the older high-osmolality ionic agents, the rate of reactions of all types is in the range 5–12% (ANSELL et al. 1980; WITTEN et al. 1973; SHEHADI 1975; KATAYAMA et al. 1990; COCHRAN et al. 2001). Most reactions in these series were mild, with moderate reactions occurring in 1–2% and severe reactions in approximately 0.10–0.15% (ANSELL et al. 1980; WITTEN et al. 1973). Mortality with the ionic agents is in the range 1 in 14,000 to 1 in 169,000 (SHEHADI 1975; KATAYAMA et al. 1990), with 1 in 75,000 an often quoted figure (HARTMAN et al. 1982).

With the newer low-osmolality nonionic agents, the reaction rates are lower, by a factor of approximately 4–5 times (KATAYAMA et al. 1990; PALMER 1988; WOLF et al. 1991; BETTMAN et al. 1997). Thus in Katayama's series of over 300,000 patients, the reaction rates for ionic and nonionic agents were overall 12.66 and 3.13%, with severe reactions in 0.22 and 0.04%, respectively (KATAYAMA et al. 1990). On the basis of a meta-analysis of all data published between 1980 and 1991, CARO et al. (1991) concluded that 80% of contrast media reactions could be prevented by using low-osmolality agents. The very low mortality means that accurate mortality figures are not yet available for the nonionic agents. In KATAYAMA et al.'s (1990) series there was no significant difference in mortality between the ionic and nonionic agents, but other data suggest a lower mortality with nonionic agents (LASSER et al. 1997).

7.2.3.2
Previous Contrast Medium Reaction

A previous reaction to an iodinated contrast medium is the most important patient factor predisposing to an acute idiosyncratic reaction (BETTMAN et al. 1997). With ionic agents, the risk of a reaction in a patient who had reacted previously has been stated to be 16–35% (WITTEN et al. 1973; SHEHADI 1975) and to be 11 times greater than the risk in a non-reactor (ANSELL et al. 1980). When a patient who previously reacted to an ionic agent is given a nonionic agent, the risk of a repeat reaction is reduced to approximately 5% (SIEGLE et al. 1991).

7.2.3.3
Asthma

Asthma is another important risk factor. SHEHADI (1975) found that 11% of asthmatics had a reaction to ionic contrast media, and ANSELL et al. (1980) stated that the risk of reaction to ionic agents was increased 5 times in an asthmatic. In patients with asthma, KATAYAMA et al. (1990) described an 8.5 times increased risk with ionic agents and a 5.8 times increased risk with nonionics. Other conditions, such as hayfever, eczema, etc., are associated with an increased risk of

reaction, but to a lesser extent than asthma (ANSELL et al. 1980; WITTEN et al. 1973; SHEHADI 1975).

7.2.3.4
Allergy

A history of allergy to foods, drugs, or other substances is associated with an increased risk of contrast medium reaction, usually by a lesser amount than a history of asthma. Thus, SHEHADI (1975) and KATAYAMA et al. (1990) found a two-fold increase in risk of a reaction, and ANSELL et al. (1980) a 4 times increase in risk of a reaction.

Allergy to foodstuffs that contain iodine, e.g., seafood, often causes particular anxiety. However, the available data suggest that allergy to seafood is no more significant than allergy to other foodstuffs (WITTEN et al. 1973; SHEHADI 1975; LEDER 1997).

Allergy to topical iodine skin preparations is a type of contact dermatitis and does not seem to predispose to acute idiosyncratic contrast medium reactions (THOMSEN and BUSH 1998).

7.2.3.5
Drugs

Whether β-blockers affect the incidence of idiosyncratic contrast medium reactions is controversial. GREENBERGER et al. (1987) reported that neither β-blockers nor calcium antagonists, given separately or together, increased the risk of reaction. Subsequently, however, LANG et al. (1991) found that β-blockers did increase the risk of reaction. It is, however, agreed that the use of β-blockers can impair the response to treatment if a reaction does occur (THOMSEN and BUSH 1998; GREENBERGER et al. 1987; LANG et al. 1991).

Patients who are receiving or have received interleukin-2 are at increased risk of adverse events following iodinated contrast media. Some of these adverse events appear to recall the side-effects of interleukin-2 (e.g. fever, nausea, vomiting, diarrhoea, pruritus, and rash) (ZUKIWSKI et al. 1990; FISHMAN et al. 1991; OLDHAM et al. 1991; CHOYKE et al. 1992). Reactions are often late, occurring more than 1 h after contrast medium, but can also occur within the first hour (CHOYKE et al. 1992).

7.2.3.6
Other Factors

Female gender has been associated with an increased risk of acute reactions (LANG et al. 1995; BETTMAN et al. 1997). Race may also increase the risk of acute reaction, with more reactions in the UK occurring in Indians and subjects of Mediterranean origin than in the indigenous white population (ANSELL et al. 1980).

7.2.4
Extravascular Administration of Iodinated Contrast Media

Acute adverse reactions to iodinated contrast media are almost always associated with intravascular administration. However, there are case reports of anaphylactoid reactions after administration of iodinated contrast media into body cavities – for example, during cystography, retrograde pyelography, arthrography, and oral administration for evaluation of the gastrointestinal tract (WEESE et al. 1993; HUGO et al. 1998; MILLER 1997; ARMSTRONG et al. 2005).

7.2.5
Prevention of Acute Idiosyncratic Reactions

In patients at increased risk of contrast medium reaction, especially if there has been a previous reaction to an iodinated contrast agent, the possibility of obtaining the necessary diagnostic information from another test, not using iodinated contrast medium (e.g., ultrasonography, magnetic resonance imaging), must be considered. If iodinated contrast medium is still deemed essential, the risk of an acute reaction can be reduced by an appropriate choice of contrast medium and pre-medication.

Because most severe reactions occur within the first 20 min after contrast medium injection (HARTMAN et al. 1982; SHEHADI 1985), patients should remain in the Radiology Department for at least this period. In high-risk subjects, monitoring for the first hour is recommended.

7.2.5.1
Choice of Contrast Medium

The single most important method of reducing the risk of idiosyncratic contrast medium reactions is to use nonionic, low-osmolality agents, which are associated with a 4–5 times lower risk of reactions (KATAYAMA et al. 1990; PALMER 1988; WOLF et al. 1991; BETTMAN et al. 1997). In many countries, nonionic agents are used for all intravascular adminis-

tration of contrast material. Where this is not possible, selective use of nonionic agents in patients at increased risk of reaction is recommended (KING 1999). The principal categories of increased risk are previous contrast medium reaction, asthma, or a history of allergy (ANSELL et al. 1980; WITTEN et al. 1973; KATAYAMA et al. 1990; MORCOS et al. 2001). When there has been a previous reaction to nonionic iodinated contrast medium, the use of a different agent may be helpful (THOMSEN and BUSH 1998; DEWACHTER et al. 2006).

7.2.5.2
Pre-medication: Possible Regimes and Evidence of Their Efficacy

To reduce the incidence of idiosyncratic contrast medium reactions, a variety of pre-medication regimes have been used. Most frequently, steroids with or without additional H1 antihistamines have been recommended, and other drugs, such as ephedrine and H2 antagonists, have also been tried.

With ionic agents, there is good evidence that steroids reduce the rate of reactions. In a randomised study of 6,763 unselected patients, LASSER et al. (1987) showed a reduction in the incidence of reactions to ionic contrast media from 9 to 6.4% when methylprednisolone was given 12 and 2 h before the contrast agent. In patients who have previously reacted to ionic contrast media, a combination of steroid and H1 antihistamine reduces the repeat reaction rate, estimated to be 16–35% without premedication (WITTEN et al. 1973; SHEHADI 1975). GREENBERGER et al. (1984) evaluated 657 procedures in 563 previous reactors using two pre-medication regimes before administering ionic contrast media. In patients given prednisone and antihistamine, the repeat reaction rate was reduced to 9.0% and the addition of ephedrine further reduced the repeat reaction rate to 3.1%. However, because of anxieties about the possible adverse effects of ephedrine in patients with hypertension or cardiovascular disease, the use of ephedrine has not been widely adopted (THOMSEN and BUSH 1998). The addition of the H2 antagonist cimetidine to the steroid, antihistamine, and ephedrine pre-medication was associated with a higher risk of reaction (GREENBERGER et al. 1985). With the ionic low-osmolality agent meglumine ioxaglate, BERTRAND et al. (1992) found that the antihistamine hydroxyzine reduced the risk of urticaria from 12.5 to 1.0% in 200 subjects.

With the nonionic, low-osmolality agents, there is less evidence of the value of pre-medication, but the available evidence does indicate that pre-medication can further reduce the incidence of reactions. In a randomised study of 1,155 unselected patients, LASSER et al. (1994) found a statistically significant decrease in the total number of reactions from 4.9 to 1.7% when patients given nonionic contrast media were pre-medicated with methylprednisolone given 12 and 2 h before the contrast agent. The number of moderate and severe reactions was also less after steroids, but the numbers were small and no statistically significant difference was found. In previous reactors, GREENBERGER and PATTERSON (1991) found that the combined use of a nonionic agent together with both prednisone and antihistamine or prednisone, antihistamine, and ephedrine reduced the repeat reaction rate to 0.5% in 181 patients. In patients who had previously reacted, or who had a history of allergy or severe cardiopulmonary disease, H1 and H2 antagonists reduced the reaction rate to 1.57% in 1,047 patients, as compared to a reaction rate of 4.37% in those who were not pre-medicated (FINK et al. 1992).

When steroid pre-medication is used, the steroids should be given at least 12 h before the contrast medium. The minimal effective time interval between steroids and contrast medium is considered unlikely to be less than 6 h (LASSER et al. 1987; MORCOS et al. 2001). To be effective, steroids require time to affect the complex processes that underlie anaphylactoid reactions. For example, steroids cause induction of the C1 esterase inhibitor, which affects the production of the mediator bradykinin. The rise in C1 esterase inhibitor levels occurs over a 12-h period (LASSER et al. 1981).

7.2.5.3
Pre-medication: Controversies

With the ionic agents, the higher risk of reaction and the stronger evidence for the value of pre-medication meant that steroid pre-medication was widely recommended and used (GREENBERGER et al. 1984; LASSER et al. 1987). With nonionic agents, the use of pre-medication is more controversial and practice is variable (DAWSON and SIDHU 1993; LASSER 1994, 1995; DORE et al. 1994, 1995; LASSER and BERRY 1994; SEYMOUR et al. 1994; COHAN et al. 1995; DAWSON 2005; RADHAKRISHNAN et al. 2005).

One point of view is that the risk of reaction with nonionic agents is very low and the evidence of the value of steroid pre-medication not sufficiently strong and therefore pre-medication is no longer warranted (DAWSON and SIDHU 1993; DAWSON 2005).

An alternative point of view is that the admittedly imperfect evidence indicates that steroid pre-medication further reduces the likelihood of a reaction to nonionic agents (GREENBERGER and PATTERSON 1991; LASSER et al. 1994; LASSER 1994; AMERICAN COLLEGE OF RADIOLOGY 2004). There is evidence that at least some acute, severe, and adverse reactions to contrast media are true allergic hypersensitivity reactions (LAROCHE et al. 1998) and high doses of steroids are used in the treatment of anaphylaxis. Their effect is attributed to the fact that they stabilise cell membranes and reduce the release of chemical mediators involved in anaphylaxis (BUSH and SWANSON 1991).

It is not possible to be dogmatic about whether patients at increased risk of reaction should receive steroid pre-medication before they are given nonionic contrast media. In emergency situations, the risk of not undertaking the investigation immediately often outweighs the possible benefit of using steroids. Radiologists may also be influenced by the setting in which they practice. While facilities for resuscitation should be available in all settings where intravascular contrast medium is administered, additional support facilities are more readily available in larger hospitals. The AMERICAN COLLEGE OF RADIOLOGY MANUAL ON CONTRAST MEDIA (2004) states that the higher the risk of reaction, the stronger the case that can be made for pre-medication. The European Society of Urogenital Radiology guidelines indicate that opinion on this topic is divided, and therefore have not issued a directive.

It must be remembered that, even with steroid pre-medication, reactions to nonionic contrast media still occur and are common in subjects with a history of allergy (FREED et al. 2001).

7.2.5.4
Pre-testing and Injection Rate

The practice of pre-testing – giving a small preliminary test dose of contrast medium intravenously before the full dose is given – has been shown to be of no value (SHEHADI 1975; FISCHER and DOUST 1972; YAMAGUCHI et al. 1991). FISCHER and DOUST (1972) found that the mortality after contrast medium administration was unaffected by pre-testing and that deaths could occur following a negative pre-test or following the pre-test itself. Yamaguchi et al. (1991) found no benefit of pre-testing either with ionic or nonionic agents.

Injection rate does not appear to have any effect on the rate of adverse reactions (Jacobs et al. 1998).

7.2.6
Summary: Iodinated Contrast Media

To reduce the risk of an acute reaction to intravascular iodinated contrast media, the important measures for all patients are as follows:
- Use nonionic contrast media.
- Keep the patient in the Radiology Department for 20 min after contrast medium injection.
- Have the drugs and equipment for resuscitation readily available.

There is an increased risk of an acute reaction to intravascular iodinated contrast media in patients with a history of
- previous generalised reaction to iodinated contrast medium, either moderate (e.g., urticaria, bronchospasm) or severe (e.g., hypotension, severe bronchospasm, pulmonary oedema, cardiovascular collapse, convulsions);
- asthma;
- allergy requiring medical treatment.

In patients with an increased risk of a reaction to intravascular iodinated contrast media
- consider whether the use of iodinated contrast medium is essential; also, whether another test (e.g. ultrasonography, magnetic resonance imaging) would give the diagnostic information needed;
- consider the use of a different iodinated agent for previous reactors to a contrast medium;
- consider pre-medication for previous reactors to iodinated contrast media and high-risk patients.

Note: Practice for the use of pre-medication is variable. If pre-medication is used, a suitable corticosteroid pre-medication regime is prednisone 30 mg orally (or methylprednisolone 32 mg orally) given 12 and 2 h before contrast medium. H2 antihistamines may also be used.

Since contrast media administered into body cavities may reach the circulation in small amounts, take the same precautions as for intravascular administration in patients at increased risk of reaction.

7.3
Gadolinium Contrast Media

7.3.1
Types of Reaction and Frequency

Adverse events following intravenous gadolinium contrast media are less common than with iodinated agents and most are minor and self-limiting (Runge 2000). Less than 1% of patients develop allergy-like or anaphylactoid reactions, and most of these are mild (Murphy et al. 1999; Li et al. 2006; Dillman et al. 2007). Anaphylactoid reactions occur within the first 30 min of contrast medium injection (Murphy et al. 1996). Only one fatal reaction definitely attributable to gadolinium has been reported (Jordan and Mintz 1995).

7.3.2
Risk Factors for Reactions

7.3.2.1
Type of Contrast Medium

There appears to be no significant difference between the incidence of reactions with the different gadolinium agents, both ionic and nonionic (Kirchin and Runge 2003).

7.3.2.2
Patient Risk Factors

Patients with a history of previous reaction to iodinated or gadolinium contrast media, or with a history of asthma or allergy, have an increased risk of acute reaction following administration of gadolinium contrast media (Nelson et al. 1995; Li et al. 2007; Dillman et al. 2007).

7.3.3
Prevention of Reactions

No evidence is available in the literature to indicate what measures should be taken to prevent a reaction to gadolinium. The measures to be taken when a patient has previously had a reaction to gadolinium or is considered to be at high risk are therefore based on principles similar to those for iodinated contrast agents (see Acr Manual 2004 and Sect. 7.3.4 below). However, pre-medication does not prevent all reactions. Even after corticosteroid and antihistamine administration, breakthrough reactions have occurred after gadolinium-based contrast agents (DILMAN et al. 2008).

7.3.4
Summary: Gadolinium Contrast Media

The risk of an acute reaction to gadolinium contrast media is very low, and much lower than the risk of a reaction to iodinated contrast media. Nonetheless, for all patients the following is recommended:

- Keep the patient in the Radiology Department for 20 min after contrast medium injection.
- Have the drugs and equipment for resuscitation readily available.

The type of contrast medium, ionic or nonionic, does not appear to affect the incidence of reactions to gadolinium agents.

In patients with a previous reaction to a gadolinium agent or who are considered at very high risk,

- consider whether the use of gadolinium contrast medium is essential. Also consider whether an unenhanced scan or other test would give the diagnostic information needed;
- choose a different gadolinium agent to that used before in previous reaction;
- consider pre-medication.

A suitable corticosteroid pre-medication regime is

- prednisolone 30 mg (or methylprednisolone 32 mg) orally given 12 and 2 h before contrast medium;
- the possible use of H2 antihistamines.

References

ACR Committee on Drugs and Contrast Media (2004) Manual on contrast media, 5th edn. American College of Radiology, Reston, VA

Ansell G, Tweedie MCK, West CR et al (1980) The current status of reactions to intravenous contrast media. Invest Radiol 15(Suppl):S32–S39

Armstrong PA, Pazona JF, Schaeffer AJ (2005) Anaphylactoid reaction after retrograde pyelography despite preoperative steroid preparation. Urology 66:880

Bertrand PR, Soyer PM, Rouleau PJ et al (1992) Comparative randomised double-blind study of hydroxyzine versus placebo as premedication before injection of iodinated contrast media. Radiology 184:383–384

Bettman MA, Heeren T, Greenfield A, Gondey C (1997) Adverse events with radiographic contrast agents: results of the SCVIR Contrast Agent Registry. Radiology 203:611–620

Bush WH, Swanson DP (1991) Acute reactions to intravascular contrast media: types, risk factors, recognition and specific treatment. Am J Roentgenol 157:1153–1161

Caro JJ, Trindade E, McGregor M (1991) The risks of death and severe nonfatal reactions with high-vs low- osmolality contrast media: a meta-analysis. Am J Roentgenol 156:825–832

Choyke PL, Miller Dl, Lotze MT et al (1992) Delayed reactions to contrast media after interleukin-2 immunotherapy. Radiology 183:111–114

Cochran ST, Bomyea K, Sayre JW (2001) Trends in adverse events after iv administration of contrast media. Am J Roentgenol 176:1385–1388

Cohan RH, Ellis JH, Dunnick NR (1995) Use of low-osmolar agents and premedication to reduce the frequency of adverse reactions to radiographic contrast media: a survey of the Society of Uroradiology. Radiology 194: 357–364

Dawson P (2005) Commentary: repeat survey of current practice regarding corticosteroid prophylaxis for patients at increased risk of adverse reaction to intravascular contrast agents. Clin Radiol 60:56–57

Dawson P, Sidhu PS (1993) Is there a role for corticosteroid prophylaxis in patients at increased risk of adverse reactions to intravascular contrast agents? Clin Radiol 48:225–226

Dewachter P, Laroche D, Mouton-Fqaivre C, Clement O (2006) Immediate and late adverse reactions to iodinated contrast media: a pharmacological point of view. Anti-Inflammatory Anti-Allergy Agents Med Chem 5:105–117

Dilman JR, Ellis JH, Cohan RC (2007) Frequency and severity of acute allergic-like reactions to gadolinium-containing IV contrast media in children and adults. Am J Roentgenol 189: 1533–1538

Dilman JR, Ellis JH, Cohan RH, Strouse PJ, Jan SC (2008) Allergic like breakthrough reactions after corticosteroid and antihistamine premedication. Am J Roentgenol 190; 187–190

Dore CJ, Sidhu PS, Dawson P (1994) Is there a role for corticosteroid prophylaxis in patients at increased risk of adverse reactions to intravascular contrast agents? Clin Radiol 49:583–584

Dore CJ, Sidhu PS, Dawson P (1995) Is there a role for corticosteroid prophylaxis in patients at increased risk of adverse reactions to intravascular contrast agents? Clin Radiol 50:198–199

Eloy R, Corot C, Belleville J (1991) Contrast media for angiography: physicochemical properties, pharmacokinetics and biocompatibility. Clin Mater 7:89–197

Fink U, Fink BK, Lissner J (1992) Adverse reactions to nonionic contrast media with special regard to high-risk patients. Eur Radiol 2:317–321

Fischer HW, Doust VL (1972) An evaluation of pretesting in the problem of serious and fatal reactions to excretory urography. Radiology 103:497–501

Fishman JE, Aberle DR, Moldawer NP et al (1991) Atypical contrast reactions associated with systemic interleukin-2 therapy. Am J Roentgenol 156:833–834

Freed KS, Leder RA, Alexander C et al (2001) Breakthrough adverse reactions to low-osmolar contrast media after steroid premedication. Am J Roentgenol 176:1389–1392

Greenberger PA, Patterson R (1991) The prevention of immediate generalised reactions to radiocontrast media in high-risk patients. J Allergy Clin Immunol 87:867–872

Greenberger PA, Patterson R, Radin RR (1984) Two pre-treatment regimens for high-risk patients receiving radiographic contrast media. J Allergy Clin Immunol 74:540–543

Greenberger PA, Patterson R, Tapio CM (1985) Prophylaxis against repeated radiocontrast media reactions in 857 cases. Arch Intern Med 145:2197–2200

Greenberger PA, Meyers SN, Kramer BL et al (1987) Effects of beta-adrenergic and calcium antagonists on the development of anaphylactoid reactions from radiographic contrast media. J Allergy Clin Immunol 80:698–702

Hartman GW, Hattery RR, Witten DM, Williamson B (1982) Mortality during excretory urography: Mayo Clinic experience. Am J Roentgenol 139:919–922

Hugo PC, Neuberg AH, Newman JS, et al. (1998) Complications of arthrography. Semin Musculoskel Radiol 2:345–348

Idee JM, Pines E, Prigent P, Corot C (2005) Allergy-like reactions to iodinated contrast agents. A critical analysis. Fundam Clin Pharmacol 19:263–281

Jacobs JE, Birnbaum BA, Langlotz CP (1998) Contrast media reactions and extravasation: relationship to intravenous injection rates. Radiology 209:411–416

Jordan RM, Mintz RD (1995) Fatal reaction to gadopentetate dimeglumine. Am J Roentgenol 164:734–744

Katayama H, Yamaguchi K, Kozuka T et al (1990) Adverse reactions to ionic and nonionic contrast media. Radiology 175:621–628

King BF (1999) Intravascular contrast media and premedication. In: Bush WH, Krecke KN, King BF, Bettman MA (eds) Radiology life support (RAD-LS): a practical approach. Arnold, New York, p 15

Kirchin MA, Runge VM (2003) Contrast agents for magnetic resonance imaging: safety update. Top Magn Reson Imag 14:426–435

Lang DM, Alpern MB, Visintainer PF, Smith ST (1991) Increased risk for anaphylactoid reaction from contrast media in patients on β-adrenergic blockers or with asthma. Ann Intern Med 115:270–276

Lang DM, Alpern MB, Visintainer PF, Smith ST (1995) Gender risk for anaphylactoid reaction to radiographic contrast media. J Allergy Clin Immunol 95:813–817

Laroche D, Aimone-Gastin I, Dubois F, et al. (1998) Mechanisms of severe, immediate reactions to iodinated contrast material. Radiology 209:183–190

Lasser EC, Farr R, Fujimagari IT (1962) The significance of protein binding of contrast media in roentgen diagnosis. Am J Roentgenol 87:338–360

Lasser EC (1987) A coherent biochemical basis for increased reactivity to contrast material in allergic patients: a novel concept. Am J Roentgenol 149:1281–1285

Lasser EC (1994) Is there a role for corticosteroid prophylaxis in patients at increased risk of adverse reactions to intravascular contrast agents? Clin Radiol 49:582–583

Lasser EC (1995) Is there a role for corticosteroid prophylaxis in patients at increased risk of adverse reactions to intravascular contrast agents? Clin Radiol 50:199

Lasser EC (2004) The radiocontrast molecule in anaphylaxis: a surprising antigen. Anaphylaxis: Novartis Foundation Symposium 257. Wiley, Chichester, pp 211–225

Lasser EC, Berry CC (1994) Is there a role for corticosteroid prophylaxis in patients at increased risk of adverse reactions to intravascular contrast agents? Clin Radiol 49:584

Lasser EC, Lang JH, Lyon SG (1981) Glucocorticoid-induced elevations of C1-esterase inhibitor: a mechanism for protection against lethal dose range contrast challenge in rabbits. Invest Radiol 16:20–23

Lasser EC, Berry CC, Talner LB et al (1987) Pretreatment with corticosteroids to alleviate reactions to intravenous contrast material. N Engl J Med 317:845–849

Lasser EC, Berry CC, Mishkin MM et al (1994) Pretreatment with corticosteroids to prevent adverse reactions to nonionic contrast media. Am J Roentgenol 162:523–526

Lasser EC, Lyon SG, Berry CC (1997) Reports on contrast media reactions: analysis of data from reports to the US Food and Drug Administration. Radiology 203:605–610

Leder R (1997) Letter. Am J Roentgenol 169:906–907

Li A, Wong CS, Wong MK et al (2006) Acute adverse reactions to magnetic resonance contrast media – gadolinium chelates. Br J Radiol 79:368–371

Miller SH (1997) Anaphylactoid reaction after oral administration of diatrizoate meglumine and diatrizoate sodium solution. Am J Roentgenol 168:959–961

Morcos SK, Thomsen HS, Webb JAW et al (2001) Prevention of generalised reactions to contrast media: a consensus report and guidelines. Eur Radiol 11:1720–1728

Morcos SK (2005). Acute serious and fatal reactions to contrast media: our current understanding. Br J Radiol 78:686–693

Murphy KJ, Brunberg JA, Cohan RH (1996) Adverse reactions to gadolinium contrast media: a review of 36 cases. Am J Roentgenol 167:847–849

Murphy KP, Szopinski KT, Cohan RH, et al. (1999) Occurrence of adverse reactions to gadolinium-based contrast material and management of patients at increased risk: a survey of the American Society of Neuroradiology Fellowship Directors. Acad Radiol 6:656–664

Nelson KL, Gifford LM, Lauber-Huber C et al (1995) Clinical safety of gadopentetate dimeglumine. Radiology 196:439–443

Oldham RK, Brogley J, Braud E (1991) Contrast medium 'recalls' interleukin-2 toxicity. J Clin Oncol 8:942–943

Palmer FJ (1988) The RACR survey of intravenous contrast media reactions: final report. Austr Radiol 32:426–428

Radhakrishnan S, Manoharan S, Fleet M (2005) Repeat survey of current practice regarding corticosteroid prophylaxis for patients at increased risk of adverse reaction to intravascular contrast agents. Clin Radiol 60:58–63

Resuscitation Council (UK) (2008) Emergency treatment of anaphylactic reactions. www.resus.org.uk

Rodriguez RM, Gueant JL, Amone-Gastin I et al (2001) Comparison of effects of ioxaglate versus iomeprol on histamine and tryptase release in patients with ischemic cardiomyopathy. Am J Cardiol 88:185–188

Runge VM (2000) Safety of approved MR contrast media for intravenous injection. J Magn Reson Imag 12:205–213

Seymour R, Halpin SF, Hardman JA et al (1994) Corticosteroid prophylaxis in patients with increased risk of adverse reactions to intravascular contrast agents: a survey of current practice in the UK. Clin Radiol 49:791–795

Shehadi WH (1975) Adverse reactions to intravascularly administered contrast media. Am J Roentgenol 124:145–152

Shehadi WH (1985) Death following intravascular administration of contrast media. Acta Radiol Diagn 26:457–461

Siegle RL, Halvorsen RA, Dillon J et al (1991) The use of iohexol in patients with previous reactions to ionic contrast material. Invest Radiol 26:411–416

Sontum PC Christiansen C, Kasparkova V, Skotland T (1998) Evidence against molecular aggregates in concentrated solutions of X-ray contrast media. Int J Pharm 169:203–212

Thomsen HS, Bush WH (1998) Adverse effects of contrast media: incidence, prevention and management. Drug Safety 19:313–324

Weese DL, Greenberg HM, Zimmern PE (1993) Contrast media reactions during voiding cystourethrography or retrograde pyelography. Urology 41:81–84

Witten DM, Hirsch FD, Hartman GW (1973) Acute reactions to urographic contrast medium. Am J Roentgenol 119:832–840

Wolf GL, Miskin MM, Roux SG et al (1991) Comparison of the rates of adverse drug reactions: ionic contrast agents, ionic agents combined with steroids and nonionic agents. Invest Radiol 26:404–410

Yamaguchi K, Katayama H, Takashima T et al (1991) Prediction of severe adverse reactions to ionic and nonionic contrast media in Japan: evaluation of prestesting. Radiology 178:363–367

Zukiwski AA, David CL, Coan J et al (1990) Increased incidence of hypersensitivity to iodine-containing radiographic contrast media after interleukin-2 administration. Cancer 65:1521–1524

Management of Acute Adverse Reactions

8

Henrik S. Thomsen

Henrik S. Thomsen
Department of Diagnostic Sciences, Faculty of Health Sciences, University of Copenhagen, DK-2200 Copenhagen N, Denmark
and
Department of Diagnostic Radiology,
Copenhagen University Hospital Herlev, 2730 Herlev, Denmark

8.1 Introduction

Improvements in the physico-chemical properties of iodinated contrast medium molecules have been followed by a significant decrease in the frequency of acute adverse reactions (POLLACK 1999; THOMSEN and MORCOS 2000). The incidence of anaphylactic reactions to gadolinium contrast media is significantly lower than to iodinated contrast media (Chaps. 7 and 23). Nonetheless, serious reactions may still occur and remain a source of concern.

A local audit in Australia demonstrated deficient acute management of anaphylactoid/anaphylactic reactions in radiology departments by both consultants and trainees (BARTLETT and BYNEVELT 2003). A poorly managed resuscitation situation and adverse outcome will be costly to practice as well as the individual in terms of financial loss and professional respect. All radiologists should be prepared to give immediate treatment for acute contrast medium reactions. Therefore, first-line management should be simple and suitable for the current era when acute adverse reactions are rare. The subsequent management of severe adverse reactions including administration of second-line drugs should be handled by the resuscitation team. The discussion of risk factors and incidence refers to iodinated contrast agents about which much more data is available. The management of acute adverse reactions is, however, identical whether they are caused by iodinated or gadolinium agents.

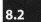

8.2
Risk Factors for Acute Reactions to Iodinated Contrast Media

A history of previous moderate or severe adverse reaction to iodinated contrast media is an important risk factor (MORCOS et al. 2001; KATAYAMA et al. 1990). In KATAYAMA et al.'s (1990) series of over 330,000 patients, there was a six-fold increase in reactions to both ionic and nonionic contrast media following a previous severe adverse reaction. Asthma is also an important risk factor with a reported six- to ten-fold increase in the risk of a severe reaction in such patients (KATAYAMA et al. 1990). Patients treated with interleukin-2 are at increased risk of adverse reactions to contrast media, whereas whether or not β-adrenergic blockers affect the incidence of idiosyncratic contrast medium reactions is controversial (LANG et al. 1991, 1993; VERVLOET and DURHAM 1998; TAYLOR 1998; FISHMAN et al. 1991; OLDHAM et al. 1990; CHOYKE et al. 1992; GREENBERGER et al. 1987). GREENBERGER et al. (1987) reported that neither β-blockers nor calcium antagonists given separately or together increased the risk of reaction. Subsequently, however, LANG et al. (1991, 1993) found that β-blockers did increase the risk of reaction. Today, β-adrenergic blockers are seldom stopped before giving intravascular contrast medium (MORCOS et al. 2001).

In patients who have had a previous severe reaction to iodinated contrast medium, most radiologists avoid giving intravascular contrast media if at all possible (MORCOS et al. 2001). If the examination is considered essential, nonionic contrast media are the agents of choice on the basis of the evidence in the literature that with nonionic agents the risk of reaction is reduced by a factor of 4–5 (KATAYAMA et al. 1990). The potential risks of the procedure should be explained to the patient, and the resuscitation team should be present when the contrast medium is given (MORCOS et al. 2001).

8.3
Acute Adverse Reactions

An acute adverse reaction is defined as an adverse event that occurs within 60 min of an injection of contrast medium. Most anaphylactic reactions occur within 20 min after intravenous injection (RESUSCITATION COUNCIL (UK) 2008). Reactions can be divided into mild, moderate, and severe. The mild reactions include flushing, nausea, arm pain, pruritus, vomiting, headache, and mild urticaria. They are usually of short duration and self-limiting, and generally require no specific treatment. Moderate reactions include more serious degrees of the above symptoms and/or moderate degrees of hypotension and bronchospasm. They usually respond readily to appropriate treatment. Severe life-threatening reactions include severe manifestations of all the symptoms included under mild and moderate reactions in addition to symptoms such as convulsions, unconsciousness, laryngeal edema, pulmonary edema, cardiac dysrhythmias and arrest, and cardiovascular and pulmonary collapse (GRAINGER 1997).

8.4
Incidence of Acute Reactions to Iodinated Contrast Media

Mild adverse reactions are encountered in as many as 15% of patients after intravenous ionic, high-osmolarity, iodine-based contrast agents (1,000–2,000 mOsm $kg^{-1}H_2O$) and up to 3% of patients after nonionic, low-osmolality contrast media (500–1,000 mOsm $kg^{-1}H_2O$). Severe and very severe reactions occur much less frequently, with an incidence of 0.22 and 0.04% (respectively) in patients after intravenous high-osmolarity contrast media and 0.04 and 0.004% in patients after low-osmolality contrast media. Thus, the incidence of contrast reactions with low-osmolarity contrast media is lower than with high-osmolarity contrast media by a factor of 5 for mild reactions and by a factor of 10 for severe reactions. Fatal reactions to both types of contrast media are exceedingly rare (1:170,000), with no difference in mortality reported between the two agents (KATAYAMA et al. 1990; THOMSEN and DORPH 1993; THOMSEN and BUSH 1998).

8.5
Mechanisms and Pathophysiology

Adverse reactions to drugs are generally classified into those that occur only in susceptible subjects and those that may occur in anyone. Reactions occurring in susceptible subjects include drug intolerance (low threshold to the normal pharmacological action of a drug), drug idiosyncrasy (a genetically determined, qualitatively abnormal reaction to a drug related to metabolic or enzyme deficiency), drug allergy (an immunologically mediated reaction, characterized by specificity, prior exposure, transferability by antibodies or lymphocytes, and recurrence on re-exposure), and pseudoallergic reactions which are the same as allergic reactions but are lacking immunological specificity (non-specific complement activation and non-specific histamine release mimicking type 1 allergic reactions) (STACUL 1999).

Although some reactions are difficult to categorize, most non-renal side effects of intravascular contrast media are considered idiosyncratic or pseudo-allergic reactions. They are unpredictable and not dose dependent, and may involve the release of histamine and other active biological mediators such as serotonin, prostaglandins, bradykinin, leukotrienes, adenosine, and endothelin (ALMEN 1994). Activation and inhibition of several enzyme systems have also been implicated. There is no conclusive evidence to indicate that reactions to iodinated contrast media are allergic in nature since antibodies against contrast media including IgE have not been consistently demonstrated (ALMEN 1994; SIEGLE 1999; LAROCHE et al. 1998).

Chemotoxic-type effects may also occur and are determined by dose, the molecular toxicity of each agent, and the physiological characteristics of the contrast agents (i.e, osmolality, viscosity, hydrophilicity, affinity to proteins, calcium-binding properties, and sodium content). Chemotoxic effects of iodinated contrast media are more likely to occur in patients who are debilitated or medically unstable. High osmolality (osmotoxicity) causes shift of fluids from the intra-cellular to the extra-cellular space, leading to cell dehydration and an increase in intra-cellular fluid viscosity precipitating cellular dysfunction (ALMEN 1994; SIEGLE 1999). Low hydrophilicity may reduce the biological tolerance to iodinated contrast media since it is associated with an increase in lipophilicity and higher affinity of the contrast medium molecule to plasma proteins and the cell membrane. High hydrophilicity of nonionic contrast media is produced by hydroxyl (–OH) groups which are symmetrically distributed, thereby offering a good coverage of the benzene ring and restricting access to lipophilic areas of the iodinated contrast molecule (ALMEN 1994; SIEGLE 1999; BONNEMANN et al. 1990).

8.6
Treatment

The vast majority of patients with severe anaphylactoid-type reactions recover if they are treated quickly and appropriately. Most patients have reactions while they are still in the radiology department, and 94–100% of severe and fatal reactions occur within 20 min of the contrast medium injection (SHEHADI 1985). The ability to assess and treat the contrast reaction effectively is an essential skill that the radiologist should have and maintain. The first-line drugs and equipment should be readily available in rooms in which either iodine- or gadolinium-based contrast agents are injected, and a list of recommended drugs and equipment is given in Chap. 29. A survey has shown that most departments have these items available (MORCOS et al. 2001).

The radiologist should remain near for at least the first critical minutes following contrast injection and should remain in the immediate vicinity for the next 30–45 min. If there is an increased risk of an adverse reaction, venous access should be left in place.

Important first-line management includes establishment of an adequate airway, oxygen supplementation, administration of intravascular physiological fluids, and measuring the blood pressure and heart rate. Talking to the patient as you check their pulse rate provides useful initial information: breathing is assessed, the possibility of a vagal reaction (bradycardia) is determined, and a rough estimate of systolic pressure is obtained (a palpable radial artery pulse approximates a systolic pressure of 80–90 mmHg).

8.6.1
Drugs, Fluid, and Oxygen

The first-line drugs and most important emergency equipment (see Chap. 29) should be available either in or just outside the room where contrast media are given.

8.6.1.1
Oxygen

Oxygen by mask at relatively high rate (6–10 l min^{-1}) is very important in the initial treatment of all severe reactions to intravascular contrast media and for other emergencies unrelated to contrast media that occur in the radiology department or angiography suite (e.g., vagal reaction, hypotension, cardiac ischemia). Hypoxia can be a major complicating factor in all these situations, and can be induced by drugs such as adrenaline used for treating reactions. A "non-rebreather" mask is optimal; nasal "prongs" are much less effective and should be avoided in an acute situation for preventing hypoxemia. Oxygen should be used for all patients; a history of chronic obstructive pulmonary disease or emphysema is not a contraindication to starting oxygen therapy for an acute reaction.

8.6.1.2
Intravascular Fluid Administration

Intravascular fluid administration is very important, and it alone has been reported to be the most effective treatment for hypotension (van Sonnenberg et al. 1987). Starting intravenous fluid early before drug treatment is the highest priority in treating hypotension. There is no evidence to support the use of colloids over crystalloids in this setting. For initial resuscitation, 0.9% saline is a suitable fluid.

8.6.1.3
Adrenaline

Adrenaline is an effective drug for treating certain serious contrast reactions. Although there are no randomised controlled trials, adrenaline is a logical treatment (Resucitation Council (UK) 2008). There is consistent anecdotal evidence supporting its use to ease breathing difficulty and restore adequate cardiac output. The α-agonist effects of adrenaline increase blood pressure and reverse peripheral vasodilatation. The vasoconstriction induced decreases angioedema and urticaria. The β-agonist actions of adrenaline reverse bronchoconstriction, produce positive inotropic and chronotropic cardiac effects (increase in strength and rate of cardiac contractions), and may increase intracellular cyclic adenosine monophosphate (AMP) (Smith and Corbascio 1970; Hoffman and Lefkowitz 1990). Increments in baseline cyclic AMP levels are generally considered to inhibit mediator release from inflammatory cells. There are β-2 adrenergic receptors on mast cells that inhibit activation.

The use of adrenaline demands careful attention (Bush and Swanson 1991). For example, in individuals with a fragile intra-cerebral or coronary circulation, the α-agonist effects of a *large* dose of adrenaline may provoke a hypertensive crisis that could produce a stroke or myocardial ischemia (Barach et al. 1984). β-Receptor sites usually respond to lower doses of adrenaline than α-sites, but if a patient is on β-blockers, the refractory response that may occur might encourage the radiologist to increase the dose of adrenaline to the point that there are unwanted α-effects. Patients with chronic asthma may simulate patients receiving β-blockers since they may have a systemic β-adrenergic hyporesponsiveness. When chronic asthmatics develop an anaphylaxis-like reaction with asthmatic symptoms requiring β-receptor stimulation, one option is to use isoproterenol as the primary adrenergic drug, combined with more conservative doses of adrenaline (Ingall et al. 1984; Bush 1996).

When possible, adrenaline should be avoided for treating a pregnant patient with severe contrast reaction and hypotension (Entman and Moise 1984). Because uterine vessels are sensitive to the α-effect of adrenaline, the combination of hypotension plus adrenaline can cause harmful sequelae to the fetus. Ephedrine is a possible alternative.

Only one concentration (1:1,000) of adrenaline should be available in the radiology department to avoid confusion under stressful emergency conditions, where ampoules of different concentrations can be misidentified. The 1:1,000 preparation should be given intramuscularly only. Intravenous administration of adrenaline by inexperienced staff can be dangerous. The intramuscular route has several benefits: (1) there is a greater margin of safety, (2) it does not require intravenous access, and (3) the intra-muscular route is easier to learn. The best site for intra-muscular injection is the antero-lateral aspect of the middle third of the thigh. The needle used for injection needs to be sufficiently long to ensure that the adrenaline is injected into the muscle (Resuscitation Council (UK) 2008). Dilution of adrenaline for intravenous use is time consuming and delays treatment. Only 43% of the participants in an Australian audit knew the recommended dose of adrenaline (Bartlett and Bynevelt 2003). This reinforces the need for a standard dose such as 0.5 mg in adults and 0.3 mg in children between 6 and 12 years old (see Chap. 29). Below 6 years of age, the Resuscitation Council in UK (2008) recommends 0.15 mg. If there is no improvement in the patient's condition, the intra-muscular adrenaline dose can be repeated at about 5 min intervals by non-specialists if the specialist resuscitation team has not arrived.

8.6.1.4
H2 Antihistamines and H2 Receptor Blockers

H2 antihistamines and H2 receptor blockers have a limited role in treating contrast media reactions. They are used primarily to reduce symptoms from skin reactions.

8.6.1.5
Corticosteroids

High-dose intravenous corticosteroids do not play a role in the first-line treatment of the acute adverse reaction. However, very high doses of corticosteroids may have an immediate stabilizing effect on cell membranes and may be used in the second-line treatment. Standard doses can be effective in reducing delayed recurrent symptoms, which can be observed for as long as 48 h after an initial reaction. It takes 6 h before corticosteroids are fully active (LASSER et al. 1977; GILLENBERGER et al. 1986).

8.6.1.6
Inhaled β-2 Adrenergic Agonists

Inhaled β-2 adrenergic agonists such as albuterol, metaproterenol, and terbutaline deliver large doses of broncho-dilating β-2 agonist drugs directly to the airways with minimal systemic absorption and, therefore, minimal cardiovascular effects.

8.6.1.7
Atropine

Atropine blocks vagal stimulation of the cardiac conduction system. Large doses of atropine (0.6–1.0 mg) are indicated, since low doses (e.g., less than 0.5 mg) of atropine can be detrimental for treating bradycardia associated with contrast-media-induced vagal reactions (BUSH and SWANSON 1991; CHAMBERLAIN et al. 1967; STANLEY and PFISTER 1976; BROWN 1990; BUSH et al. 1993).

8.6.2
Treatment of Specific Reactions

8.6.2.1
Nausea and Vomiting

Nausea and vomiting, though usually self-limited, may be the first signs of a more severe reaction. With urography using ionic, high-osmolar iodine-based contrast agents, 15–20% of fatal reactions began with nausea and vomiting (LALLI 1980). For this reason, the patient should be observed closely for systemic symptoms while intravenous access is maintained. The injection should be slowed or stopped. In severe, protracted cases, injection of an anti-emetic may be used (see Chap. 29).

8.6.2.2
Cutaneous Reactions

Treatment is usually not necessary if there are only a few scattered hives or pruritus. However, the patient should be observed closely for other systemic symptoms that may develop, and intravenous access should be maintained. Treatment should be given only if the urticaria is extensive or bothersome to the patient (see Chap. 29).

8.6.2.3
Bronchospasm

Bronchospasm without co-existing cardiovascular problems should be treated with oxygen and inhaled bronchodilators (see Chap. 29). Using a metered dose inhaler, treatment typically involves two to three deep inhalations. Adrenaline may be used if bronchospasm is not relieved by the inhaled bronchodilators.

8.6.2.4
Laryngeal Oedema

Laryngeal oedema does not respond well to inhaled β-agonists; these agents may actually worsen it. Therefore, careful clinical evaluation of the patient before beginning treatment is extremely important to differentiate laryngeal oedema from bronchospasm. Adrenaline is the primary treatment for laryngeal oedema (see Chap. 29). Oxygen supplementation is also important in the management of this condition.

8.6.2.5
Hypotension

Profound hypotension may occur without respiratory symptoms. Normal sinus rhythm and tachycardia differentiate this reaction from the so-called vagal reaction (hypotension plus sinus bradycardia). Initially, the patient's legs should be elevated, since this returns about 700 ml of blood to the central circulation (van Sonnenberg et al. 1987). Isolated hypotension is best treated first by rapid intravenous fluid replacement rather than vasopressor drugs (see Chap. 29). A total volume of up to 3,000 ml may be required to reverse the hypotension.

8.6.2.6
Vagal Reaction

Vagal reactions are characterized by the combination of prominent sinus bradycardia (pulse rate < 60 beats/min) and hypotension (systolic pressure < 80 mmHg). Although their exact cause is unknown, vagal reactions seem to be elicited or accentuated by anxiety. Proper recognition of this reaction and the associated bradycardia is vital so that the correct treatment of increasing intravascular fluid volume plus reversing the vagal stimulation is used. Elevation of the patient's legs and rapid infusion of intravenous fluids treat the vasodilatation and expanded vascular space. The bradycardia is treated by intravenous administration of atropine to block vagal stimulation of the cardiac conduction system (see Chap. 29).

8.6.2.7
Generalized Anaphylactoid Reactions

These are acute, rapidly progressing, systemic reactions characterized by multi-system involvement with pruritus, urticaria, angioedema, respiratory distress (bronchospasm and/or laryngeal edema), and profound hypotension that require prompt response. Anaphylaxis is likely when of the following three criteria are met: (1) sudden onset and rapid progression of symptoms, (2) life-threatening airway and/or breathing and/or circulation problems, and (3) skin and/or mucosal changes (flushing, urticaria, angioedema) (Resuscitation Council (UK) 2008). Recent exposure to a contrast agent supports the diagnosis. Initial treatment includes maintenance of the airway, administration of oxygen, rapid infusion of intravenous fluids, and administration of adrenergic drugs (see Chap. 29). Adrenaline is the drug of choice. Intramuscular injection of 0.5 ml of 1:1,000 adrenaline preparation is recommended in preference to intravenous administration, which requires careful electrocardiogram (ECG) monitoring and slow administration, ideally by people experienced in its use. According to the Project Team of the Resuscitation Council in the United Kingdom, adrenaline 1:1,000 should never be used intravenously because of the risk of arrhythmia, and subcutaneous administration

is not helpful in acute life-threatening situations (Project Team of the Resuscitation Council (UK) 1999; Hughes and Fitzharris 1999; Resuscitation Council (UK) 2008).

Hypoxia increases the risk of severe cardiac arrhythmias. Also, the amount of adrenaline should be limited in patients who are receiving non-cardioselective β-blocking medications (e.g., propranolol) as discussed above. Adrenaline should be avoided, if possible, in a pregnant patient experiencing an anaphylactoid reaction with hypotension. When adrenaline is contraindicated, bronchospasm can be treated with a β-2 agonist inhaler (β-2 with no α-effects).

8.7
Serum Tryptase Measurement after Acute Reactions to Contrast Agents

During anaphylaxis, tryptase is released from the mast cells into the blood. Blood tryptase levels peak at 1–2 h, and decline rapidly with a 2 h half-life. Whether or not collapse after contrast medium represented an anaphylactoid reaction may be important to future care of the patient. The UK Resuscitation Council recommends that blood samples for tryptase are taken following suspected anaphylaxis, so that the diagnosis can be established. The minimum recommendation is one sample 1–2 h after the reaction. Ideally, three samples should be obtained – the first once resuscitation is underway, the second at 1–2 h after the reaction, and the third at 24 h or during convalescence (Resuscitation Council (UK) 2008).

8.8
Be Prepared

Prompt recognition and treatment can be invaluable in blunting an adverse response of a patient to iodine- or gadolinium-based contrast agents and may prevent a reaction from becoming severe or even life threatening. Radiologists and their staff should review treatment protocols regularly (e.g., at 6–12 monthly intervals) so that each can accomplish his or her role efficiently (Bush and Swanson 1991; Gillenberger et al. 1986; Bush et al. 1993; Cohan et al. 1996; Emergency Cardiac Care Committee and Subcommittees 1992; Bartlett and Bynevelt 2003; Berden et al. 1993). Knowledge, training, and preparation are crucial for guaranteeing appropriate and effective treatment if there is an adverse contrast-related event.

References

Almen T (1994) The etiology of contrast medium reactions. Invest Radiol 29(Suppl):S37–S45

Barach EM, Nowak RM, Tennyson GL, Tomlanovich MC (1984) Epinephrine for treatment of anaphylactic shock. JAMA 251:2118–2122

Bartlett MJ, Bynevelt M (2003) Acute contrast reaction management by radiologists: a local audit study. Austr Radiol 47:363–367

Berden HJJM, Willems FF, Hendrick JMA, Pijls NH, Knape JT (1993) How frequently should basic cardiopulmonary resuscitation training be repeated to maintain adequate skills? Br J Med 306:1576–1577

Bonnemain B, Meyer D, Schaffer M, Dugast-Zrihen M (1990) New iodinated low osmolar contrast media. A revised concept of hydrophilicity. Invest Radiol 25 [Suppl]:S104-S106

Brown JH (1990) Atropine, scopolamine and antimuscarinic. In: Gilman AG, Rall TW, Nies AS, Taylor P (eds) The pharmacological basis of therapeutics. Pergamon, New York, pp 150–165

Bush WH (1996) Risk factors, prophylaxis and therapy of X-ray contrast media reactions. Adv X-Ray Contrast 3:44–53

Bush WH, Swanson DP (1991) Acute reactions to intravascular contrast media: types, risk factors, recognition, and specific treatment. Am J Roentgenol 157:1153–1161

Bush WH, McClennan BL, Swanson DP (1993) Contrast media reactions: prediction, prevention, and treatment. Postgrad Radiol 13:137–147

Chamberlain DA, Turner P, Sneddon JM (1967) Effects of atropine on heart-rate in healthy man. Lancet 2:12–15

Choyke PL, Miller DL, Leder MT et al (1992) Delayed reactions to contrast media after interleukin-2 immunotherapy. Radiology 183:111–114

Cohan RH, Leder RA, Ellis JH (1996) Treatment of adverse reactions to radiographic contrast media in adults. Radiol Clin North Am 34:1055–1060

Emergency Cardiac Care Committee and Subcommittees (1992) American Heart Association. Guidelines for cardiopulmonary resuscitation and emergency cardiac care, III: Adult Advanced Cardiac Life Support. JAMA 268:2199–2241

Entman SS, Moise KJ (1984) Anaphylaxis in pregnancy. South Med J 77:402

Fishman J, Aberle D, Moldawer N et al (1991) Atypical contrast reactions associated with systemic interleukin-2 therapy. Am J Roentgenol 156:833–834

Gillenberger PA, Halwig TM, Patterson R et al (1986) Emergency administration of a radiocontrast media in high risk patients. J Allergy Clin Immunol 77:630–635

Grainger RG (1997) Intravascular contrast media. In: Grainger RG, Allison D (eds) Grainger and Allison's diagnostic radiology: a textbook of medical imaging. Churchill Livingstone, New York, pp 40–41

Greenberger PA, Meyers SN, Kramer BL et al (1987) Effects of beta-adrenergic and calcium antagonists on the development of anaphylactoid reactions from radiographic contrast media. J Allergy Clin Immunol 80:698–702

Hoffman BB, Lefkowitz RJ (1990) Catecholamines and sympathomimetic drugs. In: Gilman AG, Rall TW, Nies AS, Taylor P (eds) The pharmacological basis of therapeutics. Pergamon, New York, pp 192–198

Hughes G, Fitzharris P (1999) Managing acute anaphylaxis, new guidelines emphasize importance of intramuscular adrenaline. Br Med J 319:1–2

Ingall M, Goldman G, Page LB (1984) Beta-blockade in stinging insect anaphylaxis (letter). JAMA 251:1432

Katayama H, Yamaguchi K, Kozuka T, Takashima T, Seez P, Matsuura K (1990) Adverse reactions to ionic and nonionic contrast media. Radiology 175:621–628

Lalli AF (1980) Contrast media reactions: data analysis and hypothesis. Radiology 134:1–12

Lang DM, Alpern MB Visintainer PF, Smith ST (1991) Increased risk for anaphylactoid reaction from contrast media in patients on β-adrenergic blockers with asthma. Ann Intern Med 115:270–276

Lang DM, Alpern MB, Visintainer PF, Smith ST (1993) Elevated risk of anaphylactoid reaction from radiographic contrast media is associated with both beta-blocker exposure and cardiovascular disorders. Arch Intern Med 153:2033–2040 (Erratum in: Arch Intern Med 1993, 153:2412)

Laroche D, Aimone-Gastin I, Dubois F et al (1998) Mechanisms of severe, immediate reactions to iodinated contrast material. Radiology 209:183–190

Lasser EC, Lang JH, Sovak M et al (1977) Steroids: theoretical and experimental basis for utilization in prevention of contrast media reactions. Radiology 125:1–9

Morcos SK, Thomsen HS, Webb JAW (2001) Prevention of generalized reactions to contrast media: a consensus report and guidelines. Eur Radiol 11:1720–1728

Oldham R, Brogley J, Braud E (1990) Contrast media"recalls" interleukin-2 toxicity (letter to the editor). J Clin Oncol 8:942

Pollack HM (1999) History of iodinated contrast media. In: Thomsen HS, Muller RN, Mattrey RF (eds) Trends in contrast media. Springer, Berlin, pp 1–19

Project Team of the Resuscitation Council (UK) (1999) Emergency medical treatment of anaphylactic reactions. J Accid Emerg Med 16:243–247

Resuscitation Council (UK) (2008) Emergency treatment of anaphylactic reactions. www.resus.org.uk

Shehadi WH (1985) Death following intravascular administration of contrast media. Acta Radiol Diagn 26:457–461

Siegle RL (1999) Mechanisms of reactions to contrast media. In: Dawson P, Cosgrove DO, Grainger RG (eds) Textbook of contrast media. Isis Medical Media, Oxford, pp 95–98

Smith NT, Corbascio A (1970) The use and misuse of pressor agents. Anesthesiology 33:58–101

Stacul F (1999) Currently available iodinated contrast media. In: Thomsen HS, Muller RN, Mattrey RF (eds) Trends in contrast media. Springer, Berlin, pp 71–72

Stanley RJ, Pfister RC (1976) Bradycardia and hypotension following use of intravenous contrast media. Radiology 121:5–7

Taylor AJN (1998) Asthma and allergy. BMJ 316:997–999

Thomsen HS, Bush WH Jr (1998) Adverse effects of contrast media. Incidence, prevention and management. Drug Saf 19:313–324

Thomsen HS, Dorph S (1993) High-osmolar and low-osmolar contrast media. An update on frequency of adverse drug reactions. Acta Radiol 34:205–209

Thomsen HS, Morcos SK (2000) Radiographic contrast media. BJU Int 86(Suppl 1):1–10

Van Sonnenberg E, Neff CC, Pfister RC (1987) Life-threatening hypotensive reactions to contrast administration: comparison of pharmacologic and fluid therapy. Radiology 162:15–19

Vervloet D, Durham S (1998) ABC of allergies: adverse reactions to drugs. BMJ 316:1511–1514

Iodinated and Gadolinium Contrast Media

Renal Adverse Effects

Contrast Medium-Induced Nephropathy

Henrik S. Thomsen

Henrik S. Thomsen
Department of Diagnostic Sciences, Faculty of Health
Sciences, University of Copenhagen, DK-2200 Copenhagen N,
Denmark
and
Department of Diagnostic Radiology,
Copenhagen University Hospital Herlev, 2730 Herlev,
Denmark

9.1
Introduction

Acute renal failure is a sudden and rapid deterioration in renal function which results in the failure of the kidney to excrete nitrogenous waste products and to maintain fluid and electrolyte homeostasis. It may be a result of intravascular administration of radiographic and magnetic resonance (MR) contrast media (see also Chap. 22). Despite increased awareness, contrast medium-induced nephropathy remains the third most common cause of hospital-acquired kidney failure, and was responsible for 11% of cases in 2002 and 12% in 1979 (Hou et al. 1983; Nash et al. 2002). The mortality rate in those cases was 14%.

The term "contrast medium-induced nephropathy" is widely used to refer to the reduction in renal function induced by contrast media. It implies impairment in renal function (an increase in serum creatinine by more than 25% or $44\,\mu$mol l^{-1} (0.5 mg dl^{-1})) that occurs within 3 days following the intravascular administration of contrast media in the absence of an alternative aetiology (Morcos et al. 1999). However, the two definitions of contrast medium-induced nephropathy – either an increase in serum creatinine by $>44\,\mu$mol l^{-1} (0.5 mg dl^{-1}), or $>25\%$ from baseline – do not reflect the same changes in kidney function. The first definition is more sensitive for detecting contrast medium-induced nephropathy in patients with advanced renal impairment, whereas the second one is more sensitive in those with better pre-existing kidney function (Thomsen and Morcos 2008). Therefore, when the results of various studies are compared, it is important to ensure that the same definition of contrast medium-induced nephropathy is used in all of them.

Contrast medium-induced nephropathy ranges in severity from asymptomatic, non-oliguric, transient renal dysfunction to oliguric, severe, acute renal failure necessitating dialysis. Serum creatinine often peaks within 3–4 days after the administration of contrast media (Morcos 1998; Katzberg 1997). Fortunately, most episodes of contrast medium-induced nephropathy are self-limited and resolve within 1–2 weeks. Many non-anuric episodes are probably undetected, because the serum creatinine is rarely measured after administration of contrast media if the patients have no symptoms, especially if they are outpatients who have received intravenous contrast medium. Permanent renal damage is very rare.

Diagnostic and interventional procedures using contrast media are performed with increasing frequency. The patient population subjected to these procedures is progressively older with more comorbid conditions (Solomon 1998). Prevention is important to avoid the substantial morbidity and even mortality that may sometimes be associated with contrast medium-induced nephropathy. Even a small decrease in renal function may greatly exacerbate morbidity and mortality caused by coexisting conditions (Gruberg et al. 2000; McCullough et al. 1997). Patients with contrast medium-induced nephropathy have a higher mortality rate (31%) than patients without it (0.6%) after primary angioplasty for acute myocardial infarction (Marenzi et al. 2004). The 30-day mortality is higher in patients with contrast medium-induced nephropathy (16.2%) than in those without (1.2%), and the difference is maintained at 1 year (23.3% vs. 3.2%) (Sadeghi et al. 2003). Sepsis, bleeding, coma, and respiratory failure are frequently observed in patients with acute renal failure. However, all this information derives from intra-arterial administration of contrast media for cardiac studies. As yet, there is no adequate information about whether contrast medium-induced nephropathy after an intravenous injection is associated with increased mortality and morbidity after 1 or more years. Also, cardiac angiography is performed on a dysfunctional heart, which may cause renal ischemia because of changes in blood pressure, whereas blood pressure changes are very infrequent in relation to intravenous injection.

9.2
Radiographic Features

A persistent nephrogram on plain radiography or computed tomography (CT) of the abdomen at 24–48 h after contrast medium injection has been described as a feature of contrast medium-induced nephropathy (Berns 1989; Love et al. 1994). However, its presence is not always associated with a reduction in renal function (Jakobsen et al. 1992; Yamazaki et al. 1997a). Also, opacification of the gall bladder is not necessarily related to the occurrence of contrast medium-induced nephropathy (Yamazaki et al. 1997b). However, if these signs are present, renal function should be assessed and the administration of further doses of contrast media should be avoided if the results are abnormal.

9.3
Incidence

Contrast medium-induced nephropathy is rare in people with normal renal function, with the incidence varying from 0 to 2% (Morcos et al. 1999; McCullough et al. 1997; Rudnick et al. 1995). In acute myocardial infarction, contrast medium-induced nephropathy occurred after primary coronary angioplasty in 13% of patients who had normal serum creatinine levels before the angioplasty (Marenzi et al. 2004). However, it is unclear whether it was the contrast medium or the cardiac dysfunction that reduced the renal function temporarily. Nearly all recent studies of contrast medium-induced nephropathy have involved arterial injection (coronary or peripheral angiography and angioplasty). Over the past 40 years, there have only been 40 studies of the effects of intravenous injection, but there have been over 3,000 studies of the effects of intra-arterial injection (Katzberg and Barrett 2007). Pre-existing renal impairment increases the frequency of contrast medium-induced nephropathy. The incidence of contrast medium-induced nephropathy ranged from 3 to 33% in several prospective controlled studies (Morcos et al. 1999; Solomon 1998; Rudnick et al. 1995; Bettmann 2005). The incidence of contrast medium-induced nephropathy varied from 3 to 45% in the control arms of prospective trials of acetylcysteine, and the contrast agent was given intra-arterially (Bettmann 2005; Sharma and Kini 2005; Solomon and duMouchel 2006; Solomon 2005). In head-to-head trials of various contrast agents administered intra-arterially, the incidence varied between 3 and 26%; the same range was found in patients with diabetic nephropathy (Thomsen et al. 2008b). The incidence is significantly higher in patients with diabetic nephropathy (19.7%) than in patients with other types of nephropathy (5.7%)

(RUDNICK et al. 1995). The most frequently used definition of contrast medium-induced nephropathy was an elevation in serum creatinine of 44 μmol l^{-1} (0.5 mg dl^{-1}) or more, particularly in the most recent studies.

The incidence of contrast medium-induced nephropathy appears to be much lower after intravenous administration. Recent studies reported 0–2% incidence of contrast medium-induced nephropathy, defined as an increase in serum creatinine level of 44 μmol l^{-1} (1.5 mg dl^{-1}) or more in an unselected group of patients with chronic kidney disease 3 and 4 (BARRETT et al. 2006; THOMSEN et al. 2008b). KUHN et al. (2008) reported a 5% incidence of contrast medium-induced nephropathy, defined as an elevation of 25% or more in serum creatinine level in patients suffering from diabetic nephropathy. In a group of cancer patients with underlying renal insufficiency receiving the contrast agent intravenously, 9.0% developed contrast medium-induced nephropathy, defined as absolute elevation of 44 μmol l^{-1} or 25% elevation in serum creatinine level, with 4.8% of patients developing irreversible renal damage (CHERUVU et al. 2007).

The long-term effects of contrast media on renal function in humans are not known.

9.4
Renal Handling of Contrast Media

After intravascular administration, contrast medium molecules move across capillary membranes (except an intact blood–brain barrier) into the interstitial extracellular space. Reverse movement from the extracellular space into the intravascular compartment occurs, and a state of equilibrium is generally reached within 2 h. Continuous elimination through the glomeruli also occurs. Less than 1% is excreted extrarenally in patients with normal renal function (THOMSEN et al. 1993). Following intravascular administration in patients with normal renal function, the elimination half-life of contrast media is about 2 h, and 75% of the administered dose is excreted in the urine within 4 h (KATZBERG 1997). After 24 h, 98% of the injected contrast medium would have been excreted. After approximately 150 min, the concentration of contrast medium decreases in a monoexponential way in patients with normal renal function, but in patients with severely reduced renal function this phase is delayed (ALMÉN et al. 1999).

9.5
Pathophysiology of Contrast Medium-Induced Nephropathy

There are three relatively distinct mechanisms or pathways *proposed* for the pathophysiology of contrast medium induced nephropathy: (1) reduction in renal perfusion (hemodynamic effects), (2) toxicity directly affecting the tubular cells, and (3) endogenous biochemical disturbances (KATZBERG 2005). Most clinical attention has focused on the hemodynamic effects of contrast media because tubular hypoxic injury is considered to play a central role in the renal dysfunction (HEYMAN et al. 2005). The mechanisms responsible for hemodynamic effects are believed to involve tubular and vascular events. The importance of direct effects of contrast media on tubular cells is debated, although evidence of a direct tubular cell toxicity of the contrast agents independent of either hemodynamic mechanisms or osmolality has been reported (HEINRICH et al. 2005). An increase in oxygen free radicals or a decrease in antioxidant enzyme activity triggered by contrast medium administration as the third potential pathway is speculative. There has been no clinical substantiation of the suggestion that the liberation of oxygen free radicals is the mechanism of contrast medium-induced nephropathy (KATZBERG 2005). The lack of understanding of the cause of contrast medium-induced nephropathy makes prevention of the condition difficult.

9.6
Predisposing Factors

The patients at highest risk for developing contrast medium-induced acute renal failure are those with pre-existing renal impairment (serum creatinine > 132 μmol l^{-1} (1.5 mg dl^{-1})), particularly when the reduction in renal function is secondary to diabetic nephropathy (MORCOS et al. 1999; RUDNICK et al. 1995). Diabetes mellitus alone without renal impairment is not a risk factor (RUDNICK et al. 1995). The degree of renal insufficiency present before the administration of contrast media to a great extent determines the severity of contrast medium-induced nephropathy. Baseline renal insufficiency in patients with acute myocardial infarction undergoing primary percutaneous coronary intervention is associated with a markedly increased mortality as well as bleeding and restenosis (SADEGHI et al.

2003). The extent to which the contrast medium contributes to the clinical deterioration is unknown, since for ethical reasons the studies did not include a control group.

Large doses of contrast media and multiple injections within 72 h increase the risk of developing contrast medium-induced nephropathy. The route of administration is also important, and contrast media are less nephrotoxic when administered intravenously than when given intra-arterially into the renal arteries or the aorta proximal to the origin of the renal blood vessels. The acute intrarenal concentration of contrast media is much higher after intra-arterial than intravenous administration.

Dehydration and congestive cardiac failure are risk factors because they are associated with a reduction in renal perfusion, which enhances the ischemic insult of the contrast media. The concurrent use of nephrotoxic drugs such as non-steroidal anti-inflammatory drugs (NSAIDs) and amino glycosides potentiates the nephrotoxic effects of contrast media. Renal dysfunction is found more frequently in patients with hypertension, hyperuricemia, or proteinuria than in patients without these conditions (Choyke et al. 1998). The type of contrast medium is also an important predisposing factor. High-osmolarity contrast media are more nephrotoxic than low- and iso-osmolarity contrast media (Morcos 1998; Katzberg 1997; Rudnick et al. 1995).

Multiple myeloma has been considered in the past to be a risk factor for contrast medium-induced nephropathy. However, if dehydration is avoided, contrast medium administration rarely leads to acute renal failure in patients with myeloma (McCarthy and Becker 1992).

9.7
Identifying Patients at Risk of Contrast Medium-Induced Nephropathy

Patients with pre-existing renal impairment are at particularly high risk of contrast medium-induced nephropathy. Serum creatinine has often been used to determine the renal function and to identify high-risk patients. Several studies have shown that, despite its many limitations, serum creatinine is a relatively satisfactory marker for identifying patients at the greatest risk of developing contrast medium-induced nephropathy because patients with severely reduced

renal function are at the greatest risk (Rudnick et al. 1995; McCullough et al. 1997; Parfrey et al. 1989; Thomsen et al. 2005, 2008a). However, renal function can be considerably reduced (Chronic Kidney Disease stage 3 (30–60 ml min^{-1}) when the serum creatinine levels are within the normal range (<132 µmol l^{-1} (1.5 mg dl^{-1})). More than 25% of older patients have normal serum creatinine levels but reduced glomerular filtration rates. Accurate determination of the glomerular filtration rate is not easy. The most precise method is the inulin clearance, and isotope methods give similar results (Blaufox et al. 1996). However, both methods are cumbersome and impractical for daily use. Also, a single determination of the glomerular filtration rate does not exclude acute renal insufficiency.

9.7.1
Validation of eGFR (Serum Creatinine) Measurements

Serum creatinine is not an ideal marker of renal function (Blaufox et al. 1996). The serum creatinine level depends on muscle mass and is not usually raised until the glomerular filtration rate has fallen by at least 50%. Endogenous serum creatinine clearance as a measure of glomerular filtration rate is also inaccurate, especially when renal function is low, because of a compensatory increase in tubular secretion of creatinine which limits its validity as a glomerular filtration marker. Radionuclide techniques are preferable (Blaufox et al. 1996) but labour intensive and, therefore, are not suitable to use in all patients receiving contrast medium. Alternatively, renal function can be estimated using specially derived predictive equations. The most accurate results are obtained with the Cockroft–Gault equation, whereas the most precise formula is the Modification of Diet in Renal Disease (MDRD) study equation (Cockroft and Gault 1976; Levey et al. 1999). However, the predictive capabilities of these formulae are suboptimal for ideal patient care (Bostrom et al. 2002). In addition, they are not useful for patients with a glomerular filtration rate above 60 ml min^{-1} (Stevens et al. 2006). Even below this level, they do not always result in the same glomerular filtration rate (Stevens et al. 2006; Band et al. 2007; Eken and Kilicaslan 2007). For instance, a 43-year-old, 70-kg male patient with a creatinine level of 132 µmol l^{-1} has a glomerular filtration level of 63 ml min^{-1} if calculated by the Cockcroft–Gault equation.

The same patient will have a glomerular filtration level of 66 ml min⁻¹ if he is African-American and 54 ml min⁻¹ if he is Caucasian, if it is calculated by the MDRD equation. Nonetheless, these equations provide a better assessment of renal function than does serum creatinine measurement.

Another possibility is to use cut-off values for serum creatinine to indicate several levels of renal impairment. However, low cut-off levels will include some patients with normal renal function and high cut-off levels will exclude some patients with renal impairment (COUCHOUD et al. 1999).

9.7.2
In Which Patients Should eGFR (Serum Creatinine) Be Measured?

A questionnaire designed to elicit a history of renal disorders as well as additional risk factors for contrast medium-induced nephropathy may be used to identify patients with normal serum creatinine in whom blood testing would be unnecessary (CHOYKE et al. 1998). The majority of patients (85%) in CHOYKE et al.'s (1998) study had normal serum creatinine values (<114 µmol l⁻¹ (1.3 mg dl⁻¹) for women, 123 µmol l⁻¹ (1.4 mg dl⁻¹) for men). All except two patients (99%) who gave negative answers to the questionnaire had serum creatinine levels <150 µmol l⁻¹ (1.7 mg dl⁻¹). There was a strong association between raised serum creatinine values and a history of renal disease, proteinuria, prior kidney surgery, hypertension, gout and diabetes. Only 6% of patients with negative answers to the six questions had abnormal serum creatinine levels.

In a study of 2,034 consecutive outpatients referred for CT examinations, only 3.2% (66 patients) had a raised serum creatinine level (>176 µmol l⁻¹ (2.0 mg dl⁻¹)) and the majority of these patients (97%) had risk factors for contrast medium-induced nephropathy (TIPPINS et al. 2000). Two of the 66 patients with a raised serum creatinine (0.1% of the total number of patients) had no identifiable risk factors. Serum creatinine was measured in a prospective study of 640 consecutive adult patients presenting to the emergency department with a clinical indication for intravenous administration of iodinated contrast medium (OLSEN and SALOMON 1996). A total of 35 (5.5%) patients had abnormal serum creatinine levels (>141 µmol l⁻¹ (1.6 mg dl⁻¹)). Of these 35 patients, 77% (27) were considered to have risk factors for renal insufficiency.

The remaining eight patients (1.3% of the total number) had no identifiable risk factors for renal insufficiency. Prospective studies where eGFR has been calculated before administration of contrast agents to consecutive patients are not yet available.

Thus, most patients at risk of contrast medium-induced nephropathy can be identified by appropriate questions, but a questionnaire does not completely exclude the presence of renal insufficiency. The Contrast Media Safety Committee of the European Society of Urogenital Radiology (ESUR) guideline recommends that serum creatinine should be measured and eGFR calculated no later than 7 days before an investigation using iodinated contrast medium if the response to any part of the questionnaire is positive, if the eGFR creatinine is known to be abnormal at the time of referral, or if contrast medium is to be given intra-arterially (see Chap. 29).

9.7.3
Risk Stratification

Risk stratification of patients to identify those susceptible to contrast medium-induced nephropathy has not been fully evaluated. On the basis of two cohorts (one derivation cohort (1993–1998) and one validation cohort (1999–2002)) of 20,479 patients, BARTHOLOMEW et al. (2004) proposed a contrast medium-induced nephropathy risk score with good predictive ability for identifying patients in whom preventive strategies are indicated. Independent variables (with weighted scores) include estimated creatinine clearance <60 ml min⁻¹ (2), urgent percutaneous coronary intervention (2), intra-aortic balloon pump use (2), diabetes mellitus (1), congestive heart failure (1), hypertension (1), peripheral vascular disease (1), and contrast volume >260 ml (1). The incidence of contrast medium-induced nephropathy after percutaneous coronary intervention increased with each unit increase in score. No patient with a score ≤1 developed contrast medium-induced nephropathy, whereas 26% of patients with a score ≥ 9 developed contrast medium-induced nephropathy.

MEHRAN et al. (2004) also developed a simple risk score for contrast medium-induced nephropathy after percutaneous coronary intervention. On the basis of a study of 8,357 patients they identified eight variables, which were assigned a weighted integer: hypotension (5); intra-aortic balloon pump (5); congestive heart failure class III/IV by New York

Heart Association classification and/or a history of pulmonary edema (5); age > 75 years (4); anemia (3); diabetes (1); contrast media volume (1 for each 100 ml) serum creatinine > 132 μmol l^{-1} (1.5 mg dl^{-1}) (4); or estimated creatinine clearance < 20 ml min^{-1} 1.73 m^2 (6), 20–40 ml min^{-1} 1.73 m^2 (4) and 40–60 ml min^{-1} 1.73 m^2 (2). In patients with a risk score ≤ 5 the risk of contrast medium-induced nephropathy was 7.5% and the risk of dialysis was 0.04%, whereas the figures for patients with a risk score ≥ 16 were 57.3 and 12.6%, respectively.

Methods of stratifying patients being given contrast media appear to have potential but need further evaluation. Currently it is not known whether they are applicable to examinations where the contrast medium is injected intravenously.

9.8
Measures to Reduce the Incidence of Contrast Medium-Induced Nephropathy

A number of measures (Table 9.1) have been recommended to reduce the incidence of contrast medium-induced nephropathy (THOMSEN 1999; MORCOS 2004,

2005). The main methods that have been used are extracellular volume expansion, administration of nonionic contrast media, and the use of a variety of drugs, all of which are discussed in this section. Other measures that have been tried include hemodialysis, hemofiltration, and use of gadolinium-based contrast media instead of iodinated agents, and they are discussed in Chaps. 10 and 22.

9.8.1
Extracellular Volume Expansion

Extracellular volume expansion is the most effective of all the measures used to prevent contrast medium-induced nephropathy (MORCOS et al. 1999; MUELLER et al. 2002; TRIVIDI et al. 2003; ALLAQABAND et al. 2002; SOLOMON et al. 1994; TAYLOR et al. 1998; THOMSEN and MORCOS 2008a). Early studies of contrast medium-induced nephropathy often described those affected as dehydrated. Intravascular volume expansion may increase kidney blood flow, reduce vasoconstriction in the kidney, reduce the dwell time of contrast medium within the kidney, improve tubular clearance of uric acid and cast material, and exert variable neurohormonal effects that reduce the rate of

Table 9.1. Current status of measures that have been proposed to decrease the risk of iodinated contrast medium-induced nephropathy (till August 2008)

Measures proven to decrease the risk	Measures for which evidence is equivocal	Measures proven to increase the risk or to have no effect
Extracellular volume expansion	Hemofiltration	Loop diuretics
Normal strength (0.9%) saline for intravenous hydration	Sodium bicarbonate intravenously	Sodium bicarbonate intravenously in large amounts
Low dose of contrast medium	Intravenous hydration in preference to controlled oral hydration	Mannitol
Low- or iso-osmolar contrast medium		Half-strength (0.45%) saline for intravenous hydration
Imaging methods not using iodinated contrast media		Iso-osmolar dimers in preference to low-osmolar monomeric contrast media
		High osmolar contrast media
		Hemodialysis
		Gadolinium-based contrast media
		Pharmacological manipulation: • Renal vasodilators • Blocking of intrarenal mediators, e.g., endothelin and adenosine • Cytoprotective drugs, e.g., acetylcysteine

contrast medium-induced nephropathy. In addition, diuresis due to effective hydration is associated with increase in intrarenal production of prostacyclin leading to vasodilation in the vulnerable region of the renal medulla.

During the last 15 years, only a few randomized trials examining prophylactic fluid therapy have been published (Table 9.2). They include patients with normal and decreased kidney function. The fluid has been administered orally, intra-arterially, and intravenously. The study sample size has varied from 18 to 1,620, but no more than 2,500 patients (in total) have participated in these trials. It is clear that forced diuresis by adding mannitol or furosemide to hypotonic saline does not work (Dussol et al. 2006; Solomon et al. 1994; Weinstein et al. 1992). The same applies to a rapid bolus of isotonic saline (250–300 ml) at the time of contrast medium exposure (Bader et al. 2004; Krasuski et al. 2003). Unrestricted access to water for 12 h prior to contrast medium administration is also on the "doesn't work" list (Trividi et al. 2003). The potentially effective measures are (1) hypotonic (0.45%) saline starting 12 h before and continuing for 12 h after contrast medium exposure at 1 ml kg^{-1} h^{-1} (Solomon et al. 1994); (2) isotonic saline 4 h before and continuing for 12 h after contrast medium exposure at 1 ml kg^{-1} h^{-1} (Mueller et al. 2002); (3) oral hydration (1,000 ml over 10 h) followed by hypotonic saline (300 ml h^{-1}) starting 0.5 h before contrast medium exposure and continuing for 6 h total (Taylor et al. 1998).

In an initial trial, Merten et al. (2004) showed that isotonic bicarbonate starting 1 h before (3 ml kg^{-1} h^{-1}) and continuing for 6 h after contrast medium exposure (1 ml kg^{-1} h^{-1}) reduced the incidence of contrast medium-induced nephropathy when compared to isotonic saline given for the same period. There were some methodological weaknesses to this trial. However, Briguori et al. (2007) reported a further trial in which patients having angiography all received acetylcysteine, with one-third also receiving isotonic bicarbonate using the Merten protocol compared to one-third each receiving 0.9% saline with or without ascorbic acid. The lowest rate of contrast medium-induced nephropathy was in the bicarbonate/acetylcysteine group, but the design of the trial did not permit an assessment of whether there was any interaction between the effects of these agents. Finally, another recent trial comparing a larger dose of bicarbonate together with acetylcysteine to saline plus acetylcysteine post angiography also found a lower rate of contrast medium-induced nephropathy in the bicarbonate group (Recio-Mayoral et al. 2007).

The interpretation of this trial is somewhat difficult given the larger amount of fluid prior to contrast medium in the bicarbonate group. If bicarbonate is used, severe alkalosis should be avoided by not using excessive doses of bicarbonate (Thomsen and Morcos 2006). The mechanism by which bicarbonate is protective is not fully understood, but it has been suggested that increasing the pH of renal medulla and urine by sodium bicarbonate may reduce the production of free radicals and protect the kidney from oxidant injury that can be associated with contrast medium-induced nephropathy (Merten et al. 2004; Bakris et al. 1990; Atkins 1986; Morcos 2005). Thus the protective effect is believed to result from antioxidant effects and scavenging of reactive free radicals rather than from better hydration than that provided by saline (Merten et al. 2004). However, there is no clinical evidence that the liberation of oxygen free radicals is the mechanism of contrast medium-induced nephropathy (Katzberg 2005).

Prolonged intravenous fluid therapy is difficult to administer for outpatient procedures. A novel fast strategy of infusing 1 l of 5% dextrose immediately before cardiac catheterization was associated with a lower rate (1.4%) of contrast medium-induced nephropathy than in the comparison group (5%) in a retrospective study of high-risk patients. Further studies are required to test this approach (Clavijo et al. 2006).

The Contrast Media Safety Committee of the ESUR recommends intravenous infusion of 0.9% saline solution at a rate of 1 ml h^{-1} kg^{-1} body weight starting 6 h before contrast medium administration and continuing for 6 h afterwards (see Chap. 29). In areas with a hot climate more fluid should be given. This regime is suitable for patients who are not in congestive heart failure and are not allowed to drink or eat before undergoing an interventional or surgical procedure. If there is no contraindication to oral administration, free fluid intake should be encouraged. At least 500 ml of water or soft drinks orally before and 2,500 ml during the 24 h following contrast medium administration is recommended. In addition, concurrent administration of nephrotoxic drugs such as gentamicin and NSAIDs should be avoided.

Mannitol and furosemide enhance the risk of contrast medium-induced nephropathy and should not be used (Solomon et al. 1994).

The disadvantages of volume expansion include its unsuitability for patients with cardiac failure and its limited use in emergency situations because fluid administration has to start several hours before contrast medium administration.

Table 9.2. Studies of prophylactic fluid therapy for prevention of contrast-induced nephropathy (adapted from Thomsen et al. 2008a)

Study	Osmolality/ route of contrast	Intervention regimen	Control regimen	Number of participants	Mean baseline kidney function	Outcome measure	Results Intervention v. Control N (%) or mean	Statistical significance
Bader et al. 2004	LOCM/IV	300 ml IV fluid during +1.5–2.0 l fluid PO (12h post)	2 l IV fluid (12h pre/12h post)	39	eGFR 110 ml min⁻¹	Mean change in GFR by contrast clearance at 48h	-34.6 v. -18.3 ml min⁻¹ 1.73 m²	$P < 0.05$
Mueller et al. 2002	LOCM/IA	1 ml kg⁻¹ h⁻¹ IV 0.9% saline (24h from morning of procedure)	1 m kg⁻¹ h⁻¹ IV 0.45% saline (24h from morning of procedure)	1,383	eGFR 84 ml min⁻¹ 50 kg lean mass	SCr increase by ≥44 µmol l⁻¹ (0.5 mg dl⁻¹) within 48h	5 (0.7%) v. 14 (2%)	$P = 0.04$
Taylor et al. 1998	Multiple/IA	75 ml h⁻¹ IV 0.45% saline (12h pre/12h post)	1 l water PO (over 10h pre), 300 ml h⁻¹ IV 0.45% saline (6h from call to lab)	36	eGFR 48 ml min⁻¹	Mean maximal change in SCr within 48h	0.21 v. 0.12 mg dl⁻¹	$P = NS$
Trivedi et al. 2003	LOCM/IA	1 ml kg⁻¹ h⁻¹ IV 0.9% saline (24h)	Unrestricted oral fluids	53	eGFR 79.6 ml min⁻¹	SCr increase by ≥44 µmol l⁻¹ (0.5 mg dl⁻¹) within 48h	1 (3.7%) v. 9 (34.6%)	$P = 0.005$
Krasuski et al. 2003	?/IA	1 ml kg⁻¹ h⁻¹ 0.45% saline (12h pre and post)	250 ml 0.9% saline (pre) and 1 ml Kg⁻¹ 0.45% saline (12h post)	63	eGFR ≈ 45 ml min⁻¹	SCr increase by ≥44 µmol l⁻¹ (0.5 mg dl⁻¹) within 48h	0 (0%) v. 4 (10.8%)	$P = NS$
Dussol et al. 2006	LOCM/IA or IV	15 ml Kg⁻¹ 0.9% saline (6h pre)	1 g per 10Kg weight salt and unrestricted water PO (2 days pre)	153	eGFR 34 ml min⁻¹ 1.73 m⁻²	SCr increase by ≥ 44 µmol l⁻¹ (0.5 mg dl⁻¹) within 48h	5 (6.6%) V. 4 (5.2%)	$P = NS$
Merten et al. 2004	LOCM/ Multiple	3 ml kg⁻¹ h⁻¹ (1h pre), 1 ml kg⁻¹ h⁻¹ (6h post) IV sodium bicarbonate 154 mmol l⁻¹	3 ml kg⁻¹ h⁻¹ (1h pre), 1 ml kg⁻¹ h⁻¹ (6h post) IV 0.9% saline	119	eGFR 41–45 ml min⁻¹ 1.73 m⁻²	SCr increase by ≥25% within 48h	1 (1.7%) v. 8 (13.6%)	$P = 0.02$
Briguori et al. 2007	IOCM/IA	3 ml kg⁻¹ h⁻¹ (1h pre), 1 ml kg⁻¹ h⁻¹ (6h post) IV sodium bicarbonate 154 mmol l⁻¹ plus NAC	1 ml kg⁻¹ h⁻¹ 0.9% saline, (12h pre and 12h post) plus NAC	220	eGFR 32–35 ml min⁻¹ 1.73 m⁻²	SCr increase by ≥25% at 48h	2 (1.9%) v. 11 (9.9%)	$P = 0.01$
Recio-Mayoral et al. 2007	LOCM/IA	5 ml kg⁻¹ h⁻¹ IV (1h pre), sodium bicarbonate 154 mmol l⁻¹ plus 2400 mg NAC, unspecified fluid at 1.5 ml kg⁻¹ h⁻¹ (12h post), plus NAC 600 mg PO q12h × 2 next day	1 ml kg⁻¹ h⁻¹ IV 0.9% saline IV (12h post) plus NAC 600 mg PO q12h × 2 next day	111	eGFR 75 ml min kg⁻¹ h⁻¹ 1.73 m²	SCr increase by ≥44 µmol l⁻¹ (0.5 mg dl⁻¹) within 3 days	1 (1.8%) v. 12 (21.8%)	$P = 0.0009$
Clavijo et al. 2006 (not an RCT)	HOCM or LOCM/IA	1 l bolus 5% dextrose in water IA before procedure	Not specified	976	eGFR 44 ml min⁻¹	SCr increase by ≥44 µmol l⁻¹ (0.5 mg dl⁻¹) between 24 and 72h post	2 (1.4%) v. 47 (5.7%)	$P = 0.03$

RCT Randomized controlled trial; *HOCM* High osmolar contrast media; *LOCM* low osmolar contrast media; *IOCM* Isoosmolar contrast media; *IA* Intraarterial; *IV* Intravenous

In conclusion, extracellular volume expansion seems to be the most effective of all the measures used to prevent CIN. The hydration regime should start before and continue for several hours after the contrast medium exposure. Normal saline offers better protection than half-strength saline. The optimal duration and intensity of fluid therapy and the possible role of bicarbonate remain to be fully established.

9.8.2
Nonionic Contrast Media

The type of contrast medium used is an important risk factor for the development of contrast medium-induced nephropathy with iso-osmolar contrast media (IOCM) and low-osmolar contrast media (LOCM) being less nephrotoxic than high-osmolar contrast agents in patients with pre-existing renal impairment (Morcos 1998; Morcos et al. 1999; Katzberg 1997; Rudnick et al. 1995 Thomsen and Morcos 2008a). Therefore low-osmolar or iso-osmolar nonionic contrast media are recommended in high-risk patients to reduce the risk of contrast medium-induced nephropathy.

The question remains as to whether LOCM or IOCM (osmolality 290 mOsm kg^{-1}) differ in terms of nephrotoxicity. A total of eight nonionic monomeric LOCM (iohexol, iomeprol, iopamidol, iopentol, ioxilan, iopromide, ioversol, iobiditrol), one ionic dimer LOCM (ioxaglate), and one nonionic dimer IOCM (iodixanol) are approved for intravascular use. Their approved use varies from country to country.

Several studies have compared LOCM with IOCM, and in most cases the contrast agents were given intra-arterially. Aspelin et al. (2003), in a randomized trial in 129 patients with moderate chronic kidney disease and diabetes mellitus, showed a significantly higher incidence of contrast medium-induced nephropathy, defined as an absolute increase in serum creatinine greater than 44 μmol l^{-1} (0.5 mg dl^{-1}), within 72 h with intra-arterial iohexol than iodixanol (26% vs. 4%). The two groups differed significantly with regard to interventional procedures and duration of diabetes, but were otherwise comparable. Using the same end point, Jo et al. (2006) did not find a significant difference overall between the IOCM iodixanol and the LOCM ionic dimer ioxaglate in 275 patients with chronic kidney disease undergoing coronary procedures; but in some subgroups, e.g., patients with diabetic nephropathy, there was a

significant difference. The other six angiographic studies have not shown any significant difference between IOCM and LOCM (Table 9.3). In a retrospective study of 225 patients with moderate to severe kidney disease, Briguori et al. (2006) could not find differences in contrast medium-induced nephropathy rates between iodixanol and the LOCM, nonionic monomer iobitridol. Neither Solomon et al. (2007) nor Wessely et al. (2008) found a difference between iopamidol and iodixanol in their prospective randomized studies of 414 and 334 patients with kidney disease, respectively.

No direct comparisons between the LOCM nonionic monomers in at risk patients have been done. However, comparisons between studies that compared a variety of LOCM with the IOCM iodixanol have raised the possibility of differences in nephrotoxic potential between the different LOCM (Bettmann 2005; Solomon and duMouchel 2006). Since the higher nephrotoxic potential of the LOCM iohexol compared to the IOCM iodixanol (Aspelin et al. 2003) was not replicated in studies using other LOCM, the possibility was raised of a difference in nephrotoxic potential between iohexol and the other nonionic monomers (Bettmann 2005; Sharma and Kini 2005; Solomon and duMouchel 2006). Solomon and duMouchel (2006) conducted a systematic analysis of published papers and the Food and Drug Administration (FDA) reports of adverse events, and found that the risk of contrast medium-induced nephropathy was higher in patients following administration of iohexol than of another nonionic monomer, iopamidol. Bettmann (2005) and Sharma and Kini (2005) analyzed control arms of studies of patients with chronic kidney disease receiving no premedication and showed that the average incidence of contrast medium-induced nephropathy after iopamidol administration was significantly lower than after iohexol, whereas the incidence after iodixanol varied from 3 to 33%. Thus it is possible that there may be a difference in the nephrotoxic potential between the various LOCM. Although there are no important differences in the physicochemical properties between the different nonionic monomeric LOCM, it may be argued that it is inappropriate to put all nonionic monomers together in any review or meta-analysis.

After intravenous injection, there seems to be no difference in the nephrotoxic potential between LOCM and IOCM (Table 9.4). Thomsen et al. (2008) reported 7% contrast medium-induced nephropathy

Table 9.3. Prospective randomized trials comparing intraarterial iso- to low-osmolality contrast media

Low osmolar CM	n	Isoosmolar CM	n	Examination	SCr μmol/l (mg/dl)	Diabetes Mellitus	Statistical result	End point	Reference
Iohexol	48	Iodixanol	54	Coronary	273 (3.1)	35%	No difference	SCr ≥ 25% from baseline	Chalmers and Jackson (1999)
Iohexol	65	Iodixanol	64	Arteriography	132 (1.5)	100%	Iodixanol superior	SCr increase ≥ 44 μmol l^{-1} (0.5 mg dl^{-1})	Aspelin et al. (2003)
Ioxaglate	135	Iodixanol	140	Coronary	117 (1.34)	48%	Iodixanol may be superior in certain subgroups	**SCr increase ≥ 44 μmol l^{-1} (0.5 mg dl^{-1})	Jo et al. (2006)
Iopamidol	204	Iodixanol	210	Coronary	128 (1.45)	41%	No difference	SCr increase ≥ 44 μmol l^{-1} (0.5 mg dl^{-1})	Solomon et al. (2007)
Iopamidol	48	Iodixanol	54	Coronary	<176 (2)	100%	No difference	SCr ≥ 25% from baseline	Hardiek et al. (2008)
Iopamidol	41	Iodixanol	46	Coronary artery stenting	CrCL < 60 ml/min	19%	No difference	SCr increase ≥ 44 μmol l^{-1} (0.5 mg dl^{-1}) or ≥25% increase from baseline	Jingwei et al. 2006
Ioxaglate	74	Iodixanol	75	Percutaneous coronary diagnostic or interventional procedures	161 (1.83)	45%	No difference	SCr increase ≥ 44 μmol l^{-1} (0.5 mg dl^{-1})	Mehran for the ICON Investigators (2006)
Iomeprol	162	Iodixanol	162	Coronary angiography	120 (1.36)	37%	No difference	SCr increase ≥ 44 μmol l^{-1} (0.5 mg dl^{-1}) or ≥25% increase from baseline	Wessely et al. (2008)

SCr Serum creatinine

Table 9.4. Prospective randomized trials comparing intravenous iso- to low-osmolality contrast media

Study	Nonionic low-osmolar CM	Nonionic iso-osmolar CM	End point	Statistical result
Carraro et al. (1998)	0/32 (Iopromide)	1/32 (Iodixanol)	50% ↑ SCr	No difference
Kolehmainen and Soiva (2003)	4/25 (Iobiditrol)	4/25 (Iodixanol)	44 mmol/L (0.5 mg dl^{-1}) ↑ SCr	No difference
Barrett et al. 2006	0/77 (Iopamidol)	2/76 (Iodixanol)	44 mmol/L (0.5 mg dl^{-1}) ↑ SCr	No difference
Thomsen et al. 2008	0/76* (Iomeprol)	5/72 (Iodixanol)	44 mmol/L (0.5 mg dl^{-1}) ↑ SCr	Iomeprol superior $p < 0.05$
Kuhn et al. 2008	7/125 (Iopamidol)	6/123 (Iodixanol)	25% ↑ SCr	No difference
Nguyn et al. 2008	10/61 (Iopromide)	3/65 (Iodixanol)	44 mmol/L (0.5 mg/dl) ↑ SCr	Iodixanol superior $p < 0.05$

after intravenous injection of 40 g I iodixanol (320 mg I ml^{-1}) and 0% contrast medium-induced nephropathy after 40 g I iomeprol (400 mg I ml^{-1}) in patients with reduced kidney function ($P < 0.05$). Also, using the same end point as in the NEPHRIC study (Aspelin et al. 2003), Barrett et al. (2006) showed a 2.6% contrast medium-induced nephropathy rate after intravenous injection of iodixanol for CT and 0% after injection of iopamidol in a randomized, multicenter trial. Kuhn et al. (2008) found no difference between iopamidol and iodixanol in patients with diabetic nephropathy. Neither did previous, smaller studies by Carraro et al. (1998) and Kolehmainen and Soiva (2003) in patients with chronic kidney disease show any difference between iodixanol and their respective comparators (iopromide and iobiditrol) (Table 9.4). On the other hand, Nguyen et al. (2008) found iopromide to be inferior to iodixanol in a randomized study of 117 patients with average GFR of 52 ml min^{-1}. It is surprising that 18.5% developed contrast medium-induced nephropathy after only 100 ml of 370 mg I ml^{-1} iopromide. In 41 patients who did not receive acetylcysteine (control arm), Tepel et al. (2000) reported a 21% rate of contrast medium-induced nephropathy after intravenous injection of 75 ml iopromide of 300 mg I ml^{-1}. In both studies the same end point ($\geq$44 µmol l^{-1} (0.5 mg dl^{-1}) was used. Pugh et al. (1993) compared iopromide and iodixanol for femoral arteriography; according to McCullough et al. (2006) they found a lower rate of contrast medium-induced nephropathy after iopromide than after iodixanol. Thus there are very conflicting results regarding iopromide, and it is impossible to draw a definite conclusion.

A number of recent reviews have recommended that the nonionic isoosmolar dimer should be used rather than the nonionic monomers in patients at risk of developing contrast medium-induced nephropathy (Gleeson and Bulugahapitaya 2004; Cavusoglu et al. 2004; Maeder et al. 2004; Nikolsky and Mehran 2003; Mitchell et al. 2004; Asif and Epstein 2004; Andrew and Berg 2004; Nicholson and Downes 2003; Erdogan and Davidson 2003). However, currently there is no conclusive evidence of a difference in the nephrotoxic potential between the various monomers and the dimer (Tables 9.3, 9.4). It is important to remember that all these agents are potentially nephrotoxic, although the risk associated with them is less than that with the old, high-osmolar contrast agents.

9.8.3
Pharmacological Manipulation

In recent years it has been claimed that various substances or drugs may protect the kidney against contrast medium-induced nephropathy. However, no intervention has proven efficacious beyond doubt. Strongly positive initial trials have often not been replicable.

Acetylcysteine is an antioxidant and scavenger of oxygen free radicals. It enhances the biologic effect of the endogenous vasodilator nitric oxide by combining with nitric oxide to form S-nitrosothiol, which is a more stable and potent vasodilator than nitric oxide. Acetylcysteine also increases the expression of nitric oxide synthase, the enzyme responsible for the endogenous production of nitric oxide in the body (SAFIRSTEIN et al. 2000). Nitric oxide is crucial to the maintenance of perfusion of the kidney, particularly in the vulnerable region of the renal medulla. Therefore, acetylcysteine might reduce the nephrotoxicity of contrast medium through antioxidant and vasodilatory effects (MESCHI et al. 2006). The results of an initial trial were dramatic, but the event rate in the controls was unexpectedly high for patients given a low-dose, intravenous, low-osmolality contrast medium (PANNU et al. 2006; FISHBANE et al. 2004; TEPEL et al. 2000; BRIGUORI et al. 2004a; MARENZI et al. 2006; LIU et al. 2005). Subsequent trials have largely involved patients with reduced kidney function having cardiac angiography. Some have shown benefit and others have not; many are limited by low power and a lack of blinding. The dose of acetylcysteine employed in most trials has not been chosen on the basis of pharmacologic principles. Two trials comparing doses of acetylcysteine have suggested that higher doses may be required, especially if higher doses of contrast medium are being employed (BRIGUORI et al. 2004b; MARENZI et al. 2006). There have been several meta-analyses of trials of acetylcysteine (ALONSO et al. 2004; PANNU et al. 2004; FISHBANE et al. 2004; LIU et al. 2005; ZAGLER et al. 2005; KISHIRSAGAR et al. 2004; BAGSHAW and GHALI 2004; BAGSHAW et al. 2006; VAITKUS and BRAR 2007; BIONDI-ZOCCAI et al. 2006). The trials included in these analyses vary. The results of meta-analysis must be interpreted with caution given the heterogeneous results of the individual trials, and the possibility of publication bias, with small negative studies under-represented (BAGSHAW et al. 2006; VAITKUS and BRAR 2007; BIONDI-ZOCCAI et al. 2006). Also, the effect of acetylcysteine on outcomes other than minor changes in serum creatinine is largely unknown. Indeed, studies in healthy volunteers have suggested that acetylcysteine might have an effect on creatinine levels unrelated to an effect on GFR (HOFFMANN et al. 2004; CURHAM 2003). POLETTI et al. (2007) found no effect of acetylsysteine when they used Cystatin C as the measure of glomerular filtration rate, but they found a significantly lower contrast medium-induced nephropathy rate in the acetylcysteine group than in the control group when they used serum creatinine as the measure of renal function. Cystatin C is not secreted by the tubular cells, whereas creatinine is. Thus there is no conclusive evidence that acetylcysteine provides consistent protection against contrast medium-induced nephropathy and its routine use for prophylaxis is not recommended.

Theophylline and aminophylline (nonselective adenosine receptors antagonists) have the potential to reduce contrast medium-induced nephropathy through antagonizing adenosine- mediated vasoconstriction. Adenosine is an important intrarenal mediator, which can induce a decrease in the glomerular filtration rate through vasoconstriction of the afferent arterioles and contraction of the mesangial cells of the glomeruli (OLDROYD et al. 2000). Adenosine also induces vasoconstriction in the renal cortex and vasodilatation in the renal medulla, increases the generation of oxygen free radical cells, and is a mediator of the tubuloglomerulo feedback (TGF) response. Clinical studies have given conflicting results. In one study, administration of 200 mg theophylline intravenously had a preventive effect (HUBER et al. 2002), but in another study 810 mg theophylline orally daily for 3 days did not offer additional protection compared to hydration alone (ERLEY et al. 1999). Recent meta-analyses found that the mean rise in serum creatinine was significantly, but only slightly, lower at 48 h after contrast medium administration among those receiving active therapy compared to placebo (IX et al. 2004; BAGSHAW and GHALI 2005). The clinical importance of this finding is not clear (THOMSEN and MORCOS 2008; GOLDENBERG and MATETZKY 2005). There was heterogeneity among studies with regard to changes in serum creatinine. There is potential for adverse effects with theophylline particularly in patients with ischemic heart disease in whom it may induce cardiac arrhythmias (MORCOS 2004). The optimal dose for prevention of contrast medium-induced nephropathy has not been established. Further studies using a selective adenosine receptor (A1) antagonist are warranted. Thus, the effectiveness of theophylline in preventing contrast medium-induced nephropathy remains uncertain.

The antioxidant ascorbic acid has been tested in two randomized trials of patients undergoing cardiac angiography (BRIGUORI et al. 2007; SPARGIAS et al. 2004). In the first study, contrast medium-induced nephropathy occurred in 11 (9%) cases given ascorbic acid compared to 23 (20%) given placebo ($p = 0.02$) (SPARGIAS et al. 2004) However, these results are difficult to interpret, as the baseline serum creatinine level was lower in the placebo group and both groups reached a similar level after contrast medium administration. In the more recent trial, ascorbic acid given with acetylcysteine and saline was associated with the same rate of contrast medium-induced nephropathy as when acetylcysteine and saline alone were given (BRIGUORI et al. 2007).

Calcium channel blockers prevent the influx of calcium ions through voltage-operated channels, thereby causing a vasorelaxant effect in all vascular beds including the kidney. In one study, 3 days' treatment with 20 mg nitrendipine prevented the development of contrast medium-induced nephropathy in patients with moderate renal impairment (NEUMAYER et al. 1989), but in another study a single dose (20 or 10 mg) given 1 h before contrast medium administration failed to prevent contrast medium-induced nephropathy (CARRARO et al. 1996). The incidence of contrast medium-induced nephropathy was 6.5% with 20 mg nitrendipine, 3.7% with 10 mg nitrendipine, and 8.3% in the control group, and the differences were not statistically insignificant. Thus the role of calcium channel blockers remains uncertain and their protective effect in patients with advanced renal impairment has not been proven. In addition, these drugs are not suitable in patients with heart failure.

The use of the vasodilators dopamine and atrial natriuretic peptide may be harmful in patients with diabetic nephropathy. The frequency of contrast medium-induced nephropathy in patients who were pretreated with either drug plus hydration was 83%, whereas the frequency in the control group, who received only hydration, was 43% (WEISBERG et al. 1994).

The selective dopamine-1 receptor agonist, fenoldopam, in contrast to dopamine, increases both cortical and medullary blood flow. Fenoldopam has the advantages of not stimulating α- and β-adrenergic receptors or dopamine-2 receptors, which can produce renal vasoconstriction. One study has shown that fenoldopam offers some protection against contrast medium-induced nephropathy (KINI et al. 2002), but two studies indicated that it offered no protection (ALLAQABAND et al. 2002; STONE et al. 2003). In addition, fenoldopam has the disadvantages that it has to be given intravenously and it induces hypotension, so regular monitoring of the blood pressure is necessary (MORCOS 2004).

Experimental studies have indicated that the potent endogenous vasoactive peptide endothelin may play an important role in mediating contrast medium-induced nephropathy (OLDROYD et al. 1995). Therefore it was suggested that endothelin antagonists (BENIGNI and REMIZZI 1999) would reduce the incidence of contrast medium-induced nephropathy in humans. However, WANG et al. (2000) found that a nonselective endothelin receptor antagonist and intravenous hydration were associated with a contrast medium-induced nephropathy rate of 56%

compared to 29% in the hydration only group. In addition, hypotension was more frequent in the treated group. WANG et al.'s (2000) study has been criticized (HAYLOR and MORCOS 2000) because the choice of a nonselective endothelin receptor antagonist, which blocks both endothelin-A and the endothelin-B receptors, was not appropriate. Endothelin-B receptors are responsible for vasodilatation and clearance of endothelin, and blocking them abolishes the vasodilatory effect and prolongs the vasoconstrictor effect of endothelin, which is released in response to contrast medium. Also, the endothelin receptor antagonist was given only 12 h after contrast medium injection so that there was no sustained drug cover.

Two studies of captopril as a prophylactic agent yielded divergent results (GUPTA et al. 1999; TOPRAK 2006; TOPRAK et al. 2003). In the first trial, serum creatinine rose by more than 0.5 mg dl^{-1} (44 μmol l^{-1}) in 2 (6%) patients given captopril for 3 days vs. 10 (29%) given placebo ($p < 0.02$) (GUPTA et al. 1999). In the second study, contrast medium-induced nephropathy was reported as occurring in five (10%) patients given captopril vs. one (3%) given placebo ($p = 0.02$) (TOPRAK 2006; TOPRAK et al. 2003).

Several other interventions have been proposed to reduce the risk of CIN, but data to support them are limited. Forced diuresis with furosemide, mannitol, dopamine, or a combination of these given at the time of the contrast exposure has been associated with similar or higher rates of contrast medium-induced nephropathy when compared to prophylactic fluids alone (SOLOMON et al. 1994; WEINSTEIN et al. 1992; STEVENS et al. 1999; GARE et al. 1999; HANS et al. 1998). Negative fluid balance might underlie some of the detrimental effects.

In summary, none of the many proposed pharmacological manipulations has been proven to be of consistent benefit (Chap. 29).

9.9
Recommendations during the Last 5 Years

In 2006, BARRETT and PARFREY (2006) reviewed the literature and recommended using intravenous saline therapy and the lowest possible dose of low-osmolality contrast media. They also indicated that NSAIDs and diuretics should be withheld for at least 24 h before and after exposure to contrast medium and that *N*-acetylcysteine was not recommended routinely, given the inconsistent results of clinical trials. Their recommendations were in accordance with ESUR guidelines from 1999 (Morcos et al. 1999). Thomsen and Morcos (2006) evaluated a plethora of reviews and guidelines on prevention of contrast medium-induced nephropathy. They concluded that guidelines should be prepared after careful study of published literature and with a thorough understanding of the subject, and recommendations should be evidence based whenever possible, relying on consistent results of well-structured, large studies. Recommending a change in clinical practice based only on a single study cannot be justified, particularly in the field of contrast medium-induced nephropathy since inconsistency of results of clinical studies is a real problem. Clinical investigation of contrast medium-induced nephropathy regularly faces the problem of finding a perfectly matching control group, as there are many variables that can influence renal function. In addition, it is important to emphasize that meta-analysis of inconsistent study results cannot offer confident recommendations about treatment (Higgins et al. 2003). There is a great need for randomized clinical trials. Guidelines should be based on proven clinical practice. In areas of contention, a consensus among experts on the subject should be sought. Guidelines should be concisely and clearly written using accurate terminology and avoiding vague recommendations. The ESUR guidelines on the prevention of contrast medium-induced nephropathy (Morcos et al. 1999), which required 3 years of preparation and involved wide consensus, remain valid in spite of the large number of new studies reported in the literature since their publication in 1999.

Summary

A major problem in the prevention of contrast medium-induced nephropathy is that the pathophysiological mechanism of the condition is not known. Current practice for preventing contrast medium-induced nephropathy still relies on identifying patients at increased risk. Estimated glomerular filtration rate has replaced serum creatinine in the routine determination of renal function. In patients with reduced renal function, the possibility of an alternative imaging method not using contrast medium should be considered. If an investigation

using iodinated contrast medium is considered essential for patient management, a number of measures that have been proved to reduce the incidence of contrast medium-induced nephropathy should be instituted. These are extracellular volume expansion, the choice of normal (0.9%) saline when intravenous hydration is used, the choice of low- or iso-osmolar nonionic contrast medium, and use of the lowest contrast medium dose consistent with a diagnostic conclusion or a therapeutic goal (see Chap. 29). Kidney function should not be used as a guide to the amount of contrast medium that can be safely given. On the basis of current knowledge, a weight-related fluid dose for hydration (e.g., $1\,ml\,kg^{-1}$ body weight h^{-1} or more) appears to be optimal. Even when the recommended measures are used, contrast medium-induced nephropathy remains a risk after administration of both iodinated and gadolinium contrast media.

Over the past 10 years, pharmacological manipulation with renal vasodilators, receptor antagonists of endogenous vasoactive mediators, and cytoprotective drugs has been widely investigated. None of the pharmacological manipulations has yet been shown to offer consistent protection against contrast medium-induced nephropathy. Therefore, pharmacological manipulation with the drugs evaluated so far cannot be recommended.

References

Allaqaband S, Tumuluri R, Malik AM et al (2002) Prospective randomized study of N-acetylcysteine, fenoldopam and saline for prevention of radiocontrast-induced nephropathy. Catheter Cardiovasc Intervent 57:279–283

Almén T, Frennby B, Sterner G (1999) Determination of glomerular filtration rate (GFR) with contrast media. In: Thomsen HS, Muller RN, Mattrey RF (eds) Trends in contrast media. Springer, Berlin, pp 81–94

Alonso A, Lau J, Jaber BL, Weintraub A, Sarnak MJ (2004) Prevention of contrast nephropathy with N-acetylcysteine in patients with chronic kidney disease: a meta-analysis of randomized controlled trials. Am J Kidney Dis 43:1–9

Andrew E, Berg KJ (2004) Nephrotoxic effects of X-ray contrast media. J Toxicol Clin Toxicol 42:325–332

Asif A, Epstein M (2004) Prevention of radiocontrast-induced nephropathy. Am J Kidney Dis 44:12–24

Aspelin P, Aubry P, Fransson S-G et al (2003) Nephrotoxic effects in high-risk patients undergoing angiography. N Engl J Med 348:491–499

Atkins JL (1986) Effect of sodium bicarbonate preloading on ischemic renal failure. Nephron 44: 70–76

Bader BD, Berger ED, Heede MB et al (2004) What is the best hydration regimen to prevent contrast media-induced nephrotoxicity? Clin Nephrol 62:1–7

Bagshaw SM, Ghali WA (2004) Acetylcysteine for prevention of contrast induced nephropathy after intravascular angiography: a systematic review and meta-analysis. BMC Med 2:38

Bagshaw SM, Ghali WM (2005) Theophylline for prevention of radiocontrast nephropathy: a systematic review and meta-analysis. Arch Intern Med 176:1087–1093

Bagshaw SM, McAlister FA, Manns BJ, Gahli WA (2006) Acetylcysteine in the prevention of contrast-induced nephropathy. Arch Intern Med 166:161–166

Bakris GL, Lass N, Habaer AO et al (1990) Radiocontrast medium induced declines in renal function. A role for oxygen free radicals. Am J Physiol 175:57–60

Band RA, Gaieski DF, Mills AM et al (2007) Discordance between serum creatinine and creatinine clearance for identification of ED patients with abdominal pain at risk for contrast induced nephropathy. Am J Emerg Med 25:268–272

Barrett BJ, Parfrey PS (2006) Preventing nephropathy induced by contrast medium. N Engl J Med 354:379–386

Barrett BJ, Katzberg RW, Thomsen HS et al (2006) Contrast induced nephropathy in patients with chronic kidney disease undergoing computed tomography: a double blind comparison of iodixanol and iopamidol. Invest Radiol 41:815–821

Bartholomew BA, Harjai KJ, Dukkipati S et al (2004) Impact of nephropathy after percutaneous coronary intervention and a method for risk stratification. Am J Cardiol 93:1515–1519

Benigni A, Remuzzi G (1999) Endothelin antagonists. Lancet 353:133–138

Berns AS (1989) Nephrotoxicity of contrast media. Kidney Int 36:730–740

Bettmann MA (2005) Contrast medium-induced nephropathy: critical review of the existing clinical evidence Nephrol Dial Transplant 20(Suppl 1):i12–i17

Biondi-Zoccai GG, Lotrionte M, Abbate A et al (2006) Compliance with QUOROM and quality of reporting over overlapping meta-analysis on the role of acetylcysteine in the prevention of contrast associated nephropathy: case study Br Med J 332:202–209

Blaufox MD, Aurell M, Bubeck B et al (1996) Report of the Radionuclide in Nephrourology Committee on renal clearance. J Nucl Med 37:1883–1890

Bostrom AG, Kronenberg F, Ritz E (2002) Predictive performance of renal function equations for patients with chronic kidney disease and normal serum creatinine levels. J Am Soc Nephrol 13:2140–2144

Briguori C, Colombo A, Airoldi F et al (2004a) N-acetylcysteine versus fenoldopam mesylate to prevent contrast agent-associated nephrotoxicity. J Am Coll Cardiol 44:762–765

Briguori C, Colombo A, Violante A et al (2004b) Standard vs. double dose of N-acetylcysteine to prevent contrast agent associated nephrotoxicity. Eur Heart J 25:206–211

Briguori C, Colombo A, Airoldi F et al (2006) Nephrotoxicity of low-osmolality versus iso-osmolality contrast agents: impact of N-acetylcysteine. Kidney Int 68:2250–2255

Briguori C, Airoldi F, D'Andrea D et al (2007) Renal insufficiency following contrast media administration trial (REMEDIAL): a randomized comparison of 3 preventive strategies. Circulation 115:1211–1217

Carraro M, Mancini W, Aretro M et al (1996) Dose effect of nitrendipine on urinary enzymes and microproteins following nonionic radiocontrast administration. Nephrol Dial Transplant 11:444–448

Carraro M, Malahan F, Antonione R et al (1998) Effects of a dimeric vs a monomeric nonionic contrast medium on renal function in patients with mild to moderate insufficiency: a double blind, randomized trail. Eur Radiol 8:144–147

Cavusoglu E, Chabra S, Marmur JD, Kini A, Sharma SK (2004) The prevention of contrast-induced nephropathy in patients undergoing percutaneous coronary intervention. Minerva Cardioangio 52:419–432

Chalmers N, Jackson RW (1999) Comparison of iodixanol and iohexol in renal impairment. Br J Radiol 72:701–703

Cheruvu B, Henning K, Mulligan J et al (2007) Iodixanol: risk of seubquent contrast nephropathy in cancer patients with underlying renal insufficiency undergoing diagnostic computed tomography examinations. J Comput Assist Tomogr 31:493–498

Choyke PL, Cady K, DePollar SL, Austin H (1998) Determination of serum creatinine prior to iodinated contrast media: is it needed in all patients? Tech Urol 4:65–69

Clavijo LC, Pinto TL, Kuchulakanti PK et al (2006) Effect of a rapid intraarterial infusion of dextrose 5% prior to coronary angiography on frequency of contrast-induced nephropathy in high-risk patients. Am J Cardiol 97:981–983

Cockroft DW, Gault MH (1976) Prediction of creatinine clearance from serum creatinine. Nephron 16:31–41

Couchoud C, Pozet N, Labeeuw M, Pouteil-Noble C (1999) Screening early renal failure: cut-off values for serum creatinine as an indicator of renal impairment. Kidney Int 55:1878–1884

Curham GC (2003) Prevention of contrast nephropathy. JAMA 289:606–608

Dussol B, Morange S, Loundoun A et al (2006) A randomized trial of saline hydration to prevent contrast nephropathy in chronic renal failure patients. Nephrol Dial Transplant 21:2120–2126

Eken C, Kilicaslan I (2007) Differences between various glomerular filtration rate calculation methods in predicting patients at risk for contrast-induced nephropathy. Am J Emerg Med 25:487 (Correspondence)

Erdogan A, Davidson CJ (2003) Recent clinical trials of iodixanol. Rev Cardiovasc Med 4(Suppl 5):S43–S50

Erley CM, Duda SH, Rehfuss D et al (1999) Prevention of radiocontrast-media-induced nephropathy in patients with pre-existing renal insufficiency by hydration in combination with the adenosine antagonist theophylline. Nephrol Dial Transplant 14:1146–1149

Fishbane S, Durham JH, Marzo K, Rudnick M (2004) N-acetylcysteine in the prevention of radiocontrast-induced nephropathy. J Am Soc Nephrol 15:251–260

Gare M, Haviv YS, Ben-Yehuda A et al (1999) The renal effect of low-dose dopamine in high-risk patients undergoing coronary angiography. J Am Coll Cardiol 34:1682–1688

Gleeson T, Bulugahapitiya S (2004) Contrast induced nephropathy. Am J Roentgenol 183:1673–1689

Goldenberg I, Matezky S (2005) Nephropathy induced by contrast media: pathogenesis, risk factors and preventive strategies. CMAJ 172:1461–1467

Gruberg L, Mintz GS, Mehran R et al (2000) The prognostic implications of further renal function deterioration with 48 h of interventional coronary procedures in patients with pre-existent chronic renal insufficiency. J Am Coll Cardiol 36:1542–1548

Gupta RK, Kapoor, Tewari S, Sinha N, Sharma RK (1999) Captopril for prevention of contrast-induced nephropathy in diabetic patients: a randomised study. Indian Heart J 51:521–536

Hans SS, Hans BA, Dhillon R, Dmuchowski C, Glover J (1998) Effect of dopamine on renal function after arteriography in patients with pre-existing renal insufficiency. Am Surg 64:432–436

Hardiek KJ, Katholi RE, Robbs RS, Katholi CE (2008) Renal effects of contrast media in diabetic patients undergoing diagnostic or interventional coronary angiography. J Diab Complications 22:171–177

Haylor JL, Morcos SK (2000) Endothelin antagonism and contrast nephropathy. Kidney Int 58:2239

Heinrich MC, Kuhlmann MK, Grgic A, Heckman M, Kramann B, Uder M (2005) Cytotoxic effects of ionic high-osmolar, nonioinic monomeric, and nonionic iso-osmolar dimeric iodinated contrast media on renal tubular cells in vitro. Radiology 235:843–849

Heyman SN, Rosenberger C, Rosen S (2005) Regional alterations in renal haemodynamics and oxygenation: a role contrast medium-induced nephropathy. Nephrol Dial Transplant 20(Suppl 1):i6–i11

Higgins JPT, Thompson SG, Deeks JJ, Altman DG (2003) Measuring inconsistency in meta-analysis. Br Med J 327:557–560

Hoffmann U, Fischereder M, Kruger B, Drobnik W, Kramer BK (2004) The value of N-acetylcysteine in the prevention of radiocontrast agent-induced nephropathy seems questionable. J Am Soc Nephrol 15:407–410

Hou SH, Bushinsky DA, Wish JB et al (1983) Hospital acquired renal insufficiency: a prospective study. Am J Med 74:243–248

Huber W, Ilgman K, Page M et al (2002) Effect of theophylline on contrast material-induced nephropathy on patients with chronic renal insufficiency: controlled, randomized, double-blinded study. Radiology 223:772–779

Ix JH, McCulloch CE, Chertow GM (2004) Theophylline for the prevention of radiocontrast nephropathy: a meta-analysis. Nephrol Dial Transplant 19:2747–2753

Jakobsen JA, Lundby B, Kristoffersen DT et al (1992) Evaluation of renal function with delayed CT after injection of non-ionic monomeric and dimeric contrast media in healthy volunteers. Radiology 182:419–424

Jingwei N, Ruiyan Z, Jiansheng Z, Xian Z, Weifeng S (2006). Safety of isoosmolar dimer during percutaneous coronary intervention. J Interv Radiol 15:327–329

Jo S-H, Youn T-J, Koo B-K et al (2006) Renal toxicity evaluation and comparison between Visipaque (iodixanol) and Hexabrix (ioxaglate) in patients with renal insufficiency undergoing coronary angiography. The RECOVER study: a randomized controlled trial. J Am Coll Cardiol 48:924–930

Katzberg WR (1997) Urography into the 21st century: new contrast media, renal handling, imaging characteristics, and nephrotoxicity. Radiology 204:297–312

Katzberg R (2005) Contrast medium-induced nephrotoxicity: which pathways? Radiology 235:752–755

Katzberg R, Barrett B (2007) Risk of contrast-induced nephropathy with intravenous administration of iodinated contrast media. Radiology 243:622–628

Kini AS, Mitre CA, Kim M et al (2002) A protocol for prevention of radiographic contrast nephropathy during percutaneous coronary intervention: effect of selective dopamine receptor agonist fenoldopam. Catheter Cardiovasc Interv 55:169–173

Kolehmainen H, Soiva M (2003) Comparison of Xenetix 300 and Visispaque 320 in patients with renal failure. Eur Radiol 13:B32–B33

Krasuski RA, Beard BM, Geoghagan JD et al (2003) Optimal timing of hydration to erase contrast-associated nephropathy: the OTHER CAN study. J Invasive Cardiol 15:699–702

Kshirsagar AV, Poole C, Mottl A et al (2004) N-acetylcysteine for the prevention of radiocontrast induced nephropathy: a metaanalysis of prospective controlled trials. J Am Soc Nephrol 15:761–769

Kuhn MJ, Chen N, Sahani DV et al (2008) The PREDICT study: a randomized double-Blind comparison of contrast-induced nephropathy after low- or isoosmolar contrast agent exposure. Am J Roentgenol 1991:151–157

Levey AS, Bosch JP, Lewis JB et al (1999) A more accurate method to estimate glomerular filtration rate from serum creatinine: a new prediction equation. Ann Intern Med 130:461–470

Liu R, Nair D, Ix J et al (2005) N-acetylcysteine and contrast-induced nephropathy: systematic review and metaanalysis. J Gen Intern Med 20:193–200

Love L, Johnson MS, Bresler ME et al (1994) The persistent computed tomography nephrogram: its significance in the diagnosis of contrast-associated nephrotoxicity. Br J Radiol 67:951–957

Maeder M, Klein M, Fehr T, Rickli H (2004) Contrast nephropathy: review focusing on prevention. J Am Coll Cardiol 44:1763–1771

Marenzi G, Lauri G, Assanelli E et al (2004) Contrast-induced nephropathy in patients undergoing primary angioplasty for acute myocardial infarction. J Am Coll Cardiol 44:1780–1785

Marenzi G, Assanelli E, Marana I et al (2006) N-acetylcysteine and contrast-induced nephropathy in primay angioplasty. N Engl J Med 354:273–278

McCarthy CS, Becker JA (1992) Multiple myeloma and contrast media. Radiology 183:519–521

McCullough PA, Wolyn R, Rocher LL et al (1997) Acute renal failure after coronary intervention: incidence, risk factors and relationship to mortality. Am J Med 103:368–375

McCullough PA, Bertrand ME, Brinker JA, Stacul F (2006) A meta-analysis of the renal safety of iso-osmolar iodixanol compared with low-osmolar contrast media. J Am Coll Cardiol 48:692–699

Mehran R, Aymong ED, Nikolsky E et al (2004) A simple risk score for prediction of contrast-induced nephropathy after percutaneous coronary intervention. Development and initial validation. J Am Coll Cardiol 44:1393–1399

Mehran R for the ICON investigators (2006) Ionic versus non-ionic contrast to obviate worsening nephropathy after angioplasty in chronic renal failure patients. Transcatheter Cardiovascular Therapies Meeting (TCT), Washington DC, 22–26 April 2006

Merten GJ, Burgess WP, Gray LV et al (2004) Prevention of contrast induced nephropathy with sodium bicarbonate: a randomized trial. JAMA 291:2328–2338

Meschi M, Detrenis S, Musini S et al (2006) Facts and fallacies concerning the prevention of contrast medium induced nephropathy. Crit Care Med 34:2060–2068

Mitchell RL, Craig JC, Webster AC (2004) Cochrane renal group report. Am J Kidney Dis 43:752–756

Morcos SK (1998) Contrast media-induced nephrotoxicity – questions and answers. Br J Radiol 71:357–365

Morcos SK (2004) Prevention of contrast media nephrotoxicity – the story so far. Clin Radiol 59:381–389

Morcos SK (2005) Prevention of contrast media-induced nephrotoxicity after angiographic procedures. J Vasc Interv Radiol 16:13–23

Morcos SK, Thomsen HS, Webb JAW and members of contrast media safety committee of the European Society of Urogenital Radiology (ESUR) (1999) Contrast media induced nephrotoxicity: a consensus report. Eur Radiol 9:1602–1613

Mueller C, Burkle G, Buerkle HJ et al (2002) Prevention of contrast media-associated nephropathy. Randomized comparison of 2 hydration regimens in 1620 patients undergoing coronary angioplasty. Arch Intern Med 162:329–336

Nash K, Hafeez A, Hou S (2002) Hospital-acquired renal insufficiency. Am J Kidney Dis 39:930–936

Neumayer HH, Junge W, Kufner A, Wenning A (1989) Prevention of radiocontrast-media-induced nephrotoxicity by calcium channel blocker nitrendipine: a prospective randomized clinical trial. Nephrol Dial Transplant 4:1030–1036

Nguyen SA, Suranyi P, Ravenel JG et al (2008) Iso-osmolality versus low-osmolality iodinated contrast medium at intravenous contrast-enhanced CT: effect on kidney function. Radiology 248:97–105

Nicholson T, Downes M (2003) Contrast nephrotoxicity and iso-osmolar contrast agents; implications of NEPHRIC. Clin Radiol 58:659–660

Nikolsky E, Mehran R (2003) Understanding the consequences of contrast-induced nephropathy. Rev Cardovasc Med 4(Suppl 5):S10–S18

Oldroyd SD, Haylor JL, Morcos SK (1995) Bosentan, an orally active endothelin antagonist: effect on the renal response to contrast media. Radiology 196:661–665

Oldroyd SD, Fang L, Haylor JL, Yates MS, El Nahas AM, Morcos SK (2000) Effects of adenosine receptor antagonists on the responses to contrast media in the isolated rat kidney. Clin Sci 98:303–311

Olsen JC, Salomon B (1996) Utility of the creatinine prior to intravenous contrast studies in the emergency department. J Emerg Med 14:543–546

Pannu N, Manns B, Lee H, Tonelli M (2004) Systematic review of the impact of N-acetylcysteine on contrast nephropathy. Kidney Int 65:1366–1374

Pannu N, Wiebe N, Tonelli M for the Alberta Kidney Disease Network (2006) Prophylaxis strategies for contrast-induced nephropathy. JAMA 295:2765–2779

Parfrey PS, Griffiths SM, Barrett BJ et al (1989) Contrast material-induced renal failure in patients with diabetes mellitus, renal insufficiency, or both: a prospective controlled study. N Engl J Med 320:143–149

Poletti PA, Saudan P, Platon A et al (2007) I.V. N-acetylcysteine and emergency CT: use of serum creatinine and Cystatin C as markers of radiocontrast nephrotoxicity. Am J Roentgenol 189:687–692

Pugh ND, Sissons GR, Ruttley et al (1993) Iodixanol in femoral arteriography (phase III): a comparative double double-blind parallel trial between iodixanol and iopromide. Clin Radiol 47:96–99

Recio-Mayoral A, Chaparro M, Pardo B et al (2007) The renoprotective effect of hydration with sodium bicarbonate plus N-acetylcystesine in patients undergoing emergency percutaneous coronary intervention: the RENO study. J Am Coll Cardiol 49:1283–1238

Rudnik MR, Goldfarb S, Wexler L et al (1995) Nephrotoxicity of ionic and nonionic contrast media in 1196 patients: a randomized trial. Kidney Int 47:254–261

Sadeghi HM, Stone GW, Grines CL et al (2003) Impact of renal insufficiency in patients undergoing primary angioplasty for acute myocardial infarction. Circulation 108:2769–2775

Safirstein R, Andrade L, Viera JM (2000) Acetylcysteine and nephrotoxic effects of radiographic contrast agents – a new use for an old drug. N Engl J Med 342:210–211

Sharma SK, Kini A (2005) Effect of nonionic radiocontrast agents on the occurrence of contrast-induced nephropathy in patients with mild-moderate chronic renal insufficiency: pooled analysis of the randomized trials. Catheter Cardiovasc Interv 65:386–393

Solomon R (1998) Contrast medium-induced acute renal failure. Kidney Int 53:230–242

Solomon R (2005) The role of osmolality in the incidence of contrast-induced nephropathy: A systematic review of angiographic contrast media in high risk patients. Kidney Int 68:2256–2263

Solomon R, DuMouchel W (2006) Contrast media and nephropathy. Findings from systematic analysis and Food and Drug Administration reports of adverse effects. Invest Radiol 41:651–660

Solomon R, Werner C, Mann D, D'Elia J, Silva P (1994) Effects of saline, mannitol and furosemide on acute decreases in renal function induced by radiocontrast agents. N Engl J Med 331:1416–1420

Solomon R, Natarajan M, Doucet S et al (2007) The cardiacangiography in renally impaired patients (CARE) study: A randomized, double blind trial of contrast-induced nephropathy (CIN) in high risk patients. Circulation 115:3189–3196

Spargias K, Alexopoulos E, Kyrzopoulos S et al (2004) Ascorbic acid prevents contrast mediated nephropathy in patients with renal dysfunction undergoing coronary angiography or intervention Circulation 110:2837–2842

Stevens MA, McCullough PA, Tobin KJ et al (1999) A prospective randomized trial of prevention measures in patients at high risk for contrast nephropathy. Results of the P.R.I.N.C.E study. J Am Coll Cardiol 33:403–411

Stevens LA, Coresh J, Greene T, Levey AS (2006) Assessing kidney function – measured and estimated glomerular filtration rate. N Engl J Med 354:2473–2483

Stone GW, McCullough PA, Tumlin JA et al (2003) CONTRAST investigators. Fenoldopam mesylate for the prevention of contrast-induced nephropathy: a randomized controlled trial. JAMA 290:2284–2291

Taylor AJ, Hotchkiss D, Morse RW, McCabe J (1998) PREPARED. Preparation for angiography in renal dysfunction: a randomized trial of inpatient vs outpatient hydration protocols for cardiac catheterization in mild-to-moderate renal dysfunction. Chest 114:1570–1574

Tepel M, Giet MVD, Schwarzfeld C et al (2000) Prevention of radiographic-contrast-agent-induced reductions in renal function by acetylcysteine. N Engl J Med 343:180–184

Thomsen HS (1999) Contrast nephropathy. In: Thomsen HS, Muller RN, Mattrey RF (eds) Trends in contrast media. Springer, Berlin, pp 103–116

Thomsen HS, Golman K, Hemmingsen L, Larsen S, Skaarup P, Svendsen O (1993) Contrast medium induced nephropathy: animal experiments. Front Eur Radiol 9:83–108

Thomsen HS, Morcos SK, Members of Contrast Media Safety Committee of European Society of Urogenital Radiology (ESUR) (2005) In which patients should serum-creatinine be measured before contrast medium administration? Eur Radiol 15:749–756

Thomsen HS, Morcos SK (2006) Contrast-medium-induced nephropathy: is there a new consensus? A review of published guidelines. Eur Radiol 16:1835–1840

Thomsen HS, Morcos SK (2008) Risk of contrast medium induced nephropathy in high risk patients undergoing MDCT – A pooled analysis of two randomized trials. Eur Radiol Epub DOI 10.1007/s00300-008-1206-4

Thomsen HS, Morcos SK, Barrett BJ (2008a) Contrast induced nephropathy: The wheel has turned 360 degrees. Acta Radiol 49: 646–657

Thomsen HS; Morcos SK, Erley CM et al (2008b) The ACTIVE trial: Comparison of the effects on renal function of iomeprol-4000 and iodixanol-320 in patients with chronic kidney disease undergoing abdominal computed tomography. Invest Radiol 43:170–178

Tippins RB, Torres WE, Baumgartner BR, Baumgarten DA (2000) Are screening serum creatinine levels necessary prior to outpatient CT examinations? Radiology 216:481–484

Toprak O(2006) Angiotension converting emzymes inhibitors and contrast-induced nephropathy. Renal Fail 28:99–100

Toprak O, Cirit M, Mayata S, Yesil M, Aslan LS (2003) The effect of pre-procedural captopril on contrast media induced nephropathy who underwenet coronary angiography. Anadolu Kardiyol Derg 3:98–103

Trivedi HS, Moore H, Nasr S et al (2003) A randomized prospective trial to assess the role of saline hydration on the development of contrast nephrotoxicity. Nephron Clin Pract 93:c29–c34

Vaitkus PT, Brar C (2007) N-acetylcysteine in the prevention of contrast induced nephropathy: publication bias perpetuated by meta-analysis. Am Heart J 153:175–280

Wang A, Holcslaw T, Bashore TM et al (2000) Exacerbation of radiocontrast nephrotoxicity by endothelin receptor antagonism. Kidney Int 57:1675–1680

Weinstein JM, Heyman S, Brezis M (1992) Potential deleterious effect of furosemide in radiocontrast nephropathy Nephron 62:413–415

Weisberg L, Kurnik PB, Kurnik RC (1994) Risk of radiocontrast nephropathy in patients with and without diabetes mellitus. Kidney Int 45:259–265

Wessely R, Koppara T, Kastrati A, Bradoric C, Schultz S, Vorpahl M, Mehilli et al (2008) Iso-osmolar vs low-osmolar contrast medium in patients with impaired renal function undergoing PCI – CONTRAST. Society for cardiovascular Angiography and Interventions Meeting (SCAI), Chicago, 1 April 2008

Yamazaki H, Matsushita M, Inoue T et al (1997a) Renal cortical retention on delayed CT after angiography and contrast associated nephropathy. Br J Radiol 70:897–902

Yamazaki H, Oi H, Matsushita M et al (1997b) Lack of correlation between gallbladder opacification in delayed CT and contrast-associated nephropathy. Eur Radiol 7:1328–1331

Zagler A, Azadpour M, Mercado C, Hennekens CH (2005) N-acetylcysteine and contrast-induced nephropathy: a meta-analysis of 13 randomized trial. Am Heart J 151:140–145

Dialysis and Contrast Media

10

Sameh K. Morcos

CONTENTS

10.1
Introduction

Contrast media-induced nephropathy remains an important cause of hospital-acquired acute renal failure. Pre-existing renal impairment, especially diabetic nephropathy and the dose of the contrast medium are major risk factors in the development of contrast nephropathy (Morcos et al. 1999; Morcos 1998, 2004). It is generally agreed that if contrast medium injection is clinically necessary prophylactic measures should be used to reduce the risk (Morcos et al. 2002). Prophylactic hemodialysis has been proposed to prevent contrast nephrotoxicity in patients with renal impairment, but has not obtained general acceptance. In addition, there is misunderstanding about

Sameh K. Morcos
Department of Diagnostic Imaging, Northern General Hospital, Sheffield Teaching Hospitals NHS Trust, Sheffield S5 7AU, UK

whether intravascular contrast medium injection in patients on dialysis should be scheduled in relation to the time of the hemodialysis session (Morcos et al. 2002). In this chapter, the use of hemodialysis and peritoneal dialysis in the elimination of water-soluble, iodinated or gadolinium-based contrast agents in patients with end-stage renal disease and the value of hemodialysis in preventing contrast media-induced nephrotoxicity in patients with pre-existing renal impairment will be discussed.

10.2
Hemodialysis in the Removal of Iodinated Contrast Media

The pharmacokinetic properties of water-soluble, iodinated contrast media are such that they are distributed in the extra cellular fluid only, protein binding is minimal, they are not metabolized and excretion is mainly by glomerular filtration. The half-life of iodinated contrast media in patients with normal, glomerular filtration rate is approximately 2 h but in patients with severe renal dysfunction it can be prolonged to over 30 h depending on the extent of renal impairment. Therefore, in patients with end-stage renal failure the plasma contrast medium concentration remains high for a long period of time. Such patients are at the risk of central nervous system reactions such as convulsions and respiratory depression. The effect on the central nervous system could be due either to contrast media or to uremia (Morcos et al. 2002). Delayed severe skin disorders including vasculitis and salivary gland swelling have also been reported in chronic renal failure patients after high-dose urography (Furukawa et al. 1996). To reduce the risk of these complications, it has been suggested that contrast media should be eliminated from the body as soon as possible.

Several factors influence the elimination of contrast media by hemodialysis (Table 10.1) (Furukawa et al. 1996; Sterner et al. 2000; Waaler et al. 1990; Udea et al. 1996; Matzkies et al. 1999; Moon et al. 1995). The first factor is the size and weight of the contrast media molecules; the smaller the solute molecule, more easily it moves across the membrane. Comparisons of dialysance *(Dialysance = blood flow rate of the hemodialysis X extraction ratio)* values of contrast media from one study to another are usually meaningless as the time period between contrast medium injection and starting dialysis, and the dialysis conditions are likely to vary from one study to another. In one study, under the same conditions the dialysance of nonionic, monomeric contrast media was slightly higher than that of ionic, dimeric contrast media, partly because of the lower molecular weight and size of the former (Furukawa et al. 1996). However, in another study the hemodialysis elimination of the nonionic monomer iohexol was similar to that of the nonionic dimer iodixanol which has a molecular mass almost twice that of the former (Sterner et al. 2000). Second, binding to the plasma proteins, which have large molecular size also decreases the efficiency of hemodialysis of contrast media. Hydrophilicity of nonionic contrast media is an important factor in determining the protein binding of their molecules. The higher the

hydrophilicity, the lower is the affinity of the molecules to proteins. The elimination by hemodialysis of the nonionic dimer iodixanol which has high hydrophilicity and very low protein binding was similar to that of the nonionic monomer iohexol (Sterner et al. 2000). The protein binding of the ionic dimer ioxaglate on the other hand is relatively high and amounts to $7.6 \pm 1.5\%$ whereas with iohexol it is $1.5 \pm 0.3\%$ determined by means of equilibrium dialysis. This difference might be partly responsible for the fact that iohexol was more easily eliminated than ioxaglate (Furukawa et al. 1996). Another possible factor is the molecular aggregation that occurs with ioxaglate, leading to the formation of large particles which are less permeable by hemodialysis. The electrical charge of the molecule also influences dialysance. Ioxaglate is almost completely dissociated in plasma and is negatively charged. As the cellulose diacetate membrane is slightly negatively charged, solutes with a negative charge such as ioxaglate move less easily across the membrane (Furukawa et al. 1996).

The degree of hepatic and renal excretion (in patients who are not anuric) may also affect the elimination rate of contrast media during hemodialysis in patients with chronic renal failure (Waaler et al. 1990; Udea et al. 1996).

The elimination of contrast media is not dependent on the pore size of the membrane during dialysis. Under clearly defined conditions, the mean clearance rate for the nonionic monomer iopromide was 108 ml min^{-1} for high- and low-flux membranes, both with a surface area of 1.3 m^2 (Matzkies et al. 1999). The clearance rate of contrast agents for polyacrylonetrile membranes is 1.5–3 times higher than that of cuprophane membranes (Matzkies et al. 2000), whereas there is no difference between polyamide and hemophane membranes (Matzkies et al. 1999).

Blood flow does not seem to have an important effect. Removal of contrast agents can be performed at low blood flow rates without loss of efficacy and this is preferable in uremic patients who are prone to develop disequilibrium syndrome because of the rapid removal of the low molecular waste products during intensive dialysis (Moon et al. 1995). The osmotic process contributes to the elimination. Greater amounts of substance are transported across the dialysis membrane when it is exposed to higher concentration. Thus, fast reduction of contrast medium concentrations can be achieved by dialysis in patients with high initial plasma levels. A short dialysis time of 2 h can be sufficient for contrast medium removal (Matzkies et al. 1999).

Table 10.1. Factors that influence the elimination of contrast media in hemodialysis

[A] Contrast media
1. Molecular size and weight.
2. Protein binding.
3. Electrical charge.
4. Hydrophilicity.
[B] Hemodialysis procedure
1. The permeability and surface area of the hemodialysis membrane.
2. Dialysis membrane material.
3. Blood flow rate.
4. Dialysate flow rate.
5. Duration of dialysis.
[C] Patient factors
1. Degree of hepatic and renal excretion.
2. Contrast medium plasma concentration.

Dialysis immediately after a procedure involving the intravascular injection of contrast material has been advocated. A prospective clinical study to evaluate this approach was carried out in ten patients on regular hemodialysis (3 times a week). The patients received between 40 and 225 ml of nonionic contrast media and were followed up with clinical and laboratory examination. No significant adverse effects were observed and no patient had clinical features that necessitated emergency dialysis. The average time interval from contrast administration to hemodialysis was 23 h (range 16–47 h). Immediate post-procedure dialysis is unwarranted as a routine practice (YOUNATHAN et al. 1994).

10.3
Elimination of Iodinated Contrast Media by Peritoneal Dialysis

Three patients with chronic renal failure (serum creatinine 389–804 µmol l^{-1}) underwent coronary angiography with iohexol. Intermittent automated peritoneal dialysis (36–60 l dialysis fluid) was able to remove 43–72% of the iohexol over 16–18 h (MOON et al. 1995). In another study, intermittent peritoneal dialysis for 64 h removed 56% of the injected meglumine diatrizoate (BROOKS and BARRY 1973). Continuous ambulatory peritoneal dialysis removed 54% (range 36–80%) of the administered dose of iopamidol 300 (30 ml) over 7 days using 8 l of dialysis fluid daily. During the same period, 27% (range: 36–80%) of the injected contrast medium was excreted in the urine (DONALLY et al. 1992). Thus, peritoneal dialysis is also effective for removing contrast agents from the body, but takes longer than hemodialysis. No side effects of the contrast agents were reported in the three studies and this is important since the residual renal function in these patients must be protected.

10.4
Elimination of Gadolinium-Based Contrast Media by Dialysis

Contrast enhanced MRI examinations are frequently required in patients with end-stage renal disease. In normal subjects, the half-life of a nonspecific extracellular gadolinium-based contrast agent is about 1.5 h and 90% of the injected dose is removed via the kidneys within the first 24 h. The elimination half-time of gadolinium-based contrast media in patients with significant reduction in renal function can be prolonged to several hours depending on the degree of renal impairment. Over 80% of the administered dose is usually excreted within 7 days in such patients. The delay in the elimination of gadolinium in patients with significant renal impairment (GFR of 30 ml min^{-1} or less) led to the recommendation of hemodialysis for these patients. The extra renal elimination of gadolinium is very small and less than 2% of the injected dose is excreted in the faeces within 5 days of injection (JOFFE et al. 1998).

Good hemodialysability and safety of MRI gadolinium-based contrast agents have been reported (JOFFE et al. 1998; OKADA et al. 2001). After three consecutive hemodialysis sessions over 6 days, 97% of the initial concentration of gadodiamide was eliminated (JOFFE et al. 1998). In another study of 70 patients, no side effects were noted (OKADA et al. 2001); this was also the case in the six patients in whom hemodialysis was performed 3 days after the contrast medium injection. A total of four routine hemodialysis sessions were required to achieve nearly complete removal of gadolinium-based contrast medium (OKADA et al. 2001).

Continuous ambulatory peritoneal dialysis for 20 days eliminated 69% of the total amount of injected gadodiamide (JOFFE et al. 1998) reflecting the low peritoneal clearance. No metabolism or transmetallation of gadodiamide occurred and there were no contrast-related adverse events. The slow removal is probably a consequence of altered apparent volume of distribution due to dialysis fluid in the peritoneal cavity and to the limitations of the peritoneum as a dialysis membrane. The peritoneal clearance of gadopentetate dimeglumine in patients undergoing continuous ambulatory peritoneal dialysis was about 5 ml per minute. No side effects were recorded during a 1-week observation period (TOMBACH et al. 2001). Injection of gadolinium-based contrast media for MRI examinations (0.1–0.3 mmol kg^{-1} BW) caused no significant change in renal function (JOFFE et al. 1998; OKADA et al. 2001; TOMBACH et al. 2001; DORSAM et al. 1995). However, currently there is a great concern about the use of MRI gadolinium-based contrast agents in patients on dialysis because of a probable causal relation between certain types of gadolinium-based contrast agents and the condition of nephrogenic systemic fibrosis (NSF). For further information, refer to Chap. 24.

10.5
Prophylactic Hemodialysis in the Prevention of Contrast Media Nephrotoxicity

A variety of approaches have been suggested to prevent contrast media nephrotoxicity, including saline hydration and administration of agents that cause increased renal blood flow or diuresis (Morcos et al. 1999; Morcos 1998, 2004). The role of hemodialysis in preventing contrast nephrotoxicity has not been proven (Morcos 2004). Several studies have demonstrated that haemodialysis does not offer any protection against contrast-induced nephropathy (Dehnharts et al. 1998; Vogt et al. 2001; Huber et al. 2002). In addition, the cost of hemodialysis and the associated risks including venous cannulation and the possibility of heparin-induced bleeding can only be justified if hemodialysis can be shown to prevent contrast medium induced nephrotoxicity (Morcos 2004).

Thirty patients with reduced renal function (mean serum creatinine concentration $212 \pm 14 \mu mol\ l^{-1}$) were randomly assigned to receive either hemodialysis for 3 h starting as soon as possible ($63 \pm 6\ min$) or conservative treatment with no hemodialysis after administration of a nonionic monomeric contrast medium (Dehnharts et al. 1998). All patients received intravenous infusion of 0.9% saline at the rate of $83\ ml\ h^{-1}$ beginning 12 h before injection of the contrast medium ($350\ mgI\ ml^{-1}$, mean dose 3 ml kg^{-1} body weight). In the control group, only the infusion of saline was continued for another 12 h after the radiographic procedure. Serum concentrations of the contrast agent and creatinine were followed for up to 14 days. Both the groups were treated with calcium channel antagonists (nitrendipine 10 mg 12 hourly). The incidence of contrast nephrotoxicity in the hemodialysis group was 53% and in the control group was 40%, so hemodialysis treatment did not decrease the incidence of contrast nephrotoxicity. Patients were hemodialysed as early as possible after contrast medium exposure, but the poor efficacy of hemodialysis in preventing contrast nephrotoxicity is related to the very rapid onset of renal injury after administration of contrast medium (Morcos 1998).

Of 113 patients with chronic renal impairment and serum creatinine above $200\ \mu mol\ l^{-1}$, 55 were randomly assigned to hemodialysis and 58 to non-hemodialysis after injection of nonionic monomeric contrast media (Vogt et al. 2001). The mean dose of contrast medium injected in the non-hemodialyis group was 143 ± 15 and $210 \pm 19\ ml$ in the hemodialysis group. The baseline serum creatinine was 316 ± 16 and $308 \pm 15 \mu mol$ l^{-1} respectively. All patients received saline infusion following the same protocol of the previous study. The hemodialysis began 30–280 min after the radiographic procedure (median time 120 min). The incidence of contrast nephrotoxicity in the hemodialysis group was 24% and in the non-hemodialysis group was 16%. There was no significant difference between the two groups in relation to clinically important events (stroke, pulmonary edema, myocardial infarction and death). The higher incidence of nephrotoxicity in the hemodialysis group could be attributed to the larger doses of contrast medium administered to these patients in comparison to the control group. In addition, hemodialysis may cause deterioration of the renal function through activation of inflammatory reactions with the release of vasoactive substances that may induce acute hypotension. Although a recent study suggested that prophylactic haemodialysis after coronary angiography (dialysis was initiated $81 \pm 32\ min$ after the angiography) is effective in improving renal outcome in patients with advanced renal impairment (creatinine clearance $13\ ml\ min^{-1}$) (Lee et al. 2007), the general consensus on the role of prophylactic haemodialysis is that performing hemodialysis immediately after administration of contrast media in patients with reduced renal function does not diminish the rate of complications, including the complication of contrast medium-induced nephrotoxicity (Rodby 2007; Cruz et al. 2006).

10.6
Conclusion

Hemo- and peritoneal dialysis are effective for eliminating iodinated or gadolinium-based contrast media. Relating the time of the contrast medium injection to the dialysis schedule is unnecessary. Hemodialysis does not offer any protection against contrast medium-induced nephrotoxicity. There is as yet no convincing evidence to show that hemodialysis prevents the development of nephrogenic systemic fibrosis. However, the least stable gadolinium-based contrast agents are contraindicated in patients on dialysis or with severely reduced renal function (Chap. 24).

References

Brooks MH, Barry KG (1973) Removal of iodinated contrast material by peritoneal dialysis. Nephron 12:10–14

Cruz DN, Perazella MA, Bellomo R, Corradi V, de Cal M, Kuang D, Ocampo C, Nalesso F, Ronco C (2006) Extracorporeal blood purification therapies for prevention of radiocontrast-induced nephropathy: a systematic review. Am J Kidney Dis 48:361–371

Dehnarts T, Keller E, Gondolf K, Schiffner T, Pavenstadt H, Schollmeyer P (1998) Effect of haemodialysis after contrast medium administration in patients with renal insufficiency. Nephrol Dial Transplant 13:358–362

Donally PK, Burwell N, McBurney A, Ward JW, Wals J, Warkin EM (1992) Clearance of iopamidol, a nonionic contrast medium, by CAPD in patients with end-stage renal failure. Br J Radiol 65:1108–1113

Dörsam J, Knopp MV, Schad L, Peische S, Carl S, Oesingmann N (1995) Elimination of gadolinium-DTPA by peritoneal dialysis. Nephrol Dial Transplant 10:1228–1230

Furukawa T, Ueda J, Takahashi S, Sajaguchi K (1996) Elimination of low-osmolality contrast media by haemodialysis. Acta Radiol 37:966–971

Huber W, Jeschke B, Kreymann B, Henning M, Page M, Salmhofer H, Eckel F, Schmidt U, Umgelter A, Schweigart U, Classen M (2002) Haemodialysis for the prevention of contrast-induced nephropathy. Outcome of 31 patients with severely impaired renal function, comparison with patients at similar risk and review. Invest Radiol 37:471–481

Joffe P, Thomsen HS, Meusel M (1998) The pharmacokinetics of gadodiamide in patients with severe renal insufficiency treated conservatively or undergoing hemodialysis or continuously ambulatory peritoneal dialysis. Acad Radiol 5:491–502

Lee PT, Chou KJ, Liu CP, Mar CY, Chen CL, Hsu CY, Fang HC, Chung HM (2007) Renal protection for coronary angiography in advanced renal failure patients by prophylactic hemodialysis. A randomized controlled trial. JACC 50:1015–1020

Matzkies FK, Tombach B, Kisters K, Schuhmann G, Hohage H, Schaefer RM (1999) Clearance of iopromide during haemodialysis with high and low flux membranes. Acta Radiol 40:220–223

Matzkies FK, Reinecke H, Tombach B, Koeneke J, Hohage H, Kisters K, Schaefer RM (2000) Reduced iopromide elimination in hemodialysis with cuprophan membranes. Acta Radiol 41:671–673

Moon SS, Back S E, Kurkus J, Nilsson-Ehle P (1995) Haemodialysis for elimination of the nonionic contrast medium iohexol after angiography in patients with impaired renal function. Nephron 70:430–437

Morcos SK, Thomsen HS, Webb JAW and members of the Contrast Media Safety Committee of the European Society of Urogenital Radiology (ESUR) (1999) Contrast media induced nephrotoxicity: a consensus report. Eur Radiol 9:1602–1613

Morcos SK (1998) Contrast media induced nephrotoxicity-questions and answers. Br J Radiol 71:357–365

Morcos SK (2004) Prevention of contrast media induced nephrotoxicity-the story so far. Clin Radiol 59:381–389

Morcos SK, Thomsen HS, Webb JAW and members of the Contrast Media Safety Committee of the European Society of Urogenital Radiology (ESUR) (2002) Dialysis and contrast media. Eur Radiol 12:3026–3030

Okada S, Katagiri K, Kumazaki T, Yokoyama H (2001) Safety of gadolinium contrast agents in haemodialysis patients. Acta Radiol 42:339–341

Rodby RA (2007) Preventing complications of radiographic contrast media: is there a role for dialysis? Semin Dial 20:19–23

Sterner G, Frennby B, Mansson S, Ohisson A, Prutz KG, Almen T (2000) Assessing residual renal function and efficiency of hemodialysis- an application for urographic contrast media. Nephron 85:324–333

Tombach B, Bremer C, Reimer P, Kisers K, Schaefer R M, Greens V, Heindel W (2001) Renal tolerance of a neutral gadolinium chelate (gadobutrol) in patients with chronic renal failure. Results of a randomized study. Radiology 218:651–652

Ueda J, Furukawa T, Takahashi S, Sakaguchi K (1996) Elimination of ioversol by hemodialysis. Acta Radiol 37:826–829

Vogt B, Ferrari P, Schonholzer C, Marti HP, Mohaupt M, Wiederkehr M, Cereghetti C, Serra A, Huynh-Do U, Uehlinger D, Frey FJ (2001) Pre-emptive haemodialysis after radiocontrast media in patients with renal insufficiency is potentially harmful. A J Med 111:692–698

Waaler A, Svaland M, Fauchald P, Jakobsen JA, Kolmannskog F, Berg KJ (1990) Elimination of iohexol, a low osmolar nonionic contrast medium, by haemodialysis in patients with chronic renal failure. Nephron 56:81–85

Younathan CM, Kaude JV, Cook MD, Shaw GS, Peterson JC (1994) Dialysis is not indicated immediately after administration of non ionic contrast agents in patients with end-stage renal disease treated by maintenance dialysis. AJR 163:969–971

Non-Insulin-Dependent Diabetes and Contrast Media

11

JUDITH A.W. WEBB

CONTENTS

JUDITH A.W. WEBB
Department of Diagnostic Radiology, St Bartholomew's
Hospital, West Smithfield, London EC1A 7BE, UK

11.1 Introduction

In the 1990s, there was anxiety about the risk of lactic acidosis if intravascular iodinated contrast media caused nephrotoxicity in non-insulin-dependent diabetic patients on metformin. Guidelines from the European Society of Urogenital Radiology (ESUR) published in 1999 indicated that metformin administration should be stopped from the time of contrast medium administration for 48 h and only restarted when serum creatinine had been shown to be normal (THOMSEN et al. 1999). Since 1999, new data on the risk of metformin-associated lactic acidosis have become available and clinical practice for prescribing metformin to diabetic patients with impaired renal function has changed.

11.2 Metformin: Action and Pharmacokinetics

Metformin (dimethylbiguanide) was introduced in 1957 for the treatment of non-insulin-dependent diabetes mellitus (NIDDM). It is regarded as a drug of first choice in adults with NIDDM not controlled by diet and exercise (BOLEN et al. 2007) and is the most widely prescribed oral agent in diabetes (HOLSTEIN and STUMVOLL 2005). It may also be used in combination with sulphonylurea or insulin.

Metformin lowers the blood glucose, principally by increasing the insulin sensitivity of the tissues. This results in increased glucose uptake by muscle and decreased gluconeogenesis in the liver with reduced liver glucose output (SIRTORI and PASIK 1994; DUNN and PETERS 1995; BAILEY and TURNER 1996).

About 40–60% of orally ingested metformin is absorbed from the gut, largely from the small bowel (Sirtori and Pasik 1994; Dunn and Peters 1995; Bailey and Turner 1996). Metformin is not bound to plasma protein or metabolised. Renal excretion is rapid, with 90% excreted in the first 12 h. Excretion is by both glomerular filtration and tubular secretion (Bailey and Turner 1996). The mean plasma elimination half-life is between 4 and 8.7 h in patients with normal renal function and elimination is prolonged in renal impairment (Dunn and Peters 1995). In a study of pharmacokinetics, metformin clearance was reduced by 23–33% in mild renal impairment, and by 74–78% in moderate or severe renal impairment (Sambol et al. 1995). During metformin treatment, blood lactate increases slightly, within the normal range, and this is largely cleared by the liver (Bailey and Turner 1996).

11.3
Lactic Acidosis Associated with Biguanide Agents

The most important side effect of the biguanides is lactic acidosis which occurs when lactic acid accumulates in the blood faster than it can be removed. It is characterised by a blood pH less than 7.25 and lactic acid levels greater than 5 mmol l^{-1}.

The biguanide agent phenformin was introduced in the late 1950s. It is metabolised by the liver, and was associated with an unacceptable risk of lactic acidosis, resulting in its withdrawal in 1977.

Metformin has been estimated to have a risk of inducing lactic acidosis ten to twenty times less than phenformin (Bailey and Turner 1996). Nonetheless, lactic acidosis is considered to be an important adverse effect of metformin and various contraindications to metformin use have been recommended to reduce the risk of lactic acidosis. An important contraindication to metformin treatment is renal impairment, in which decreased metformin excretion can lead to blood metformin levels many times greater than the therapeutic level (Sirtori and Pasik 1994). Threshold serum creatinine levels, which have been recommended as exclusion criteria for metformin, are greater than or equal to 132 µmol l^{-1} (1.5 mg dl^{-1}) for men and 124 µmol l^{-1} (1.4 mg dl^{-1}) for women (Bailey and Turner 1996).

Other contraindications to metformin treatment are conditions which may predispose to lactic acidosis by causing hypoxia and/or reduced peripheral perfusion, such as heart failure, respiratory failure, or severe infection, or conditions which impair liver metabolism, such as liver disease or alcohol abuse (Bailey and Turner 1996).

11.4
Recent Data on the Risk of Metformin-Associated Lactic Acidosis and Changes in Metformin Prescribing Practice

A recent Cochrane review showed that the risk of lactic acidosis in diabetic patients on metformin was 6.3 cases per 100,000 patient years (Salpeter et al. 2006). Both this and another review (the COSMIC approach study) indicated that there was no significant difference in the incidence of lactic acidosis between metformin and sulphonylurea (Salpeter et al. 2006; Cryer et al. 2005). Most patients in these studies only received metformin in the absence of recognised contraindications. Almost all patients on metformin, who have developed lactic acidosis, either had one of the recognised contraindications to metformin or had received doses greater than those recommended (Sirtori and Pasik 1994).

As the safety of metformin has been increasingly recognised, some of the contraindications to its use have been disregarded in clinical practice. In a review of more than 2,500 patients in whom a variety of contraindications were not applied, only one case of lactic acidosis was reported (Holstein and Stumvoll 2005). It has been suggested that 'mild renal impairment', including patients with CKD3, is no longer a contraindication to the use of metformin (Holstein and Stumvoll 2005; Shaw et al. 2007). Rachmani et al. (2002) proposed that metformin could even be prescribed up to a serum creatinine level of 220 µmol l^{-1}). However, a GFR of less than 40 ml min^{-1} 1.73 m^{-2} is still generally regarded to be an absolute contraindication to metformin (Holstein and Stumvoll 2005; Shaw et al. 2007).

11.5
Lactic Acidosis After Intravascular Iodinated Contrast Media in NIDDM Patients on Metformin

Anxiety about diabetic patients on metformin, who receive intravascular iodinated contrast media, relates to the potential nephrotoxicity of these agents in diabetic patients. Intravascular iodinated contrast media are recognised to be nephrotoxic in diabetic patients with impaired renal function, with diabetics with renal impairment having a higher risk of nephrotoxicity than non-diabetic patients with the same degree of renal impairment (PARFREY et al. 1989; RUDNICK et al. 1995; McCULLOUGH et al. 2006). However, the risk of contrast medium nephrotoxicity is very low in diabetics with normal renal function (PARFREY et al. 1989; RUDNICK et al. 1995). If renal function declines after contrast medium administration, metformin can accumulate, with the risk of lactic acidosis.

Other factors which increase the risk of nephrotoxicity include dehydration, the use of high-osmolar ionic contrast agents, use of contrast medium doses over 100 ml and intra-arterial contrast medium administration (McCULLOUGH et al. 2006).

11.6
Evolution of Guidelines for Using Iodinated Contrast Media in NIDDM Patients on Metformin

The withdrawal of phenformin caused a temporary decline in the use of metformin, but from the late 1980s metformin was increasingly used in Europe. In late 1994, metformin was approved for use in the US. Shortly after this, letters appeared in *Radiology* drawing attention to restrictions in the metformin package insert. This stated that metformin should be stopped for 48 h before and 48 h after contrast medium administration, and should be restarted only after serum creatinine had been measured and shown to be normal (DACHMAN 1995; ROTTER 1995). This protocol was widely adopted.

The new guideline was however attacked as being unnecessarily restrictive (RASULI et al. 1996; DUDDY 1998; CHERRYMAN et al. 1998; McCARTNEY et al. 1999; NAWAZ et al. 1998). When McCARTNEY et al. reviewed the 120 cases of metformin-associated lactic acidosis in the literature in 1999, they found 18 cases which had occurred after intravascular iodinated contrast media. Of these, only one (or perhaps two) had normal serum creatinine. Many also had intercurrent illness and/or liver dysfunction (McCARTNEY et al. 1999).

It subsequently emerged that the manufacturers' recommendation to stop metformin 48 h before contrast medium was based only on theoretical considerations of drug kinetics (RASULI et al. 1998). In 1998, the FDA authorised a change in the package insert stating that metformin should be stopped only for

the 48 h following contrast medium administration (BETTMAN 2002). This is the recommendation followed in the current ESUR guidelines (THOMSEN et al. 1999).

As the safety of metformin has been increasingly recognised, the need to measure serum creatinine after metformin has been withheld for 48 h in patients who are clinically well, has been questioned (BETTMAN 2002; THOMSEN 2006). The most recent guidelines from the UK Royal College of Radiologists recommend that if less than 100 ml of iodinated contrast medium is to be given intravenously to a patient on metformin with normal renal function, no special precautions are needed and it is not even necessary to stop metformin (ROYAL COLLEGE OF RADIOLOGISTS 2005).

11.7
Reliability of Serum Creatinine and eGFR Estimations for Assessing Renal Function in Diabetic Patients

If the protocol for using intravascular iodinated contrast medium in diabetics on metformin who have normal renal function is to be relaxed, it is important that renal function is measured accurately. A normal serum creatinine level does not necessarily indicate a normal glomerular filtration rate (GFR). This is particularly the case in patients with a low muscle mass, who can have a markedly reduced GFR despite a serum creatinine in the 'normal' range.

Various methods of estimating GFR from serum creatinine levels (eGFR) are now available. These give a more accurate indication of renal function in diabetics with CKD 2 and 3 than does serum creatinine (NEW et al. 2007; FONTSERE et al. 2006). However, in diabetics with normal renal function or with hyperfiltration they are less satisfactory and may even underestimate GFR (FONTSERE et al. 2006).

Recent data using GFR estimation as well as serum creatinine measurement have shown that metformin is now being prescribed to a significant number of patients with reduced GFR. For example, in over 5,000 diabetics, 67% of those with CKD 3 (GFR 30–59 ml min^{-1} 1.73 m^{-2}) had a serum creatinine less than 120 $\mu mol\ l^{-1}$ (NEW et al. 2006). In another study, a majority of patients prescribed metformin within the serum creatinine range of 130–150 $\mu mol\ l^{-1}$ had CKD3 (SHAW et al. 2007). In over 7,500 diabetic patients, it was noted that a serum creatinine level equal to or greater than 120 $\mu mol\ l^{-1}$ had only a sensitivity of

45.3% for identifying patients with CKD3, with a specificity of 100% (Middleton et al. 2006).

11.8
Gadolinium Contrast Media

There are no specific safety data available for the use of gadolinium contrast agents in diabetics on metformin. Although nephrotoxicity following gadolinium contrast media has been reported (Thomsen 2004), it is a very rare occurrence when approved doses are not exceeded.

No special precautions are necessary if patients with NIDDM on metformin receive intravascular gadolinium contrast agents.

11.9
Metformin for the Treatment of Polycystic Ovaries

In polycystic ovary syndrome (PCO), there is reduced insulin sensitivity. Initial reports that metformin could reduce the symptoms of the condition and induce ovulation were encouraging (Lord 2003). Although more recent reviews suggest that metformin is no better than the oral contraceptive pill for reducing PCO symptoms and that it is less effective than clomiphene for ovulation induction (Balen and Rutherford 2007; Legro et al. 2007), metformin is still prescribed in patients with PCO.

Polycystic ovary syndrome is not associated with reduced renal function or with an increased risk of nephrotoxicity. Therefore, no special precautions need to be taken in PCO patients on metformin who receive intravascular iodinated contrast media.

11.10
Guidelines on Metformin for Diabetic Patients Receiving Intravascular Contrast Media

11.10.1
Iodinated Agents

All patients should be well hydrated before contrast medium administration and should receive the smallest dose of a nonionic contrast medium consistent with a diagnostic result.

Before administration of intravascular iodinated contrast medium, all patients should have an assessment of renal function, preferably with eGFR estimation as well as serum creatinine measurement.

11.10.1.1
Patients with eGFR equal to or greater than 60 ml min^{-1} 1.73 m^{-2} (CKD 1 and 2)

The patient can continue to take metformin normally.

11.10.1.2
Patients with eGFR 30–59 ml min^{-1} 1.73 m^{-2} (CKD 3)

Imaging not using an iodinated contrast medium should be considered.

If it is clinically essential to use iodinated contrast medium, all precautions to reduce the risk of contrast medium nephrotoxicity should be taken: intravenous hydration, use of a nonionic contrast medium in the lowest dose consistent with a diagnostic result, and avoidance of nephrotoxic drugs (see Chap. 29.3).

Metformin should be stopped 48 h before contrast medium administration. Metformin can be restarted 48 h after contrast medium, provided there has been no deterioriation in serum creatinine/eGFR.

It is to be noted that metformin should not be prescribed to patients with GFR less than 40 ml min^{-1} 1.73 m^{-2}. In some countries, it is contraindicated to prescribe metformin to patients with abnormal se-creatinine levels.

11.10.1.3
Patients with eGFR less than 30 ml min^{-1} (CKD 4 and 5), or with an intercurrent illness causing hypoxia or impaired liver function.

When the GFR is less than 30 ml min^{-1}, or when there is serious intercurrent illness likely to cause lactic acidosis, metformin is contraindicated and alternative diabetic medication should be used.

In diabetic patients with CKD 4 and 5, the risk of contrast medium nephrotoxicity is significant and intravascular iodinated contrast media should be avoided if possible.

process, with fibrosis and adjacent muscle atrophy detected at the injection site by 8 weeks.

Early detection is important to avoid the acute inflammatory response which peaks at 24–48 h after extravasation (COHAN et al. 1990b). While COHAN et al. (1990b) found that ionic contrast media were more toxic than nonionic agents, no difference was found by JACOBS et al. (1998). The presence of meglumine as a cation may also play a role in the cytotoxicity of ionic contrast media (KIM et al. 1990).

15.2.4.3
Volume

The third factor is the volume of extravasated contrast medium. Although severe skin lesions have been described following an extravasation of less than 15 mL, the majority occurred with large-volume extravasations (UPTON et al. 1979).

15.2.4.4
Compression

The fourth factor is the mechanical compression caused by large-volume extravasations that may lead to compartment syndromes (POND et al. 1992; YOUNG 1994; MEMOLO et al. 1993; BENSON et al. 1996). Infection at the extravasated site may increase the severity of local lesions.

15.2.4.5
Indwelling Lines

Extravasation from indwelling intravenous lines is often due to phlebitis that develops in the veins that have been cannulated (COHAN et al. 1996). Thrombosis increases vascular resistance in the same way as an injection does. Other mechanisms include the inadequate placement of the catheter in the vein, multiple punctures of the same vein, and high injection pressure, which can break the vessel wall.

15.3
Clinical Picture

The presentation of extravasation of the iodinated and MRI contrast media varies from minor erythema and swelling to tissue necrosis associated with progressive edema and skin ulceration. The injuries may heal or rarely lead to long-term sequelae including hypoesthesia, marked weakness, and pain (FEDERLE et al.

1998). Symptoms of extravasation are very variable and many patients complain of stinging or burning pain. Although unconscious patients, the elderly and infant children cannot complain of pain, others, who are able to complain, do not experience any discomfort and remain asymptomatic. On physical examination, the extravasation site appears swollen, red and tender. Most extravasation injuries resolve spontaneously in 2–4 days. At the initial examination, it is not possible to predict whether the extravasation injury will resolve or will result in ulceration, or necrosis and damage to soft tissue. A number of clinical findings suggest severe injury and justify seeking the advice of a surgeon. These include skin blistering, altered tissue perfusion, paresthesiae, and increasing or persistent pain after 4 h (COHAN et al. 1996). Extravasation may also result in acute compartmental syndromes producing tense and dusky forearms, with swelling and diminished arterial pulses. Compartmental syndromes may necessitate emergency fasciotomy to relieve neurovascular compromise (POND et al. 1992; YOUNG 1994; MEMOLO et al. 1993; BENSON et al. 1996).

Extravasation injuries must be distinguished from other local reactions to injected fluid, including hypersensitivity reactions and local irritative effects of iodinated contrast agents on the vessel wall. In these reactions, edema and erythema are absent and the catheter is well positioned in the vein. Transient, local pain has been reported in 2–5% of patients following intravenous administration of ionic contrast material while delayed arm pain at or above the injection site has been reported in 0.1–14.0% of patients who received iodinated contrast material (SHEHADI 1975; McCULLOGH et al. 1989). The duration of pain may be as long as several days (mean, 3 days; range, 1–30 days) and may progress to phlebitis in rare cases (PANTO and DAVIES 1986). Similar features may also be observed with extravasation of high-osmolar contrast agents.

Extravasated gadolinium contrast media are better tolerated than conventional ionic radiographic contrast media and produce a zone of signal void on short relaxation time MR images because of the high local concentration (CARRIER et al. 1993).

The presence of a trained nurse or physician beside the patient during contrast medium injection would be ideal for early detection, but exposure to ionizing radiation makes such close observation difficult. New devices for detection of extravasation are currently under evaluation. In a study (BIRNBAUM et al. 1999) of 500 patients, an extravasation detection accessory (EDA) had a sensitivity of 100% and a specificity of 98% for detecting clinically relevant extravasation (>10 mL). The device was easy to use, safe, and accurate for the monitoring of intravenous injections for extravasation, and could prove especially useful in high flow rate CT applications. Other devices are currently being evaluated.

15.4
Treatment

There is no consensus about the best approach for the management of extravasation (COHAN et al. 1996; FEDERLE et al. 1998; PARK et al. 1993; KATAYAMA et al. 1990; YUCHA et al. 1994). The methods described in the following sections have been used:

15.4.1
Elevation of the Affected Limb

Elevation is often useful to reduce the edema by decreasing the hydrostatic pressure in the capillaries.

15.4.2
Topical Application of Heat Or Cold

Heat produces vasodilatation and thus resorption of extravasated fluid and edema, while cold produces vasoconstriction and limits inflammation. The immediate application of warm compresses reduced the volume of extravasated fluid in healthy volunteers (HASTINGS-TOLSMA et al. 1993). In an experimental study, application of cold compresses was associated with a decrease in the size of skin ulcers produced by extravasation of iothalamate and diatrizoate (ELAM et al. 1991) No significant difference was found at the injection site in untreated rats, rats treated with warmth, and rats treated with cooling (COHAN et al. 1990a). In patients, cooling can easily be produced with ice packs placed at the injection site for 15-60 min three times a day for 1-3 days or until symptoms resolve.

15.4.3
Prevention of Secondary Infection

Applications of silver sulfadiazine ointment are recommended by many plastic surgeons if blistering is evident (HECKLER 1989).

15.4.4
Hyaluronidase and other Drugs

Local subcutaneous injection of hyaluronidase, which breaks down connective tissue, has frequently been used in patients with large extravasation of high- or low-osmolality contrast medium and of chemotherapeutic agents (LAURIE et al. 1984). It should be administered within 1 h of the extravasation. Dose recommendation is variable, and efficacy has not been convincingly shown. Some animal and clinical studies suggest a beneficial effect (COHAN et al. 1996; HECKLER 1989; LAURIE et al. 1984), while McALISTER and PALMER (1971) reported a deleterious effect.

Corticosteroids, vasodilators, and a variety of other agents have been proposed for treating extravasation, but most studies failed to demonstrate any value of these agents or did not evaluate extravasation of contrast media.

15.4.5
Surgery

Most plastic surgeons believe that the majority of extravasation injuries heal without surgery and recommend a conservative policy (COHAN et al. 1990a). Surgical drainage or emergency suction applied within 6 h can be effective (LOTH and JONES 1988) and the use of emergency suction alone or combined with saline flushing has also been helpful (GAULT 1993; VANDEWEYER et al. 2000).

15.4.6
Aspiration of Fluid from the Extravasation Site

Aspiration of fluid from the extravasation site is controversial, as it usually removes only a small amount of extravasated fluid and carries a risk of infection.

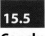

15.5
Conclusion

Extravasation of contrast material is a frequent complication of enhanced imaging studies and large volume extravasation may result in severe damage. Early identification is important and conservative management is effective in most cases. A guideline can be found in Chap. 29.

References

Ayre-Smith G (1982) Tissue necrosis following extravasation of contrast media. J Can Assoc Radiol 33:104

Benson LS, Sathy MJ, Port RB (1996) Forearm compartment syndrome due to automated injection of computed tomography contrast material. J Orthop Trauma 10:433–436

Birnbaum BA, Nelson RC, Chezmar JL, Glick SN (1999) Extravasation detection accessory: clinical evaluation in 500 patients. Radiology 212:431–438

Carrier DA, Ford JJ, Hayman LA (1993) MR appearance of extravasated gadolinium contrast medium. AJNR 14:363–364

Cochran ST, Bomyea K, Sayre JW (2001) Trends in adverse events after IV administration of contrast media. AJR 176:1385–1388

Cohan RH, Dunnick NR, Leder RA, Baker ME (1990a) Extravasation of nonionic contrast media: efficacy of conservative treatment. Radiology 174:65–67

Cohan RH, Leder RA, Bolick D, et al (1990b) Extravascular extravasation of radiographic contrast media: effects of conventional and low-osmolar contrast agents in the rat thigh. Invest Radiol 25:504–510

Cohan RH, Leder RA, Herzberg AJ, et al (1991) Extravascular toxicity of two magnetic resonance contrast agents: preliminary experience in the rat. Invest Radiol 26:224–226

Cohan RH, Ellis JH, Garner WL (1996) Extravasation of radiographic contrast material: recognition, prevention, and treatment. Radiology 200:593–604

Cohan RH, Bullard MA, Ellis JH, Jan SC et al (1997) Local reactions after injection of iodinated contrast material: detection, management, and outcome. Acad Radiol 4:711–718

Elam EA, Dorr RT, Lagel KE, Pond GD (1991) Cutaneous ulceration due to contrast extravasation: experimental assessment of injury and potential antidotes. Invest Radiol 26:13–16

Federle MP, Chang PJ, Confer S, Ozgun B (1998) Frequency and effects of extravasation of ionic and nonionic CT contrast media during rapid bolus injection. Radiology 206:637–640

Gault DT (1993) Extravasation injuries. Br J Plast Surg 46:91–96

Gothlin J (1972) The comparative frequency of extravasal injection at phlebography with steel and plastic cannulas. Clin Radiol 23:183–184

Hastings-Tolsma TM, Yucha CB, Tompkins J, Robson L, Szeverenyi N (1993) Effect of warm and cold applications on the resolution of IV infiltrations. Res Nurs Health 16:171–178

Heckler FR (1989) Current thoughts on extravasation injuries. Clin Plast Surg 16:557–563

Jacobs JE, Birnbaum BA, Langlotz CP (1998) Contrast media reactions and extravasation: relationship to intravenous injection rates. Radiology 209:411–416

Kaste SC, Young CW (1996) Safe use of power injectors with central and peripheral venous access devices for pediatric CT. Pediatr Radiol 26:499–501

Katayama H, Yamaguchi K, Kozuka T, Takashima T, Seez P, Mattsuura K (1990). Adverse reactions to ionic and nonionic contrast media: a report from the Japanese Committee on the Safety of Contrast Media. Radiology 175:621–628

Kim SH, Park JH, Kim YI, Kim CW, Han MC (1990) Experimental tissue damage after subcutaneous injection of water-soluble contrast media. Invest Radiol 25:678–685

Laurie WS, Wilson L, Kernahan A, Bauer S, Vistnes DLM (1984) Intravenous extravasation injuries: the effectiveness of hyaluronidase in their treatment. Ann Plast Surg 13:191–194

Loth TS, Jones DEC (1988) Extravasations of radiographic contrast material in the upper extremity. J Hand Surg 13:395–398

McAlister WH, Palmer K (1971) The histologic effects of four commonly used contrast media for excretory urography and an attempt to modify the responses. Radiology 99:511–516

McCullogh M, Davies P, Richardson R (1989) A large trial of intravenous Conray 325 and Niopam 300 to assess immediate and delayed reactions. Br J Radiol 62:260–265

Memolo M Dyer R, Zagoria RJ (1993) Extravasation injury with nonionic contrast material. AJR 160:203

Miles SG, Rasmussen JF, Litwiller T (1990) Safe use of an intravenous power injector for CT: experience and protocol. Radiology 176:69–70

Panto PN, Davies P (1986) Delayed reactions to urographic contrast media. Br J Radiol 59:41–44

Park KS, Kim SH, Park JH, Han MC, Kim DY, Kim SJ (1993) Methods for mitigating soft-tissue injury after subcutaneous injection of water-soluble contrast media. Invest Radiol 28:332–334

Pond GD, Dorr RT (1993) Extravasation injury with nonionic contrast material. AJR 160:203–204

Pond GD, Dorr RT, McAleese KA (1992) Skin ulceration from extravasation of low-osmolar contrast medium: a complication of automation. AJR 158:915–916

Runge VM, Dickey KM, Williams NM, Peng X (2002) Local tissue toxicity in response to extravascular extravasation of magnetic resonance contrast media. Invest Radiol 37:393–398

Shedadi WH (1975) Adverse reactions to intra-vascularly administered contrast media: a comprehensive study based on a prospective survey. Radiology 124:145–152

Sistrom CL, Gay SB, Peffley L (1991) Extravasation of iopamidol and iohexol during contrast-enhanced CT: report of 28 cases. Radiology 176:65–67

Upton J, Mulliken JB, Murray JE (1979) Major intravenous extravasation injuries. Am J Surg 137:497–506

Vandeweyer E, Heymans O, Deraemaecker R (2000) Extravasation injuries and emergency suction as treatment. Plast Reconstr Surg 105:109–110

Wang C, Cohan RH, Ellis JH, Adusumilli S, Dunnick NR (2007) Frequency, management, and outcome of extravasation of nonionic iodinated contrast medium in 69 657 intravenous injections. Radiology 243:80–87

Young RA (1994) Injury due to extravasation of nonionic contrast material (letter). AJR 162:1499

Yucha CB, Hastings-Tolsma TM, Szeverenyi N (1994) Effect of elevation on intravenous extravasations. J Intraven Nurs 17:231–234

Iodinated Contrast Media

Late Adverse Reactions

16

Fulvio Stacul

CONTENTS

16.1
Introduction

Late adverse reactions to intravascular iodinated contrast media are defined as reactions occurring between 1 h and 1 week after contrast medium injection. They were first recognized in the mid-1980s (PANTO and DAVIES 1986) and since then have been widely studied, particularly the reactions to low osmolality contrast media. However, many aspects remain controversial and there is widespread uncertainty among radiologists about the incidence, significance and management of late reactions.

16.2
Reaction Type and Severity

In reports of late reactions, the symptoms most commonly described are headache, skin rash, itching, nausea, dizziness, urticaria, fever, arm pain and gastrointestinal disturbances. When late reactions to enhanced and unenhanced CT were compared, only skin reactions occurred more frequently in the group who received contrast medium (nonionic monomer or dimer) (SCHILD 1996; SCHILD et al. 2006; YASUDA and MUNECHIKA 1998) and skin reactions appear to account for the majority of true late reactions. The types of late skin reactions and their relative frequencies are similar to those which occur with many other drugs (BIGBY et al. 1986). Maculopapular rash is observed in more than 50% of the affected patients (HOSOYA et al. 2000). Other frequently occurring skin reactions are angioedema, urticaria, erythema, macular exanthema and scaling skin eruption (BIGBY et al. 1986; CHRISTIANSEN et al. 2000; KANNY et al. 2005; RYDBERG et al. 1998; SUTTON et al. 2001, 2003; VERNASSIERE et al. 2004). Lesser-known delayed skin reactions have been discussed by BÖHM and SCHILD (2006).

In most cases, skin reactions are mild or moderate, i.e. they may cause discomfort and may require specific treatment (steroids, antihistamines, topical emollients) (HOSOYA et al. 2000; MUNECHIKA et al. 2003; RYDBERG et al. 1998; SUTTON et al. 2001, 2003). Depending on their site, these reactions cause some disturbance to the patient, the most troublesome being those affecting the palms, soles of the feet or face (SUTTON et al. 2001). Severe delayed reactions needing hospital treatment and/or leading to persistent disability or death have been reported, but are very rare. In the eight cases CHRISTIANSEN et al. (2000) collected from the literature, four had underlying serious

FULVIO STACUL
Dept. of Radiology, Ospedale Maggiore, 34134 Trieste, Italy

medical conditions (GOODFELLOW et al. 1986; REYNOLDS et al. 1993; SADI et al. 1995; SAVILL et al. 1988) and there are only a few other case reports of serious reactions (ATASOY et al. 2003; CONROY et al. 1994; LAFITTE et al. 2004; ROSADO et al. 2001; VAVRICKA et al. 2002).

A number of pathophysiological mechanisms have been proposed for late skin reactions. Although the pathogenesis is still not fully understood, it appears that many are type IV hypersensitivity reactions, i.e. they are T-cell mediated (BROCKOW et al. 2005; CHRISTIANSEN et al. 2000; CHRISTIANSEN 2002; KANNY et al. 2005). The skin reactions often show typical features of late hypersensitivity, including exanthematous rash, positive skin tests and lymphocyte rich dermal perivascular infiltrate, sometimes accompanied by eosinophils on skin biopsy.

If there is doubt about whether contrast medium is responsible for the skin reaction, skin testing (patch and delayed intradermal tests) may be attempted (AKIYAMA et al. 1998; BÖHM and SCHILD 2006; BROCKOW et al. 1999, 2005; COURVOISIER and BIRCHER 1998; GALL et al. 1999; KANNY et al. 2001, 2005; SCHICK et al. 1996; SEDANO et al. 2001; WATANABE et al. 1999). However, the low negative predictive value of such tests should be borne in mind (BROCKOW et al. 2005; VERNASSIERE et al. 2004). Moreover, it remains to be established if skin testing is also a suitable tool for selection of an alternative contrast medium (BROCKOW et al. 2005). Unfortunately, cross-sensitivity to different contrast media is frequent and occurs among ionic and nonionic, and monomeric and dimeric agents (KANNY et al. 2005).

16.3

Frequency

Determining the true frequency of late adverse reactions to contrast media from the literature is difficult. First, a variety of different methodologies have been used, with different methods of data collection (questionnaires, patient interviews in person or by phone), different starting points (at a variety of times from 30 min after contrast medium injection) and different data collection periods (from 1 to 7 days).

A further problem is the fact that the greater the time interval between the contrast medium injection and the onset of symptoms, the more difficult it is to be sure that the symptoms are contrast medium induced. This has been highlighted by the studies on "background noise" by several investigators who have shown a high incidence of late symptoms after radiological investigations not using contrast medium. In one study, late adverse reactions occurred in 12.4% of patients who had contrast medium enhanced CT, and in 10.3% who had unenhanced CT (YASUDA and MUNECHIKA 1998), and in another study approximately 50% of late adverse reactions were found to be unrelated to contrast media (BEYER-ENKE and ZEITLER 1993). UEDA et al. (2001) reported late reactions in 8.4% of patients having enhanced CT, and in 7.9% having plain CT. SCHILD (1996) reported more late adverse reactions following plain CT than enhanced CT, with the exception of skin reactions which were more common after enhanced CT. More recently, SCHILD et al. (2006) considered 895 patients who underwent CT following the injection of a dimeric agent, following injection of a monomeric agent or without contrast material injection. They found that the overall rates of delayed reactions were comparable in all the three study groups (53.1, 50.8, and 48.4%, respectively), and again skin reactions were more common after enhanced CT.

The frequency of late adverse reactions to nonionic monomers has been reported to be between 0.52 and 50.8% (BARTOLUCCI et al. 2000; CHOYKE et al. 1992; COCHRAN et al. 1993; HIGASHI and KATAYAMA 1990; HOSOYA et al. 2000; MIKKONEN et al. 1995; MUNECHIKA et al. 2003; PEDERSEN et al. 1998; RYDBERG et al. 1998; SCHILD et al. 2006; UEDA et al. 2001; YASUDA and MUNECHIKA 1998; YOSHIKAWA 1992). Several studies suggest that the incidence in the 1- to 24-h period is 4% or less (BEYER-ENKE and ZEITLER 1993; CHOYKE et al. 1992; PEDERSEN et al. 1998) and in four large studies the frequency of late skin reactions was 1–3% over a period of 7 days (HOSOYA et al. 2000; MUNECHIKA et al. 1999; RYDBERG et al. 1998; YASUDA and MUNECHIKA 1998). There do not appear to be significant differences in the incidence of late reactions between ionic and nonionic agents (MCCULLOUGH et al. 1989; PANTO and DAVIES 1986; PEDERSEN et al. 1998; YAMAGUCHI et al. 1992), nor between the different nonionic monomers (PANTO and DAVIES 1986; PEDERSEN et al. 1998; YAMAGUCHI et al. 1992). No significant differences have been found between the nonionic monomers and the ionic dimer ioxaglate either (BERTRAND et al. 1995; MIKKONEN et al. 1995; OI et al. 1997).

The available evidence suggests that late skin reactions are more common with nonionic dimers. In two studies conducted by the same group, the nonionic dimer iodixanol caused more late skin reactions than either the ionic dimer ioxaglate or the nonionic monomers iopamidol and iomeprol (SUTTON et al. 2001, 2003). SCHILD et al. (2006) did not find significant difference in the overall incidence of delayed reactions between the nonionic dimer iotrolan and the nonionic monomer iopromide, but they found a higher incidence of cutaneous symptoms (itching or skin rash) in the dimeric group. In another study, the frequency of late skin reactions with iodixanol was similar to that with nonionic monomer, but more of the iodixanol patients were treated with hydrocortisone or antihistamine (RYDBERG et al. 1998). FRANSSON et al. (1996), however, found no difference in the frequency of late skin reactions between iodixanol and ioxaglate. The nonionic dimer iotrolan was withdrawn in 1995 because of the high incidence of late reactions, particularly skin reactions, initially reported from Japan but subsequently also from the USA (HOSOYA et al. 2000; NIENDORF 1996).

16.4
Reaction Onset and Duration

Late skin reactions after contrast medium develop within 1–7 days, with the majority occurring within the first 3 days (HOSOYA et al. 2000). Most reactions are self-limiting and resolve by 7 days, with up to three-quarters resolving within 3 days (HOSOYA et al. 2000; YOSHIKAWA 1992).

16.5
Predisposing Factors

A number of factors appear to predispose a person to the development of late adverse reactions. A previous reaction to contrast medium is an important predisposing factor, increasing the risk by a factor of 1.7–3.3 (HOSOYA et al. 2000; MIKKONEN et al. 1995; YOSHIKAWA 1992). However, there is no evidence that patients with a previous late reaction are at increased risk for a subsequent immediate anaphylactic reaction (HOSOYA et al. 2000; YAMAGUGHI et al. 1992; YOSHIKAWA 1992). A history of allergy is a further risk factor (HIGASHI and KATAYAMA 1990; HOSOYA et al. 2000; MUNECHIKA et al. 1999, 2003; OI et al. 1997; SCHILD et al. 2006; YOSHIKAWA 1992), increasing the likelihood of a reaction approximately two-fold. A history of drug and contact allergy especially seems to predispose to late skin reactions after contrast medium exposure (AOKI and TAKEMURA 2002; KANNY et al. 2005; VERNASSIERE et al. 2004). A seasonal variation in the incidence of late skin reactions has been described with 45% of the reactions occurring in the period April to June in Finland (MIKKONEN et al. 2000). A relation to the pollen season and/or to the possible photosensitizing effect of contrast media has been postulated. A significantly higher incidence of late adverse reactions during the pollen season was confirmed by MUNECHIKA et al. (2003). Females are more likely to develop late adverse reactions than males (BARTOLUCCI et al. 2000; HIGASHI and KATAYAMA 1990; HOSOYA et al. 2000; MIKKONEN et al. 1995; OI et al. 1997; SCHILD et al. 2006). Coexisting diseases also appear to predispose to late reactions, especially renal disease, but also cardiac and liver disease and diabetes mellitus (BARTOLUCCI et al. 2000; HOSOYA et al. 2000; MIKKONEN et al. 1995). Some of the most severe skin reactions reported occurred in patients with systemic lupus erythematosus or in patients who were taking hydralazine, which induces a lupus-like syndrome in some patients (GOODFELLOW et al. 1986; REYNOLDS et al. 1993; SAVILL et al. 1988). Bone marrow transplantation patients were reported to be another risk group for severe contrast medium induced skin eruptions (VAVRICKA et al. 2002).

The increased incidence of late reactions to contrast media in patients who have received interleukin-2 (IL-2) immunotherapy is well documented, with an increased frequency of two to four times (CHOYKE et al. 1992; FISHMAN et al. 1991; OLDHAM et al. 1990; SHULMAN et al. 1993; ZUKIWSKI et al. 1990). Skin rash, pruritus and flu-like syndrome were all more frequent in patients who had received IL-2 (CHOYKE et al. 1992).

16.6
Prophylaxis

In view of the infrequent and self-limiting nature of the great majority of late reactions, it does not seem appropriate to warn patients with no special risk factors about the possibility of a late reaction. However, it is recommended that patients who have had a previous late skin reaction after contrast medium administration, who suffer from major drug or contact allergy or who have received interleukin-2 are warned about the possibility of a late skin reaction and told to contact a physician if they have a problem.

If patients who have previously had a late skin reaction to iodinated contrast medium require further contrast medium, it is recommended that an alternative contrast medium is chosen and steroid prophylaxis is given (WATANABE et al. 1999). However, because of frequent cross-reactivity among different contrast media, change of contrast agent is no guarantee against a repeat reaction (BROCKOW et al. 2005).

Conclusion

Late adverse reactions to iodinated contrast media have been recognized for 20 years. They are mainly mild or moderate skin reactions which develop from 1 h to 7 days after contrast medium administration and usually resolve within 3–7 days. The majority of these cutaneous reactions are T-cell mediated allergic reactions. A simple guideline was produced by the ESUR Contrast Media Safety Committee (WEBB et al. 2003) and can be found in Chap. 29.

References

Akiyama M, Nakada T, Sueki H et al (1998) Drug eruption caused by nonionic iodinated X-ray contrast media. Acad Radiol 5(Suppl 1):S159–S161

Aoki Y, Takemura T (2002) Allergies correlated to adverse reactions induced by nonionic monomeric and ionic dimeric contrast media for contrast enhanced CT examination. Radiol Technol 58:1245–1251

Atasoy M, Erdem T, Sari RF (2003) A case of acute generalized exanthematous pustulosis (AGEP) possibly induced by iohexol. J Dermatol 30:723–726

Bartolucci F, Cecarini M, Gabrielli G et al (2000) Reazioni tardive a un mezzo di contrasto radiologico (iopamidolo–Bracco). Radiol Med 100:273–278

Bertrand P, Delhommais A, Alison D, Rouleau P (1995) Immediate and delayed tolerance of iohexol and ioxaglate in lower limb phlebography: a double-blind comparative study in humans. Acad Radiol 2:683–686

Beyer-Enke SA, Zeitler E (1993) Late adverse reactions to nonionic contrast media: a cohort analytic study. Eur Radiol 3:237–241

Bigby M, Jick S, Jick H, Arndt K (1986) Drug induced cutaneous reactions. A report from the Boston Collaborative Drug Surveillance Program on 15,438 consecutive inpatients, 1975–1982. JAMA 256:3358–3363

Böhm I, Schild HH (2006) A practical guide to diagnose lesser-known immediate and delayed contrast media-induced adverse cutaneous reactions. Eur Radiol 16:1570–1579

Brockow E, Becker EW, Worret W-I, Ring J (1999) Late skin test reactions to radiocontrast medium. J Allergy Clin Immunol 104:1107–1108

Brockow K, Christiansen C, Kanny G et al (2005) Management of hypersensitivity reactions to iodinated contrast media. Allergy 60:150–158

Choyke PL, Miller DL, Lotze MT et al (1992) Delayed reactions to contrast media after Interleukin-2 immunotherapy. Radiology 183:111–114

Christiansen C (2002) Late-onset allergy-like reactions to X-ray contrast media. Curr Opin Allergy Clin Immunol 2:333–339

Christiansen C, Pichler WJ, Skotland T (2000) Delayed allergy-like reactions to X-ray contrast media: mechanistic considerations. Eur Radiol 10:1965–1975

Cochran ST, Cugley AL, Kiourmehr F (1993) Delayed reactions in patients receiving nonionic contrast media. Adv X-Ray Contrast 1:61–62

Conroy RM, Bjartveit K, Sheppick A et al (1994) Iodixanol in intravenous urography: a comparison of iodixanol 270 mg I/ml, iodixanol 320 mg I/ml and iopamidol 300 mg I/ml (NIOPAM). Clin Radiol 49:337–340

Courvoisier S, Bircher AJ (1998) Delayed-type hypersensitivity to a nonionic, radiopaque contrast medium. Allergy 53: 1221–1224

Fishman JE, Aberle DR, Moldawer NP et al (1991) Atypical contrast reactions associated with systemic interleukin-2 therapy. Am J Roentgenol 156:833–834

Fransson SG, Stenport G, Andersson M (1996) Immediate and late adverse reactions in coronary angiography. A comparison between iodixanol and ioxaglate. Acta Radiol 37:218–222

Gall H, Pillekamp H, Peter R-U (1999) Late-type allergy to the X-ray contrast medium Solutrast (iopamidol). Contact Dermatitis 40:248–250

Goodfellow T, Holdstock GE, Brunton FJ, Bamforth J (1986) Fatal acute vasculitis after high-dose urography with iohexol. Br J Radiol 59:620–621

Higashi TS, Katayama M (1990) The delayed adverse reactions of low osmolar contrast media. Nippon Igaku Hoshasen Gakkai Zasshi – Nippon Acta Radiol 50:1359–1366

Hosoya T, Yamaguchi K, Akutzu T et al (2000) Delayed adverse reactions to iodinated contrast media and their risk factors. Radiat Med 18:39–45

Kanny G, Marie B, Hoen B et al (2001) Delayed adverse reaction to sodium ioxaglic acid-meglumine. Eur J Dermatol 11:134–137

Kanny G, Pichler WJ, Morisset M et al (2005) T cell-mediated reactions to iodinated contrast media: evaluation by skin and lymphocyte activation tests. J Allergy Clin Immunol 115:179–185

Laffitte E, Nevadov Beck M, Hofer M et al (2004) Severe Stevens-Johnson syndrome induced by contrast medium iopentol (Imagopaque). Br J Dermatol 150:376–378

McCullough M, Davies P, Richardson R (1989) A large trial of intravenous Conray 325 and Niopam 300 to assess immediate and delayed reactions. Br J Radiol 62:260–265

Mikkonen R, Kontkann T, Kivisaari L (1995) Acute and late adverse reactions to low-osmolal contrast media. Acta Radiol 36:72–76

Mikkonen R, Vehmas T, Granlund H, Kivisaari L (2000) Seasonal variation in the occurrence of late adverse skin reactions to iodine-based contrast media. Acta Radiol 41:390–393

Munechika H, Hiramatsu M, Nakamura H et al (1999) Large-scale study of delayed adverse events to nonionic contrast medium, iohexol: incidence and risk factors of adverse events following non-interventional radiography. Eur Radiol 9(Suppl 1):S440

Munechika H, Hiramatsu Y, Kudo S et al (2003) A prospective survey of delayed adverse reactions to iohexol in urography and computed tomography. Eur Radiol 13:185–194

Niendorf HP (1996) Delayed allergy-like reactions to X-ray contrast media. Problem statement exemplified with iotrolan (Isovist) 280. Eur Radiol 6 [Suppl 3]:S8–S10

Oi H, Yamazaki H, Matsushita M (1997) Delayed vs. immediate adverse reactions to ionic and nonionic low-osmolality contrast media. Radiat Med 15:23–27

Oldham RK, Brogley J, Braud E (1990) Contrast medium "recalls" interleukin-2 toxicity. J Clin Oncol 8:942–943

Panto PN, Davies P (1986) Delayed reactions to urographic contrast media. Br J Radiol 59:41–44

Pedersen SH, Svaland MG, Reiss A-L, Andrew E (1998) Late allergy-like reactions following vascular administration of radiography contrast media. Acta Radiol 39:344–348

Reynolds NJ, Wallington TB, Burton JL (1993) Hydralazine predisposes to acute cutaneous vasculitis following urography with iopamidol. Br J Dermatol 129:82–85

Rosado A, Canto G, Veleiro B, Rodriguez J (2001) Toxic epidermal necrolysis after repeated injections of iohexol. Am J Roentgenol 176:262–263

Rydberg J, Charles J, Aspelin P (1998) Frequency of late allergy-like adverse reactions following injection of intravascular nonionic contrast media. A retrospective study comparing a nonionic monomeric contrast medium with a nonionic dimeric contrast medium. Acta Radiol 39:219–222

Sadi AM, Toda T, Kiyuna M et al (1995) An autopsy case of malignant lymphoma with Lyell's syndrome. J Dermatol 22:594–599

Savill JS, Barrie R, Ghosh S et al (1988) Fatal Stevens-Johnson syndrome following urography with iopamidol in systemic lupus erythematosus. Postgrad Med J 64:392–394

Schick E, Weber L, Gall H (1996) Delayed hypersensitivity reaction to the nonionic contrast medium iopromide. Contact Dermatitis 35:312

Schild HH (1996) Delayed allergy-like reactions in patients: monomeric and dimeric contrast media compared with plain CT. Eur Radiol 6 (Insert to Issue 5: Delayed allergy-like reactions to X-ray contrast media):9–10

Schild HH, Kuhl CK, Hübner-Steiner U et al (2006) Adverse events after unhenhanced and monomeric and dimeric contrast-enhanced CT: a prospective randomized controlled trial. Radiology 240: 56–64

Sedano E, Vega JM, Rebollo S et al (2001) Delayed exanthema to nonionic contrast medium. Allergy 56:1015–1016

Shulman KL, Thompson JA, Benyunes MC et al (1993) Adverse reactions to intravenous contrast media in patients treated with interleukin-2. J Immunother 13:208–212

Sutton AGC, Finn P, Grech ED et al (2001) Early and late reactions after the use of iopamidol 340, ioxaglate 320 and iodixanol 320 in cardiac catheterization. Am Heart J 141:677–683

Sutton AGC, Finn P, Campbell PG et al (2003) Early and late reactions following the use of iopamidol 340, iomeprol 350 and iodixanol 320 in cardiac catheterization. J Invas Cardiol 15:133–138

Ueda S, Mori H, Matsumoto S et al (2001) True delayed adverse reactions to nonionic contrast media: does it really exist? Eur Radiol 11(Suppl 1):377

Vavricka SR, Halter J, Furrer K et al (2002) Contrast media triggering cutaneous graft-versus-host disease. Bone Marrow Transplant 29:899–901

Vernassiere C, Trechot P, Commun N et al (2004) Low negative predictive value of skin tests in investigating delayed reactions to radio-contrast media. Contact Dermatitis 50:359–366

Watanabe H, Sueki H, Nakada T et al (1999) Multiple fixed drug eruption caused by iomeprol (Iomeron), a nonionic contrast medium. Dermatology 198:291–294

Webb JAW, Stacul F, Thomsen HS et al (2003) Late adverse reactions to intravascular iodinated contrast media. Eur Radiol 13:181–184

Yamaguchi K, Takanashi I, Kanauchi T et al (1992) A retrospective survey of delayed adverse reactions to ionic and nonionic contrast media. Nippon Igaku Hoshasen Gakkai Zasshi – Nippon Acta Radiol 52:1565–1570

Yasuda R, Munechika H (1998) Delayed adverse reactions to nonionic monomeric contrast-enhanced media. Invest Radiol 33:1–5

Yoshikawa H (1992) Late adverse reactions to nonionic contrast media. Radiology 183:737–740

Zukiwski AA, David CL, Coan J et al (1990) Increased incidence of hypersensitivity to iodine-containing radiographic contrast media after interleukin-2 administration. Cancer 65:1521–1524

Peter Aspelin, Fulvio Stacul, and Sameh K. Morcos

CONTENTS

Peter Aspelin
Division of Radiology, Center for Surgical Sciences,
Karolinska Institute, Huddinge University Hospital,
14186 Stockholm, Sweden
Fulvio Stacul
Institute of Radiology, Ospedale di Cattinara,
34149 Trieste, Italy
Sameh K. Morcos
Department of Diagnostic Imaging, Northern General
Hospital, Sheffield Teaching Hospitals NHS Trust,
Sheffield S5 7AU, UK

17.1
Introduction

Iodinated contrast media are widely used either to visualize blood vessels (angiography) or to enhance the density of the parenchyma of different organs. In both instances, they are administered intravascularly and ideally their effects on blood and endothelium should be minimal. However, all contrast media have some effects on the endothelium, blood, and its constituents. There is a vast literature on these effects both in vitro and in vivo. The present chapter summarizes the effects from a clinical perspective in order to clarify whether there are important differences between the types of iodinated contrast media in current clinical use.

Iodinated contrast media may be either ionic or nonionic and they all produce various effects on blood components. These effects are thought to be caused by the chemical nature of contrast media, their electrical charge, and by the viscosity and the osmolality of the solution in which they are given. Different contrast media have varying effects on the many components of the blood.

The hematologic effects of iodinated contrast media have been divided into the following categories: red blood cells, white blood cells, endothelium, platelets, coagulation, and fibrinolysis.

17.2
Red Blood Cells

The effect of contrast media on red blood cells can be divided into the effects on morphology, aggregation, and rheology (flow properties of the blood). When iodinated contrast media come into contact with red blood cells, the normal discoid shape of the red blood cells changes (ASPELIN et al. 1980; NASH and MEISELMAN 1991). Two changes caused by extraction of water may occur: either shrinkage of the red blood cells producing a dessicocyte, or changes in shape called echinocyte or stomatocyte deformation.

17.2.1
Red Cell Morphology

Dessicocyte formation is an in vitro effect of dehydration of the red blood cell and is proportional to the osmolality of the contrast media to which it is exposed (ASPELIN et al. 1980). It is observed only in a fraction of red blood cells if exposed to almost undiluted high-osmolar contrast medium.

Echinocyte formation in vitro is dependent on the chemotoxicity (including electrical charge, pH, or salt concentration) (CHRONOS et al. 1993) and not on the osmolality of the contrast agent. All contrast media including the iso-osmolar dimers may induce some degree of echinocyte formation (HARDEMAN et al. 1991; ASPELIN et al. 1987).

17.2.2
Red Blood Cell Aggregation

Contrast media in vitro cause disaggregation of red blood cell rouleaux and not aggregation as sometimes believed (ASPELIN et al. 1987). The reason for the misunderstanding could be that contrast media make red cells more rigid causing precapillary stasis, which can be mistaken for increased red blood cell aggregation (ASPELIN and SCHMID-SCHÖNBEIN 1978; ASPELIN 1992).

17.2.3
Blood Rheology

The combined effect of the dessicocyte, echinocyte, and stomatocyte is reduced plasticity of the red blood cells as compared with normal red blood cells (ASPELIN and SCHMID-SCHÖNBEIN 1978; ASPELIN 1992; LOSCO et al. 2001). Plasticity is essential for the smooth flow of red blood cells through small capillaries and when it is lost there is a decrease in blood flow especially after intra-arterial injections (DAWSON et al. 1983; LE MIGNON et al. 1988; STRICKLAND et al. 1992b; PUGH 1996). Pure echinocyte and stomatocyte formation without any dehydration of red blood cells produces only minor rheological change (ASPELIN et al. 1980; NASH and MEISELMAN 1991). However, the overall in vivo effect is a mixture of the effect of contrast media on red blood cell morphology, rigidity, viscosity, and vascular tone. Contrast media can induce both vasoconstriction and vasodilatation in different organs (MORCOS et al. 1998; MILLS et al. 1980; ALMÉN et al. 1980; LISS et al. 1996). In the pulmonary circulation, contrast media can induce red cell rigidity and pulmonary arterial vasoconstriction, leading to an increase in pulmonary vascular resistance (PUGH 1996; MORCOS et al. 1998; MILLS et al. 1980; ALMÉN et al. 1980). In the kidney, contrast media can reduce the blood flow in the vasa recta in the medulla (LISS et al. 1996). It is not clear whether this effect is mainly caused by stasis due to vasoconstriction or by increased red blood cell aggregation in vivo. The morphological red cell changes may also affect the capacity for oxygen delivery and pH buffering (GALTUNG et al. 2002). However, these effects have not been proven to be of importance in clinical studies (STRICKLAND et al. 1992a).

The overall effect of contrast media on red blood cells has not been shown to be of clinical importance.

17.3
White Blood Cells

The function of the white blood cells is mainly host defense, but their interactions with the endothelial cells and platelets are also important. White blood cells must be able to adhere to the endothelium and migrate through the vessel wall in order to phagocytize and inactivate toxic products. This involves adherence, chemotaxis, degranulation, and phagocytosis. In vitro studies have shown that all these processes are affected by contrast media.

17.3.1
Phagocytosis

Contrast media reduce the ability of white blood cells to exhibit phagocytosis (RASMUSSEN et al. 1988, 1992b; RASMUSSEN 1998). This effect has been studied only with ionic, high-osmolar contrast media. It may also be caused by calcium chelating agents in the solution. The clinical importance of these in vitro observations is not known.

17.3.2
Chemotaxis, Granulocyte Adherence, and Inflammation

Contrast media have been shown in vitro to inhibit the chemotoxic response of white blood cells. In vivo studies have not shown this finding to be significant (RASMUSSEN et al. 1992c). All contrast media decrease the adherence property of white blood cells (RASMUSSEN et al. 1992a; BARANI et al. 2002; BLANN et al. 2001; ZHAN et al. 1998). Contrast media may interfere with the inflammatory response of white blood cells in the body (HERNANZ-SCHULMAN et al. 2000; FANNING et al. 2002; LASKEY and GELLMAN 2003).

There are no clinical data to suggest that any of these interactions between contrast media and white blood cells are of clinical importance.

17.4
Endothelium

Endothelial cells contribute to the regulation of many aspects of vascular homeostasis, including coagulation, fibrinolysis, and platelet function. In addition, they are important modulators of vascular tone, primarily by the regulated secretion and rapid clearance of powerful vasoactive mediators such as prostacyclin, nitric oxide, endothelin, and adenosine. The endothelium also controls solute permeability and leukocyte movement during the generation of inflammatory and immune responses (PEARSON 1991).

Endothelial cells are exposed transiently to high concentrations of contrast media following intravascular administration. The endothelial effects of contrast media may contribute to the hemodynamic disturbances, thrombosis, and pulmonary edema associated with the intravascular use of these agents.

Modulation of the production of endothelial vasoactive substances plays an important role in mediating the hemodynamic effects of contrast media particularly in the kidney (MORCOS 1998). Contrast media can increase the release and expression of the potent vasoconstrictor peptide endothelin by the endothelial cells (OLDROYD and MORCOS 2000). In addition, contrast media may decrease the endothelial production of nitric oxide by reducing the activity of the enzyme nitric oxide synthase which is responsible for the endogenous synthesis of this vasodilator (SCHWARTZ et al. 1994; HEYMAN et al. 1998). How contrast media increase the release of endothelin or reduce the production of nitric oxide is not fully understood.

Contrast media, particularly high-osmolality ionic agents, have cytostatic and cytotoxic effects on endothelial cells which may precipitate thrombosis (BARSTAD et al. 1996; WILSON and SAGE 1994; LAERUM 1983; MORGAN and BETTMANN 1989; FAUSER et al. 2001; GABELMAN et al. 2001; SUMIMURA et al. 2003). In addition, contrast media can induce apoptosis (programmed cell death) of endothelial cells (ZHANG et al. 2000). An increase in the frequency of apoptosis in the endothelium may alter vascular homeostasis including coagulant and thrombotic properties, permeability and tone of the blood vessel wall, as well as vessel growth and angiogenesis (ZHANG et al. 2000).

The biocompatibility of contrast media is influenced both by osmolality and chemical structure, particularly the presence of carboxyl groups in the molecules of the ionic agents. In nonionic media, the absence of carboxyl groups and the presence of many hydroxyl groups that increase hydrophilicity markedly improve biocompatibility and significantly reduce cytotoxicity (HEPTINSTALL et al. 1998; ELOY et al. 1991; LABARTHE et al. 2003; ALBANESE et al. 1995). Ionic contrast media, in particular high-osmolar agents, have greater effects on enzymes and higher affinity to proteins and lipids in comparison to nonionic media, and can induce injury to cell membranes and interfere with cell metabolism (KRAUSE and NIEHUES 1996; DAWSON 1996). In addition, contrast media can penetrate endothelial cells, forming dense granules on the luminal surface and pinocytotic vesicles (NORDBY et al. 1989).

Ionic contrast media may increase vascular endothelial permeability leading to pulmonary edema (MORCOS 2003; FURUTA et al. 2001, 2002; SENDO et al. 2000; TOMINAGA et al. 2001; EMERY et al. 2001). Subclinical pulmonary edema without obvious signs or symptoms of respiratory distress is thought to be common after intravascular use of contrast media but its true incidence is difficult to establish (IDÉE et al. 2002). Pulmonary edema produced by contrast media could also be responsible for the increase in the pulmonary vascular resistance (PVR) caused by these agents (MORCOS 2003). Experimental studies have shown that ioxaglate induced the largest increase in PVR of the isolated rat lung preparation and more marked pulmonary edema compared to other classes of contrast media (FURUTA et al. 2001, 2002; SENDO et al. 2000; TOMINAGA et al. 2001; EMERY et al. 2001). However, these experimental observations have not been confirmed in larger clinical studies (IDÉE et al. 2002).

The endothelial effect of high-osmolar ionic contrast media is of clinical importance in phlebography because of the increased frequency of thrombosis after the procedure.

Platelets

Briefly, platelets adhere to exposed collagen, von Willebrand factor, and fibrinogen at the site of arterial injury (adhesion step). Adherent platelets are then activated by mediators such as thrombin, collagen, adenosine diphosphate (ADP), serotonin, etc. (activation step). Activated platelets degranulate and secrete chemotaxins, clotting factors, and vasoconstrictors, thereby promoting thrombin generation, vasospasm, and additional platelet accumulation (aggregation step) (FERGUSON et al. 2000; BECKER 2001). Therefore, when the interaction of contrast media with platelets is assessed, each step of platelet physiology should be evaluated separately.

17.5.1
Experimental Effects

17.5.1.1
Platelet Adhesion

GRABOWSKI et al. (1991a, b) showed that in vitro platelet adhesion/aggregation was inhibited in the order diatrizoate > ioxaglate > iohexol > saline. However, these effects were rapidly diminished because of hemodilution. In a baboon study (MARKOU et al. 2001), contrast media were found to inhibit platelet deposition on stents in the order ioxaglate > iohexol = iodixanol > saline. Thus, all contrast media inhibit platelet adhesion, with ionic agents being more potent than nonionic ones.

17.5.1.2
Platelet Activation by Thrombin

In vitro platelet activation by thrombin was inhibited by low-osmolar ionic contrast media, whereas nonionic monomeric and dimeric contrast media did not affect it (LI and GABRIEL 1997).

17.5.1.3
Direct Platelet Activation

Direct activation of platelets (i.e., degranulation and release of the procoagulant content of dense bodies and α-granules) was induced in vitro by nonionic monomeric contrast media. Lesser activation was caused by high-osmolar ionic contrast media and there was no activation by low-osmolar ionic and nonionic dimeric contrast media (CHRONOS et al. 1993; COROT et al. 1996). CHRONOS et al. (1993) showed that blood from patients anticoagulated with heparin and pretreated with aspirin in preparation for percutaneous coronary angioplasty (PTCA) showed the same pattern of nonionic monomeric contrast-medium-induced platelet activation as normal subjects.

17.5.1.4
Platelet Aggregation

An inhibitory effect of contrast media on platelet aggregation was first described by ZIR et al. (1974) and has been widely investigated since. Both high- and low-osmolar ionic contrast media inhibit in vitro platelet aggregation (induced by mediators such as thrombin, ADP, or collagen) more than nonionic agents (monomeric or dimeric) (HEPTINSTALL et al. 1998; ELOY et al. 1991). Potentiation of the antithrombotic effects of clopidogrel, an antiaggregant drug, has been found in rats with an ionic low-osmolar contrast medium but not with a nonionic monomer (LABARTHE et al. 2003).

17.5.2
Clinical Pharmacology Studies

Clinical pharmacology studies comparing the different categories of contrast media, however, led to more equivocal conclusions than in vitro or animal studies.

In one study of patients, no significant platelet activation (P-selectin expression) was found following left ventriculography or coronary angiography with iohexol (ALBANESE et al. 1995). Similarly, ARORA et al. (1991) and BRZOKO et al. (1997) did not find a significant difference between ionic and nonionic contrast media when platelet degranulation markers were measured in peripheral venous samples. POLANOWSKA et al. (1992) reported an increase in the venous level of β-thromboglobulin following arteriography with a high-osmolar contrast agent.

Conversely, in another study (JUNG et al. 2002), following cardiac catheterization, no platelet activation was found with ioxaglate, whereas serotonin release was detected following injection of a nonionic monomer. Most of these studies, with the exception of that of ALBANESE et al. (1995), evaluated peripheral venous and not local blood samples. It is known that arterial catheterization itself may activate platelets.

With respect to platelet aggregation, most clinical pharmacology studies have shown a higher antiaggregatory effect for ionic agents than nonionic monomers, as confirmed by DALBY et al. (2002) and ELOY et al. (1991). However, one study did not show a difference between these categories of contrast media (STORMORKEN et al. 1986).

The clinical impact of these in vitro and experimental in vivo changes is debatable and is discussed in the section on coagulation.

In summary, there are no clinical data to suggest that the effect of nonionic contrast media on platelets induces increased coagulation. The mechanisms responsible for the effects of contrast media on platelets are still unclear and clinically significant effects have not been shown.

17.6
Coagulation

17.6.1
In Vitro Effects of Contrast Media

All contrast media inhibit blood coagulation but to different extents. Prothrombin time, reptilase time, activated partial thromboplastin time, and recalcification clotting time are significantly increased in proportion to the dose of the contrast media (ELOY et al. 1991). Comparison of assays of fibropeptide A and thrombin–antithrombin complex between ionic agents (both monomeric and dimeric) and nonionic monomers showed that coagulation times were shorter for nonionic monomers, but were always longer than in the controls (IDÉE et al. 2002; COROT et al. 1989; ENGELHART et al. 1988; GRABOWSKI et al. 1991a, b; PARVEZ and MONCADA 1986; PARVEZ and VIK 1991; RASULI et al. 1989).

The ionic dimer ioxaglate shows an anticoagulant activity similar to that of the ionic monomers (ELOY et al. 1991). In one study, the nonionic dimer iodixanol was found significantly less anticoagulant than the nonionic monomer iohexol (COROT et al. 1996), while in another study it was reported that iodixanol affects the bleeding time similar to nonionic monomers (MELTON et al. 1995). However, the precise mechanisms responsible for this inhibition are still unclear. It has been suggested that the main factors are inhibition of activation of factor X, which leads to the formation of thrombin from prothrombin (ELOY et al. 1991; FAY and PARKER 1998; IDÉE and COROT 1999) and inhibition of fibrin polymerization (STORMORKEN et al. 1986; FAY and PARKER 1998; DAWSON et al. 1986; DAWSON 1999). AL DIERI et al. (2001, 2003) showed that ioxaglate blocks feedback activation of factors V and VIII, significantly inhibits platelet-dependent thrombin generation, and boosts the effect of abciximab, whereas iodixanol does not. Interference with the assembly of fibrin monomers by contrast media results in poor fibrin stabilization of clots (CHRONOS et al. 1993; ENGELHART et al. 1988).

Therefore, ionic monomers and dimers have similar anticoagulant activity in vitro, which is more pronounced than that of nonionic monomers and dimers. Nonionic monomers probably have more anticoagulant effect than nonionic dimers.

17.6.2
Clinical Trials

Clinical data are less easy to evaluate because of patient-related and procedure-related variability (state of the hemostatic system, condition of the vessel wall, use of guidewires, catheters, balloons, stents). Because of the rapid clearance of contrast media, their anticoagulant effect is local rather than systemic and their effect may be not significant if measured in distant peripheral blood vessels.

Following the in vitro observation by ROBERTSON (1987) of more frequent clot formation in blood contaminated syringes with nonionic monomers than with ionic agents, a few case reports of thrombotic complications in diagnostic angiography with nonionic monomers have been published (BASHORE et al. 1988; GROLLMAN et al. 1988; MILLET and SESTIER 1989). However, trials have shown no clinical evidence of significant differences in thrombotic complications when ionic agents are compared to nonionic monomers for coronary angiography (DAVIDSON et al. 1990; SCHRADER 1998).

Randomized trials comparing ioxaglate to nonionic monomers during PTCA have produced conflicting results (PIESSENS et al. 1993; GRINES et al. 1996; ESPLUGAS et al. 1991; MALEKIANPUR et al. 1998; SCHRADER et al. 1999; FLEISCH et al. 1999; DANZI et al. 2003). In the two studies with the largest number of patients, one showed no significant difference between ioxaglate and iomeprol in the incidence of sudden vessel occlusion (SCHRADER et al. 1999), whereas the other showed a trend toward less thromboembolic complications with ioxaglate compared to ioversol (FLEISCH et al. 1999). SCHELLER et al. (2001) reported that patients undergoing stent placement had fewer acute and subacute stent occlusions when imaged using ioxaglate (vs. multiple nonionic agents). However, DANZI et al. (2003) reported that nonionic monomers (iopamidol and iopromide) did not adversely affect stent patency when compared to ioxaglate. The considerable periprocedural use of antiplatelet agents may explain their results. A meta-analysis comparing nonionic monomers to ioxaglate showed a significant reduction of coronary vessel abrupt occlusions with ioxaglate (CUCHERAT and LEIZOROVICZ 1999). Iodixanol was compared to ioxaglate in three trials. In one, no significant differences with regard to major adverse cardiac events (MACE) were detected (BERTRAND et al. 2000). In the second, high-risk patient group, less abrupt vessel occlusions ($p = 0.05$) were found with iodixanol (DAVIDSON et al. 2000). This difference was more significant in patients who did not receive GpIIb/IIIa blockers. In the third, no significant differences between the two media were found and there was no clear advantage with the use of an ionic contrast agent in a large population of patients undergoing percutaneous coronary intervention for both stable and unstable coronary artery disease (SUTTON et al. 2002).

17.6.3
Contrast Media Interactions with Angiographic Devices

Interactions of contrast media with angiographic devices have been investigated both in vitro and in vivo. The syringe material greatly influenced the possibility of clot formation in syringes containing contrast media and blood. Glass was a more powerful activator of coagulation than plastic, and among the plastic syringes those made of styrene acrylonitrile activated coagulation more than those made of polypropylene. Furthermore, clots formed only in situations where there was very poor angiographic technique (DAWSON et al. 1986).

Teflon-coated catheters and guidewires are more thrombogenic than polyurethane materials and much more than polyethylene materials (DAWSON 1999). IDÉE and COROT (1999) comprehensively reviewed the many factors influencing clotting in catheters, including the length of the procedure, blood/catheter contact time, volume of blood in the catheter, size and type of the catheter, type of contrast material, and degree of blood/contrast medium mixture in the catheter. Some of these factors are difficult to control or standardize in clinical studies.

Therefore, catheter and guidewire materials probably play a significant role in clinical studies of contrast media and coagulation. The use of equipment with technically improved surfaces will probably largely overcome this problem.

17.7
Fibrinolysis

Contrast media impede fibrinolysis and delay the onset of lysis by recombinant tissue-type plasminogen activator (rt-PA), urokinase, and streptokinase (DEHMER et al. 1995). This effect is reduced by increasing the concentration of the lysis agent. Contrast media cause fibrin to form in long/thin fibrils, which have a lower mass/length ratio and are more resistant to fibrinolysis (GABRIEL et al. 1991; PARVEZ et al. 1982). In vitro studies have shown that diatrizoate and iohexol delay the onset of lysis induced by all lysis agents. However, ioxaglate delayed the onset of lysis by rt-PA and urokinase but not by streptokinase (DEHMER et al. 1995). Another in vitro study showed that thrombi formed with iodixanol and iohexol are larger and more resistant to thrombolysis when compared to thrombi formed with ioxaglate (JONES and GOODAL 2003). In vivo studies in dogs showed that alteplase-induced thrombolysis could be delayed by iohexol and amidotrizoate, whereas ioxaglate had no significant effect (PISLARU et al. 1998). In a small group of patients undergoing pulmonary angiography, iohexol significantly increased plasma levels of PAI-1, an inhibitor of t-PA and urokinase, while ioxaglate did not (VAN BEEK et al. 1994). Other effects on fibrinolysis caused by interactions of contrast media with concomitantly given drugs are described in more detail in Chap. 20.

Conclusion

All contrast agents may alter the morphology and function of red blood cells. However, the overall effect of contrast media on red cells has not been shown to be of clinical importance. Similarly, the effect on white blood cells has not been shown to be clinically important.

In vitro studies have shown that nonionic monomers cause more activation of platelets than ionic contrast media. Iso-osmolar dimeric contrast media have not been shown to activate platelet function. Clinical studies have not confirmed these in vitro observations.

Contrast media have cytostatic, cytotoxic, and apoptotic effects on endothelial cells. These effects are more evident with ionic contrast media, in particular high-osmolar agents, than with nonionic media. Contrast media-induced endothelial injury may play a role in the pathophysiology of the effects of contrast media. These include hemodynamic effects, thrombosis, and contrast media-induced pulmonary edema.

The risk of thrombosis induced by contrast media relates to the combined effect on platelets, endothelial cells, and coagulation factors. In clinical practice, high-osmolar contrast media can induce thrombosis after intravenous injection, mainly because of endothelial injury produced by high osmolality. This effect is less with nonionic low-osmolar and iso-osmolar contrast media.

All contrast media have anticoagulant properties, and ionic media are more anticoagulant than nonionic compounds. Acute and subacute thrombus formation remains a topic of debate, including the use of low-osmolar ionic contrast media in preference to low-osmolar nonionic contrast media in coronary interventions. However, the general consensus is that a good angiographic technique is the most important factor in reducing thrombotic complications. Drugs and interventional devices that decrease the risk of thromboembolic complications during interventional procedures minimize the importance of the effects of contrast media (AGUIRRE et al. 1997).

References

Aguirre FV, Simoons ML, Ferguson JJ et al (1997) Impact of contrast media on clinical outcomes following percutaneous coronary interventions with platelet glycoprotein IIb/

IIIa inhibition: meta-analysis of clinical trials with abciximab. Abstract. Circulation 96(Suppl 1):161

Albanese JR, Venditto JA, Patel GC, Ambrose JA (1995) Effects of ionic and nonionic contrast media on in vitro and in vivo platelet activation. Am J Cardiol 76:1059–1063

Al Dieri R, de Muinck E, Hemker C, Beguin S (2001) An ionic contrast agent inhibits platelet-dependent thrombin generation and boots the effect of abciximab. Thromb Haemost 85:944–945

Al Dieri R, Beguin S, Hemker C (2003) The ionic contrast medium ioxaglate interferes with thrombin-mediated feedback activation of factor V, factor VIII and platelets. J Thromb Haemost 1:269–274

Almén T, Aspelin P, Nilsson P (1980) Aortic and pulmonary arterial pressure after injection of contrast media into the right atrium of the rabbit. Comparison between metrizoate, ioxaglate and iohexol. Acta Radiol [Suppl] 362:37–41

Arora R, Khandelwal M, Gopal A (1991) In vivo effects of nonionic and ionic contrast media on beta-thromboglobulin and fibrinopeptide levels. J Am Coll Cardiol 17:1533–1536

Aspelin P (1992) Contrast media and red blood cell aggregation: interaction dangerous or harmless from a clinical view – an overview. Clin Hemorheol 12:401–406

Aspelin P, Schmid-Schönbein H (1978) Effect of ionic and nonionic contrast media on red cell aggregation in vitro. Acta Radiol Diagn (Stockh) 19:766–784

Aspelin P, Stöhr-Liessen M, Almén T (1980) Effect of Iohexol on human erythrocytes. I. Changes of red cell morphology in vitro. Acta Radiol [Suppl] 362:117–122

Aspelin P, Nilsson PE, Schmid-Schonbein H, Schroder S, Simon R (1987) Effect of four nonionic contrast media on red blood cells in vitro. III. Deformability. Acta Radiol [Suppl] 370:89–91

Barani J, Gottsater A, Mattiasson I, Lindblad B (2002) Platelet and leukocyte activation during aortoiliac angiography and angioplasty. Eur J Vasc Endovasc Surg 23:220–225

Barstad RM, Buchmann MS, Hamers MJ et al (1996) Effects of ionic and nonionic contrast media on endothelium and on arterial thrombus formation. Acta Radiol 37:954–961

Bashore TM, Davidson CK, Mark DB (1988) Iopamidol use in the cardiac catheterization laboratory: a retrospective analysis of 3313 patients. Cardiology 5:60–100

Becker RC (2001) Markers of platelet activation and thrombin generation. Cardiovasc Toxicol 1:141–145

Bertrand ME, Esplugas E, Piessens J, Rasch W (2000) Influence of a nonionic, iso-osmolar contrast medium (iodixanol) versus an ionic, low-osmolar contrast medium (ioxaglate) on major adverse cardiac events in patients undergoing percutaneous transluminal coronary angioplasty: a multicenter, randomized, double-blind study. Visipaque in percutaneous transluminal coronary angioplasty VIP Trial Investigators. Circulation 101:131–136

Blann AD, Adams R, Ashleigh R, Naser S, Kirkpatrick U, McCollum CN (2001) Changes in endothelial, leucocyte and platelet markers following contrast medium injection during angiography in patients with peripheral artery disease. Br J Radiol 74:811–817

Brzosko M, Cyrylowski L, Brzosko I, Domanski Z, Fiedorowicz-Fabrycy I (1997). Effects of ionic and nonionic contrast media on platelet function as evaluated by plasma concentration on beta-thromboglobulin. Br J Radiol 70:1239–1244

Chronos NAF, Goodall AH, Wilson DJ, Sigwart U, Buller NP (1993) Profound platelet degranulation is an important side effect of some types of contrast media used in interventional cardiology. Circulation 88:2035–2044

Corot C, Perrin JM, Belleville J, Amiel M, Eloy R (1989) Effect of iodinated contrast media on blood clotting. Invest Radiol 24:390–393

Corot C, Chronos N, Sabattier V (1996) In vitro comparison of the effects of contrast media on coagulation and platelet activation. Blood Coagul Fibrinolysis 7:602–608

Cucherat M, Leizorovicz A (1999) Effects of nonionic contrast media on abrupt vessel closure and ischaemic complications after angioplasty. A meta-analysis. Abstract. Am J Cardiol [Suppl] 84:98P

Dalby MCD, Davidson SJ, Burman JF, Clague J, Sigwart U, Davies SW (2002) Systemic platelet effects of contrast media: implications for cardiologic research and clinical practice. Am Heart J 143:E1

Danzi GB, Capuano C, Sesana M, Predolini S, Baglini R (2003) Nonionic low-osmolar contrast media have no impact on major adverse cardiac events in patients undergoing coronary stenting with appropriate antiplatelet therapy. Catheter Cardiovasc Interv 60:477–482

Davidson CJ, Mark DB, Pieper KS et al (1990) Thrombotic and cardiovascular complications related to nonionic contrast media during cardiac catheterization: analysis of 8517 patients. Am J Cardiol 65:1481–1484

Davidson CJ, Laskey WK, Hermiller JB et al (2000) Randomized trial of contrast media utilization in high-risk PTCA. The COURT trial. Circulation 101:2172–2177

Dawson P (1996) X-ray contrast-enhancing agents. Eur J Radiol 23:172–177

Dawson P (1999) Contrast media interactions with endothelium and the blood. In: Dawson P, Cosgrove DO, Grainger RG (eds) Textbook of contrast media. Dunitz, London, pp 191–209

Dawson P, Harrison M, Weisblatt E (1983) Effect of contrast media on red cell filtrability and morphology. Br J Radiol 56:707–710

Dawson P, Hawitt P, Mackle IJ, Machin SJ, Amin S, Bradshaw A (1986) Contrast, coagulation and fibrinolysis. Invest Radiol 21:248–252

Dehmer GJ, Gresalfi N, Daly D, Oberhardt B, Tate DA (1995) Impairment of fibrinolysis by streptokinase, urokinase and recombinant tissue-type plasminogen activator in the presence of radiographic contrast agents. J Am Coll Cardiol 25:1069–1075

Eloy R, Corot C, Belleville J (1991) Contrast media for angiography: physicochemical properties, pharmacokinetics and biocompatibility. Clin Mater 7:89–197

Emery CJ, Fang L, Laude EA, Morcos SK (2001) Effects of radiographic contrast media on pulmonary vascular resistance of normoxic and chronically hypoxic pulmonary hypertensive rats. Br J Radiol 74:1109–1117

Engelhart JA, Smith DC, Maloney MD, Westengard JC, Bull BS (1988) A technique for estimating the probability of clots in blood/contrast agent mixtures. Invest Radiol 23:923–927

Esplugas E, Cequier A, Jara F et al (1991) Risk of thrombosis during coronary angioplasty with low osmolality contrast media. Am J Cardiol 68:1020–1024

Fanning NF, Manning BJ, Buckley J, Redmond HP (2002) Iodinated contrast media induced neutrophil apoptosis through a mitochondrial and caspase mediated pathway. Br J Radiol 75:861–873

Fauser C, Ullisch EV, Kubler W, Haller C (2001) Differential effects of radiocontrast agents on human umbilical vein endothelial cells: cytotoxicity and modulators of thrombogenicity. Eur J Med Res 6:465–472

Fay WP, Parker AC (1998) Effects of radiographic contrast agents on thrombin formation and activity. Thromb Haemost 80:266–272

Ferguson JJ, Quinn M, Moake JL (2000). Platelet physiology. In: Ferguson JJ, Chronos NA, Harrington RA (eds) Antiplatelet therapy in clinical practice. Dunitz, London, pp 5–34

Fleisch M, Mulhauser B, Garachemani A et al (1999) Impact of ionic (ioxaglate) and nonionic (ioversol) contrast media on PTCA-related complications. J Am Coll Cardiol 33(Suppl A): 85A (abstract 1188–1192)

Furuta W, Sendo T, Kataoka Y, Oishi R (2001) Morphologic degeneration of human microvascular endothelial cells induced by iodinated contrast media. Acad Radiol 8:158–161

Furuta W, Yamauchi A, Dohgu S et al (2002) Contrast media increase vascular endothelial permeability by inhibiting nitric oxide production. Invest Radiol 37:13–19

Gabelmann A, Haberstroh J, Weyrich G (2001) Ionic and nonionic contrast agent-mediated endothelial injury. Quantitative analysis of cell proliferation during endothelial repair. Acta Radiol 42:422–425

Gabriel DA, Jones MR, Reece NS, Boothroyd E, Bashore T (1991) Platelet and fibrin modification by radiographic contrast media. Circ Res 68:881–887

Galtung HK, Sörlundsengen V, Sakariassen KS, Benestad H (2002) Effect of radiologic contrast media on cell volume regulatory mechanisms in human red blood cells. Acad Radiol 9:878–885

Grines CL, Schreiber TL, Savas V et al (1996) A randomized trial of low osmolar ionic versus nonionic contrast media in patients with myocardial infarction or unstable angina undergoing percutaneous transluminal coronary angioplasty. J Am Coll Cardiol 27:1381–1386

Grabowski EF, Kaplan KL, Halpern EF (1991a) Anticoagulant effects of nonionic versus ionic contrast media in angiography syringes. Invest Radiol 26:417–421

Grabowski EF, Rodriquez M, McDonnel SL (1991b) Platelet adhesion/aggregation and endothelial cell function in flowing blood: effect of contrast media. Semin Hematol 28(Suppl 7):60–65

Grollman JH Jr, Liu CK, Astone RA, Lurie MD (1988) Thromboembolic complications in coronary angiography associated with the use of nonionic contrast medium. Cathet Cardiovasc Diagn 14:159–164

Hardeman MR, Goedhart P, Koen IY (1991) The effect of low-osmolar ionic and nonionic contrast media on human blood viscosity, erythrocyte morphology, and aggregation behavior. Invest Radiol 26:810–819

Heptinstall S, White A, Edwards N et al (1998) Differential effects of three radiographic contrast media on platelet aggregation and degranulation: implications for clinical practice? Br J Haematol 103:1023–1030

Hernanz-Schulman M, Vanholder R, Waterloos M-A, Hakim R, Schulman G (2000) Effect of radiographic contrast agents on leukocyte metabolic response. Pediatr Radiol 30:361–368

Heyman S, Goldfarb M, Carmeli F, Shina A, Rahmilewitz D, Brezis M (1998) Effects of radiocontrast agents on intrarenal nitric oxide (NO) and NO synthase activity. Exp Nephrol 6:557–562

Idée J-M, Corot C (1999) Thrombotic risk associated with use of iodinated contrast media in interventional cardiology: pathophysiology and clinical aspects. Fundam Clin Pharmacol 13:613–623

Idée J-M, Prigent P, Corot C (2002) Effects of ioxaglate on cultured microvascular endothelial cells: do all in vitro studies actually reflect clinical situations? Acad Radiol 9:98–100

Jones CI, Goodal AH (2003) Differential effects of the iodinated contrast agents Ioxaglate, Iohexol and Iodixanol on thrombus formation and fibrinolysis. Thromb Res 112: 65–71

Jung F, Spitzer SG, Pindur G (2002) Effect of an ionic compared to a nonionic X-ray contrast agent on platelets and coagulation during diagnostic cardiac catheterisation. Pathophysiol Haemost Thromb 32:121–126

Krause W, Niehues D (1996) Biochemical characterization of X-ray contrast media. Invest Radiol 31:30–42

Labarthe B, Idée JM, Burnett R, Corot C (2003) In vivo comparative antithrombotic effect of ioxaglate and iohexol and interaction with the platelet antiaggregant clopidogrel. Invest Radiol 38:34–43

Laerum F (1983) Acute damage to human endothelial cells by brief exposure to contrast media in vitro. Radiology 147:681–684

Laskey WK, Gellman J (2003) Inflammatory markers increase following exposure to radiographic contrast media. Acta Radiol 44:498–503

Le Mignon MM, Ducret MN, Bonnemain B, Donadieu AM (1988) Effect of contrast media on whole blood filtrability. Acta Radiol 29:593–597

Li X, Gabriel DA (1997) Differences between contrast media in the inhibition of platelet activation by specific platelet agonists. Acad Radiol 4:108–114

Liss P, Nygren A, Olsson U, Ulfendahl HR, Erikson U (1996) Effects of contrast media and mannitol on renal medullary blood flow and red cell aggregation in the rat kidney. Kidney Int 49:1268–1275

Losco P, Nash G, Stone P, Ventre J (2001) Comparison of the effects of radiographic contrast media on dehydration and filterability of red blood cells from donors homozygous for hemoglobin A or hemoglobin S. Am J Hematol 68:149–158

Malekianpour M, Bonan R, Lespérance J, Gosselin G, Hudon G, Doucet S (1998) Comparison of ionic and nonionic low osmolar contrast media in relation to thrombotic complications of angioplasty in patients with unstable angina. Am Heart J 135:1067–1075

Markou CP, Chronos NAF, Hanson SR (2001) Antithromotic effects of ionic and nonionic contrast media in nonhuman primates. Thromb Haemost 85:488–493

Melton LG, Muga KM, Gabriel DA (1995) Effect of contrast media on in vitro bleeding time: assessment by a hollow fiber instrument. Acad Radiol 2:239–243

Millet PJ, Sestier F (1989) Thromboembolic complications with nonionic contrast media. Cathet Cardiovasc Diagn 17:192

Mills SR, Jackson BF, Older RA, Heaston DK, Moore AV (1980) The incidence, aetiologies and avoidance of complications of pulmonary angiography in a large series. Radiology 136:295–299

Morcos SK (1998) Contrast media-induced nephrotoxicity-questions and answers. Br J Radiol 71:357–365

Morcos SK (2003) Effects of radiographic contrast media on the lung. Br J Radiol 76:290–295

Morcos SK, Dawson P, Pearson JD et al (1998) The haemodynamic effects of iodinated water soluble radiographic contrast media: a review. Eur J Radiol 29:31–46

Morgan DML, Bettmann MA (1989) Effects of X-ray contrast media and radiation on human vascular endothelial cells in vitro. Cardiovasc Intervent Radiol 12:154–160

Nash GB, Meiselman HJ (1991) Effect of dehydration on the viscoelastic behaviour of red cells. Blood Cells 17:517–522

Nordby A, Thorstensen K, Halgunset J, Haugen OA, Solberg S (1989) Effects on the ATP content of cultured cells after radiographic contrast media exposure – evidence for accumulation of contrast media in cultured cells. Acta Radiol 30:541–547

Oldroyd SD, Morcos SK (2000) Endothelin: what does the radiologist need to know? Br J Radiol 73:1246–1251

Parvez Z, Moncada R (1986) Nonionic contrast medium: effects on blood coagulation and complement activation in vitro. Angiology 37:358–364

Parvez Z, Vik H (1991) Nonionic contrast media and blood clotting. A critical review. Invest Radiol 26(Suppl 1): S103–S106; discussion S107–S109

Parvez Z, Moncada R, Messmore HL, Fareed J (1982) Ionic and nonionic contrast media interaction with anticoagulant drugs. Acta Radiol Diagn (Stockh) 23:401–404

Pearson JD (1991) Endothelial cell biology. Radiology 179: 9–14

Piessens JH, Stammen F, Vrolix MC et al (1993) Effects of an ionic versus a nonionic low osmolar contrast agent on the thrombotic complications of coronary angioplasty. Cathet Cardiovasc Diagn 28:99–105

Pislaru S, Pislaru C, Szilard M, Arnout J, van der Werf F (1998) In vivo effects of contrast media on coronary thrombolysis. J Am Coll Cardiol 32:1102–1108

Polanowska R, Wilczynska m, Slawinski W, Goch JH, Augustiniak W, Cierniewski CS (1992) Changes in platelet activity and tissue plasminogène activator during arteriography in patients with chronic limb ischaemia. Thromb Res 65:663–665

Pugh N (1996) Haemodynamic and rheological effects of contrast media: the role of viscosity and osmolality. Eur Radiol 6(Suppl 2):S13–S15

Rasmussen F (1998) The influence of radiographic contrast media on some granulocyte functions. Acta Radiol [Suppl] 419:7–35

Rasmussen F, Georgsen J, Grunnet N (1988) Influence of radiographic contrast media on phagocytosis. Acta Radiol 29:589–592

Rasmussen F, Antonsen S, Georgsen J (1992a) Granulocyte adherence is inhibited by radiographic contrast media in vitro. Acta Radiol 33:379–383

Rasmussen F, Georgsen J, Antonsen S, Grunnet N (1992b) Phagocytic properties of granulocytes after intravenous injection of ioxaglate or iohexol. Acta Radiol 33:271–274

Rasmussen F, Georgsen J, Pedersen JO, Antonsen S (1992c) Granulocyte chemotaxis before and after urography. Influence of four different contrast media. Acta Radiol 33:164–168

Rasuli P, McLeish WA, Hammond DI (1989) Anticoagulant effects of contrast materials: in vitro study of iohexol, ioxaglate and diatrizoate. Am J Roentgenol 152:309–311

Robertson HJF (1987) Blood clot formation in angiographic syringes containing nonionic contrast media. Radiology 163:621–622

Scheller B, Hennen B, Pohl A, Schieffer H, Markwirth T (2001) Acute and subacute stent occlusion: risk reduction by ionic contrast media. Eur Heart J 22:385–391

Schrader R (1998) Thrombogenic potential of nonionic contrast media, fact or fiction? Eur J Radiol 23(Suppl 1):S10–S13

Schrader R, Esch I, Ensslen R et al (1999) A randomized trial comparing the impact of a nonionic (iomeprol) versus an ionic (ioxaglate) low osmolar contrast medium on abrupt vessel closure and ischaemic complications after coronary angioplasty. J Am Coll Cardiol 33:395–402

Schwartz D, Blum M, Peer G et al (1994) Role of nitric oxide (EDRF) in radiocontrast acute renal failure in rats. Am J Physiol 267:F374–F379

Sendo T, Kataoka Y, Takeda Y, Furuta W, Oishi R (2000) Nitric oxide protects against contrast media-induced pulmonary vascular permeability in rats. Invest Radiol 35:472–478

Stormorken H, Skalpe IO, Testart MC (1986) Effects of various contrast media on coagulation, fibrinolysis and platelet function. An in vitro and in vivo study. Invest Radiol 21:348–354

Strickland NH, Rampling MW, Dawson P, Martin G (1992a) Contrast media-induced effects on blood rheology and their importance in angiography. Clin Radiol 45:240–242

Strickland N, Rampling M, Dawson P, Martin G (1992b) The effects of contrast media on the rheological properties of blood. Clin Hemorheol 12:369–379

Sumimura T, Sendo T, Itoh Y et al (2003) Calcium-dependent injury of human microvascular endothelial cells induced by variety of iodinated radiographic contrast media. Invest Radiol 38:366–374

Sutton AGC, Ashton VJ, Campbell PG, Price DJA, Hall JA, de Belder MA (2002) A randomized prospective trial of ioxaglate 320 (Hexabrix) vs iodixanol 320 (Visipaque) in patients undergoing percutaneous coronary intervention. Catheter Cardiovasc Interv 57:346–352

Tominaga K, Kataoka Y, Sendo T, Furuta W, Niizeki M, Oishi AR (2001) Contrast media-induced pulmonary vascular hyperpermeability is aggravated in a rat climacterium model. Invest Radiol 36:131–135

Van Beek EJR, Levi M, Reekers JA, Hack CE, Buller HR, ten Cate JW (1994) Increased plasma levels of PAI-1 after administration of nonionic contrast medium in patients undergoing pulmonary angiography. Radiology 193:821–823

Wilson AJ, Sage MR (1994) Cytochemical studies on contrast medium-induced blood-brain-barrier damage. Invest Radiol 29(Suppl 2):S105–S107

Zhan X, Agrawal DK, Thorpe PE (1998) Effect of iodinated contrast media on neutrophil adhesion to cultured endothelial cells. J Vasc Interv Radiol 9:808–816. Erratum in: J Vasc Interv Radiol 9:889, 1998

Zhang H, Holt CM, Malik N, Shepherd L, Morcos SK (2000) Effects of radiographic contrast media on proliferation and apoptosis of human vascular endothelial cells. Br J Radiol 73:1034–1041

Zir LM, Carvalho AC, Hawthorne JW, Colman RW, Lees RS (1974) Effect of contrast agents on platelet aggregation and ^{14}C-serotonin release. N Engl J Med 291:134–135

Effect on Thyroid Function

18

Aart J. van der Molen

CONTENTS

Aart J. van der Molen
Department of Radiology, C-2S, Leiden University Medical
Center, PO Box 9600, 2300 RC Leiden, The Netherlands

18.1
Introduction

The two main reasons for the development of thyrotoxicosis are Graves' disease and thyroid autonomy. In Graves' disease, thyroid stimulating autoantibodies enhance iodine uptake and thyroid hormone synthesis. In thyroid autonomy, the autonomous tissue is not under the control of thyroid stimulating hormone (TSH) and, if subjected to high iodine loads, produces and secretes excessive thyroid hormone with or without a concomitant decrease in TSH.

From time to time, the issue of "contrast medium-induced thyrotoxicosis" is brought to the attention of radiologists. Since contrast medium solutions contain some free iodide, contrast media may induce thyrotoxicosis in the above-mentioned patient groups. Iodine deficiency is an important factor in the development of thyroid autonomy and goiter. Therefore, iodine-induced thyrotoxicosis is more commonly seen in areas where the iodine intake is low.

18.2
Terminology

The terms *iodine* and *iodide* are often used interchangeably. Iodine is often used in the generic sense as in "iodine deficiency" or in describing diseases like "iodine-induced thyrotoxicosis". Iodide refers to the metabolically important, nonorganic free form that can be present in excess because of a number of factors. Iodine enters the body in the form of iodide or iodate ions. Iodate is rapidly converted to iodide, which can be trapped and organically bound in the thyroid gland.

The term *hyperthyroidism* is used to describe excessive secretion of thyroid hormone from the thyroid gland, which may or may not become clinically symptomatic. *Thyrotoxicosis* is the preferred term for the clinical syndrome caused by excess thyroid hormone. This excess can come from both endogenous and exogenous sources of iodide.

18.3
Iodine Deficiency Areas

As iodine deficiency is an important factor in the development of thyroid autonomy and multinodular goiter, in iodine-deficient areas the number of patients at risk for iodine-induced thyrotoxicosis is higher. Important geographical differences in iodine intake still exist because of differences in national laws, fortification programs (e.g., iodized salt), and awareness. Global WHO data covering 92% of the world's population show that prevalence is intimately related to iodized salt intake, which is highest in the Americas. Therefore, prevalence of iodine deficiency in the general population in the Americas (9.8%) is significantly lower than in Europe (56.9%), which has the highest prevalence worldwide (DE BENOIST et al. 2003). In 2002, the International Council for Control of Iodine Deficiency Disorders (ICCIDD) designated European countries with sufficient or likely sufficient and deficient or likely deficient iodine nutrition status (Table 18.1) (VITTI et al. 2003). More than 60% of nearly 600 million Europeans live in iodine-deficient countries, which include countries such as Germany, France, Belgium, Italy, and Spain.

18.4
Free Iodide

According to the quality control regulations for production of water-soluble contrast media, the content of free iodide per milliliter is far below the total amount of (organically bound) iodine per mililiter. In a bottle with a contrast medium concentration of 300 mgI ml^{-1}, the upper limit of free iodide is generally below 50 µg ml^{-1} directly after production and below 90 µg ml^{-1} after 3–5 years of shelf-life. In most products, the actual content of free iodide is below 1/10th of these upper limits, depending on the time between production and use. For instance, a 150-ml dose of a contrast medium containing 10 µg ml^{-1} provides 1,500 µg free iodide, equivalent to 10 times the recommended daily intake in adults.

Table 18.1. Iodine nutrition status in Europe by country as designated by the International Council for Control of Iodine Deficiency Disorders (ICCIDD) (VITTI et al. 2003)

Sufficient	Likely sufficient	Deficient	Likely deficient
Austria	Iceland	Belgium	Albania
Bosnia	Luxembourg	Denmark	
Bulgaria	Norway	France	
Croatia	Sweden	Germany	
Cyprus		Greece	
Czech Republic		Hungary	
Finland		Ireland	
Macedonia		Italy	
Netherlands		Montenegro	
Poland		Romania	
Portugal		Slovenia	
Slovak Republic		Spain	
Serbia			
Switzerland			
UK			

In addition, it was shown (RENDL and SALLER 2001) that iodinated contrast media molecules can be deiodinated in the body. The resulting amount of free iodide depends on the time that the contrast medium is circulating and is 0.01–0.15% (1 h–1 week circulation time) of the amount of the organically bound iodine administered. Biliary contrast media circulate longer and are metabolized at a greater rate, resulting in the release of a significant amount of free iodide in the circulation. Therefore, the effects of biliary contrast media on the thyroid may be greater, and persist longer than for the other water-soluble media.

18.5
Effect of Contrast Media on Thyroid Function in Normal, Euthyroid Patients

In an older review (HEHRMANN et al. 1996), it was reported that within 21 days of administration of large doses of contrast medium, there is a small decrease followed by an increase within normal limits in free thyroxine (T_4) and a decrease followed by a rapid increase (<5 days) within normal limits in TSH. More recently, in 102 euthyroid patients who underwent coronary angiography (Fassbender et al. 2001a) subgroup analyses showed small increases in TSH in small glands but decreases in larger glands. Also, a discrete increase in free T_4 was seen in patients with large glands and low-normal TSH values. Another study of 22 patients specifically evaluated the early time period after contrast medium administration (Gartner and Weissel 2004). There were increases in TSH 3–5 days after contrast administration, with increases outside the normal range (18%) in patients with basal high-normal TSH values. Thyroid hormone levels were unchanged. This suggests transient subclinical hypothyroidism, a condition more frequently seen in patients with autoimmune (Hashimoto) thyroiditis (Roberts and Ladenson 2004). Thus, in most normal euthyroid patients no changes in thyroid functional parameters are seen, although transient subclinical hypothyroidism or hyperthyroidism may sometimes occur. However, administration of contrast media to a population of geriatric patients may lead to long-lasting subclinical hyperthyroidism with increased free T_4 and decreased TSH for as long as 8 weeks post injection (Conn et al. 1996). This is thought to be caused by undiagnosed autonomous nodules in the thyroid glands of these elderly patients.

18.6
Contrast Medium-Induced Thyrotoxicosis

18.6.1
Mechanism of Contrast Medium-Induced Thyrotoxicosis

Iodine is an essential requirement for thyroid hormone synthesis. The recommended daily intake for adults is about 150 µg. The thyroid gland has intrinsic regulatory mechanisms that maintain thyroid function even in the presence of iodide excess. When large amounts of iodide are given to subjects with normal thyroid function, the synthesis of thyroid hormones decreases transiently for about 2 days. This acute inhibitory effect of iodide on thyroid hormone synthesis is called the Wolff–Chaikoff effect and is due to increased iodide concentration. Escape from, or adaptation to, the acute Wolff–Chaikoff effect is produced by a blockage in the thyroid iodide trap. This reduces the intrathyroidal iodide concen-

tration because of a decrease in the sodium iodide symporter (NIS) mRNA and protein expression.

Excess iodide ingestion also reduces the release of thyroxine (T_4) and tri-iodothyronine (T_3) from the thyroid. This results in small decreases in serum T_4 and T_3 concentrations, with compensatory increases in basal and thyrotropin release hormone (TRH)-stimulated thyrotropin (TSH) concentrations. All values remain in the normal range (Roti and Uberti 2001).

Iodine-induced hyperthyroidism is not a single etiologic entity. It may occur in patients with a variety of underlying thyroid diseases, the most important of which are Graves' disease and multinodular goiters in patients who live in areas of iodine deficiency. Rare causes of hyperthyroidism include the presence of ectopic thyroid tissue (e.g., in the tongue or thorax), or abnormal autoregulation of thyroid tissue, which can occur in patients with well-differentiated papillary and follicular thyroid carcinoma or its metastases (Roti and Uberti 2001). The exact pathophysiology and epidemiology of the complete spectrum of iodine-induced hyperthyroidism goes beyond the scope of this chapter, and has been reviewed elsewhere (Braverman 1994; Stanbury et al. 1998).

In addition to contrast media, other sources of iodide excess include disinfectants, secretolytic agents, the iodine-containing antiarrhythmic amiodarone, eye drops and ointments, seaweed, multivitamin preparations, skin ointments, toothpaste, etc. (Hehrmann et al. 1996).

18.6.2
Biochemical Diagnosis of Hyperthyroidism

Hyperthyroidism is defined as elevation of plasma free thyroxine (FT_4) or total tri-iodothyronine (T_3) level and suppression of TSH level (Martin and Deam 1996).

18.6.3
Prevalence of Contrast Medium-Induced Thyrotoxicosis

Little is known about the true prevalence of iodine-induced thyrotoxicosis caused by the contrast medium. It was calculated (Rendl and Saller 2001) that in an iodine-deficient country, 38 cases of thyrotoxic crisis (the most severe form of thyrotoxicosis) due to contrast media are seen per year, while in the same year about 5 million contrast-enhanced studies are performed (0.0008%). Two large studies in unselected populations in an iodine-deficient area showed a prevalence of 0.25–0.34% (NOLTE et al. 1996; HINTZE et al. 1999), while in an iodine-sufficient area this figure is 10-fold lower at 0.028% (DE BRUIN 1994). In an iodine-deficient Computed Tomography (CT) population, the percentage of latent and overt hyperthyroidism is estimated as 5.8 and 0.8%, respectively (SAAM et al. 2005).

18.6.4
Clinical Symptoms of Thyrotoxicosis

Hyperthyroidism caused by the free iodide in contrast media is usually self-limiting, but in rare cases (and in the presence of risk factors) the free iodide can lead to clinically significant thyrotoxicosis. Hyperthyroidism occurs more frequently in the elderly, so the diagnosis may not be apparent, particularly in the presence of cognitive impairment (MARTIN and DEAM 1996). Clinically, it cannot be differentiated from other forms of thyrotoxicosis and, depending on the underlying risk factors, may give rise to symptoms such as weight loss, nervousness, easy fatigability, intolerance to heat, hyperkinesia, periodic paralysis, palpitations, and cardiac arrhythmias.

The most important manifestations of thyrotoxicosis are cardiovascular. It can aggravate pre-existing cardiac diseases and can also lead to atrial fibrillation, congestive heart failure, worsening of angina, thromboembolism, and, rarely, death. In the absence of pre-existing cardiac disease, treatment of thyrotoxicosis usually returns cardiac function to normal (DUNN et al. 1998).

Palpitations are probably the most common cardiac symptom. They are caused by either sinus tachycardia or the development of supraventricular tachycardia, usually atrial fibrillation. Atrial fibrillation occurs in 15–20% of patients with hyperthyroidism, compared with less than 1% of euthyroid adults. Angina is another common symptom. It usually occurs in patients with known coronary disease, but angina from coronary spasm in previously healthy patients has also been reported. Dyspnea on exertion, pulmonary edema, and other signs of heart failure can also occur, particularly if cardiomyopathy has developed.

Thromboembolic events complicating atrial fibrillation may be the presenting symptom of thyrotoxicosis (DUNN et al. 1998; ROTI and UBERTI 2001). Tachycardia is the most common sign of thyrotoxicosis at physical examination, occurring in more than 40% of patients on initial presentation. Other signs of a hyperdynamic circulation, such as systolic hypertension and prominent cardiac pulsations, are frequent.

18.6.5
Clinical Studies on Contrast Medium-Induced Thyrotoxicosis

There are very few studies dealing with the development of thyrotoxicosis following injection of contrast media. Patient populations and results may differ depending on whether the study is performed in iodine-deficient or iodine-sufficient areas.

A number of studies have been undertaken in areas without iodine deficiency. One study showed no effect on serum T_4, T_3, or FT_4 index up to 56 days after cardiac catheterization using meglumine ioxaglate (GRAINGER and PENNINGTON 1981). Seven patients with multinodular goiter of a cohort of 24,600 CT scans performed over a 3-year period needed hospital admission because of clinically severe iodine-induced hyperthyroidism following administration of a total dose of 3–12 mg free iodide in nonionic contrast media (DE BRUIN 1994). After CT of the thyroid using 100 ml iohexol, 8 of 22 patients with thyroid disease had a temporary change in thyroid function. Four patients showed increases in TSH levels, while in a further four, temporary hyperthyroidism developed over a period of 1 month (NYGAARD et al. 1998). In geriatric populations, iodine-induced thyrotoxicosis following contrast radiography with iopamidol 370 mgI ml^{-1} was the cause in 7 of 28 cases of hyperthyroidism seen over 20 months (MARTIN et al. 1993). Although the condition appeared self-limited, it was associated with increased patient morbidity and prolonged hospital stay. In another study from the same group of 60 patients with hyperthyroidism over the age of 70 years, 23% had been exposed to iodinated contrast media within the previous 6 months. In 62% of the patients hyperthyroidism was not suspected at admission (MARTIN and DEAM 1996).

In an iodine-deficient area, the prevalence and pathogenesis of thyrotoxicosis following contrast media administration was evaluated between 1971 and 1979 (STIEDLE 1989). In 89 (15%) of 663 patients with thyrotoxicosis, the condition could be related to iodine-containing contrast media. The majority (95%) occurred after 12 weeks. Goiter was present in 63% of the patients and most of them were elderly. In a large study in unselected patients, only two of 788 developed hyperthyroidism within 12 weeks of coronary angiography (HINTZE et al. 1999). Administration of nonionic iodinated contrast medium to 102 euthyroid patients did not lead to hyperthyroidism in any patient despite the large number of nodularly transformed glands and patients with goiter (FASSBENDER et al. 2001a). The same study showed that thyroid morphology at ultrasound was not a prognostic factor for the development of hyperthyroidism.

Thus, iodine-induced thyrotoxicosis does not seem to be clinically relevant in unselected patient populations or in euthyroid patients. It seems to be relevant only in patients with previous thyroid disease or in patients at risk, especially in areas of iodine deficiency and in geriatric populations.

18.7

Prevention and Prophylaxis of Contrast Media-Induced Thyrotoxicosis

Prevention of iodine-induced thyrotoxicosis in patients at high risk is important because treatment with thyrostatic drugs is hindered by the high iodide levels in the blood, and there are more complications associated with treatment than in other forms of thyrotoxicosis.

In patients with risk factors, a strong indication for administering iodinated contrast medium is essential. If there is manifest hyperthyroidism, administration of contrast media is contraindicated as stated in the drug package insert. In other patients at increased risk, diagnostically equivalent alternative imaging modalities not requiring iodinated contrast media should be considered, e.g., ultrasound, magnetic resonance imaging (MRI), scintigraphy, or unenhanced CT.

In thyroid autonomy, the amount of autonomous tissue is one of the key determinants of the risk of iodine-induced hyperthyroidism. The results of a previous technetium scintigram have been used to quantify the amount of autonomous tissue to stratify risk (EMRICH et al. 1993; HEHRMANN et al. 1996; FRICKE et al. 2004). However, this indication for scintigraphy has fallen somewhat into disuse as very sensitive TSH assays have become generally available more recently. To reduce the incidence of iodine-induced thyrotoxicosis further, it has been suggested that prophylactic drugs could be administered, starting well before the examination. The subject of medical prophylaxis is controversial, and recommendations are related to the presence or absence of iodine deficiency.

A number of indications and regimens have been suggested. Prophylaxis by perchlorate has been recommended only in cardiac patients with a goiter and subnormal levels of TSH (VAN GULDENER et al. 1998). In a prospective randomized study in high-risk subjects with autonomy, prophylaxis with either perchlorate or thiamazole prevented only small increases in circulating thyroid hormone levels, but was not able to prevent hyperthyroidism completely and combination therapy was advised (NOLTE et al. 1996). Administration of perchlorate and a thioamide-class drug to elderly patients with suppressed serum TSH and/or palpable goiter has been suggested (LAWRENCE et al. 1999). It has been recommended that this combination be started the day before and continued for 2 weeks after contrast medium administration in patients with thyroid autonomy (HEHRMANN et al. 1996; LAWRENCE et al. 1999; RENDL and SALLER 2001), but others restrict its use to patients with high Tc-uptake levels (JOSEPH 1995). A sample combination protocol for prophylaxis is summarized in Table 18.2

An alternative strategy is to monitor high-risk patients closely, using biochemical tests (NYGAARD et al. 1998). In euthyroid, not-at-risk patients, iodine-induced hyperthyroidism after coronary angiography was rare and therefore prophylactic therapy was not considered necessary (HINTZE et al. 1999). The risk of side effects from medical prophylaxis in these patients is probably greater than the risk of developing iodine-induced thyrotoxicosis.

Table 18.2. Sample combination regimen for prophylaxis of contrast medium-induced thyrotoxicosis

Elective contrast-enhanced studies:		
Sodium perchlorate	300 mg 3 times daily	Start the day before and continue for 8–14 days
Thiamazole	30 mg once daily	Start the day before and continue for 14 days
Emergency contrast-enhanced studies:		
Sodium perchlorate	800 mg once daily	Directly prior to examination
		Continue with 3 × 300 mg for 8–14 days
Thiamazole	30 mg once daily	Directly prior to exam and continue for 14 days

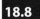

18.8
Nuclear Medicine Studies and Contrast Media

For a long time it has been known that giving iodinated contrast media interferes with both diagnostic scintigraphy and radioiodine treatment. It is believed that the reduced uptake of the radioactive tracer is due to the amount of inorganic free iodide in the contrast medium solution, which can range from 1 to 20 μg ml⁻¹ (Coel et al. 1975; Laurie et al. 1992).

18.8.1
Effect of Contrast Media on Thyroid Scintigraphy

In nuclear medicine literature, an interval of 3–6 weeks is advocated after intravascular (water-soluble) contrast medium administration before scintigraphy, depending on the indication for the study and on whether the patient is euthyroid or hyperthyroid (Wilson and O'mara 1997; Martin and Sandler 2003). To avoid nondiagnostic studies, some hospitals use an interval as long as 3 months. As biliary contrast agents are metabolized and excreted more slowly, a longer interval of 2 months applies. For reasons of consistency and simplicity, a conservative period of 2 months for all types of water-soluble contrast media is recommended (Chap. 29; van der Molen et al. 2004).

18.8.2
Effect of Contrast Media on Radioiodine Treatment

Before radioiodine treatment with ¹³¹I, excess iodine should be avoided. Nuclear medicine literature and a European Association of Nuclear Medicine guideline advise that iodinated water-soluble contrast media should be withheld 1–2 months before radioiodine treatment (Tuttle et al. 2003; European Association of Nuclear Medicine 2003), although some hospitals use even longer periods. Also, in preparation of patients, iodine-containing antiseptics (e.g., povidone-iodine) should not be used 2 weeks prior to radioiodine treatment (Tuttle et al. 2003). It seems advisable to have a period of 2 months between giving iodinated water-soluble contrast media and undertaking radioiodine treatment (see Chap. 29)

(van der Molen et al. 2004). Because of slower metabolism and excretion, biliary contrast agents should be withheld for a longer period of 3–4 months.

18.9
Effect of Impaired Renal Function

Water-soluble iodinated contrast medium molecules are almost completely eliminated from the body within 24 h after injection in patients with normal renal function. In patients with a decreased glomerular filtration rate (GFR), elimination is delayed and a longer period of interference with nuclear medicine studies can be expected. There is, however, no evidence of an increased risk of contrast medium-induced thyrotoxicosis in patients with severely reduced renal function (GFR <20 ml min⁻¹). There is no evidence in the literature to suggest that deiodination and the resulting thyrotoxicosis occur in patients with end-stage renal failure.

18.10
Nonvascular Routes of Administration

Very little data exists on the administration of iodinated contrast media by other routes. Most information concerns contrast administration during endoscopic retrograde cholangiopancreatography (ERCP). Administration of iodinated contrast agents into the biliary and pancreatic ducts during ERCP led to significant increases of serum levels of total iodine and free iodide and of urinary iodine excretion, which returned to normal in 2–3 weeks in one study (Mann et al. 1994). Levels of TSH, free T_4, and free T_3 remained unchanged and no hyperthyroidism occurred. However, even a small amount of contrast medium given enterally can be associated with thyroid stimulation (Fassbender et al. 2001b). A decrease of TSH as well as an increase in total T_3, free T_4, and urinary iodine excretion was reported after ERCP, especially in patients with multinodular goiter. However, clinical symptoms of hyperthyroidism did not occur. A third study concluded that routine measurement of TSH and thyroid hormone levels before ERCP is not indicated, given the relatively low iodine load administered during the procedure (Mönig et al. 1999).

18.11

Conclusions

In patients without risk factors, contrast medium-induced thyrotoxicosis is very rare. Therefore, it is not necessary to routinely assess thyroid function or morphology before injection of contrast media. However, a small group of patients are at increased risk and radiologists should be aware of the potential effects on thyroid function associated with administration of iodinated contrast media. The history and physical examination are important, and risk factors should always be communicated to the radiologist via the request form.

Patients with Graves' disease and multinodular goiter with thyroid autonomy are at increased risk of developing thyrotoxicosis after administration of an iodinated contrast medium. In at-risk patients, the prevalence of contrast medium-induced thyrotoxicosis is significantly higher in iodine-deficient areas (RENDL and SALLER 2001). Also, iodine-induced thyrotoxicosis has been reported to occur more frequently in the elderly (CONN et al. 1996). Clinically, this thyrotoxicosis is most relevant in patients with an associated cardiovascular risk (DUNN et al. 1998). Nowadays, this geriatric population is exposed to diagnostic imaging including imaging-guided intervention more frequently than in the past because of major technological advances and increased longevity. Although thyroid stimulation is more common in these patients (even following nonvascular administration of contrast medium), the literature does not unequivocally prove an increased incidence of clinically relevant thyrotoxicosis in the elderly.

Nonetheless, in high-risk patients, knowledge of thyroid function (at least TSH) before a contrast-enhanced study is helpful. All high-risk patients should be monitored closely after the injection of an iodinated contrast medium, preferably by endocrinologists (NYGAARD et al. 1998). Selected patients (e.g., the elderly patient with multinodular goiter and concomitant cardiac disease) may benefit from prophylactic thyrostatic therapy. In patients with established hyperthyroidism, administration of iodinated contrast media is contraindicated. It is not advisable to use intravenous cholangiographic media in patients at risk (RENDL and SALLER 2001).

A more frequently observed problem in clinical practice is a decreased uptake of radioactive technetium and/or iodine in nuclear medicine studies following exposure to iodinated contrast agents. This has compromised the diagnosis of thyroid disorders and treatment of thyroid carcinoma. When urgent treatment is essential, gadolinium-based contrast media up to 0.3 mmol kg^{-1} body weight may be used in diagnostic studies (THOMSEN et al. 2002; CHRISTENSEN et al. 2000). However, this will seldom result in satisfactory radiographic or CT examinations and this practice should certainly be avoided in patients with reduced kidney function.

References

Braverman LE (1994) Iodine and the thyroid: 33 years of study. Thyroid 4:351–356

Christensen CR, Glowniak JV, Brown PH et al (2000) The effect of gadolinium contrast media on radioiodine uptake by the thyroid gland. J Nucl Med Technol 28:41–44

Coel M, Talner B, Lang H (1975) Mechanism of radioactive iodine uptake depression following intravenous urography. Br J Radiol 48:146–147

Conn JJ, Sebastian MJ, Deam D et al (1996) A prospective study of the effect of ionic media on thyroid function. Thyroid 6:107–110

De Benoist B, Andersson M, Takkouche B et al (2003) Prevalence of iodine deficiency worldwide. Lancet 362:1859–1860

De Bruin TW (1994) Iodide induced hyperthyroidism with computed tomography contrast fluids (letter). Lancet 343:1160–1161

Dunn JT, Semigran MJ, Delange F (1998) The prevention and management of iodine-induced hyperthyroidism and its cardiac features. Thyroid 8:101–106

Emrich D, Erlenmaier U, Pohl M et al (1993) Determination of the autonomously functioning volume of the thyroid. Eur J Nucl Med 20:410–414

European Association of Nuclear Medicine (2003) EANM procedure guidelines for therapy with iodine-131. Eur J Nucl Med 30:BP27–BP31

Fassbender WJ, Schlüter S, Stracke H et al (2001a) Schilddrüsenfunktion nach Gabe jodhaltigen Röntgenkontrastmittels bei Koronar-angiographie – eine prospektive Untersuchung euthyroider Patienten. Z Kardiol 90:751–759

Fassbender WJ, Vogel C, Doppl W et al (2001b) Thyroid function, thyroid immunoglobulin status, and urinary iodine excretion after enteral contrast-agent administration by endoscopic retrograde cholangiopancreatography. Endoscopy 33:245–252

Fricke E, Fricke H, Esdorn E, et al (2004). Scintigraphy for risk stratification of iodine-induced thyrotoxicosis in patients receiving contrast agent for coronary angiography: a prospective study of patients with low thyrotropin. J Clin Endocrinol Metab 89:6092–6096

Gartner W, Weissel M (2004) Do iodine-containing contrast media induce clinically relevant changes in thyroid function parameters of euthyroid patients within the first week? Thyroid 14:521–524

Grainger RG, Pennington GW (1981) A study of the effect of sodium/meglumine ioxaglate (Hexabrix) on thyroid function. Br J Radiol 54:768–772

Hehrmann R, Klein D, Mayer D et al (1996) Hyperthyreoserisiko bei Kontrastmitteluntersuchungen. Aktuel Radiol 6:243–248

Hintze G, Blombach O, Fink H et al (1999) Risk of iodine-induced thyrotoxicosis after coronary angiography: an investigation in 788 unselected subjects. Eur J Endocrinol 140:264–267

Joseph K (1995) Leser fragen – Experten Antworten. Welche Empfehlungen zur Prophylaxe liegen vor für Patienten mit erhöhtem Hyperthyreoserisiko, wenn eine Untersuchung mit jodhaltigen Kontrastmitteln durchgeführt werden müß? Internist 36:1014–1015

Laurie AJ, Lyon SG, Lasser EC (1992) Contrast material iodides: potential effects on radioactive iodine thyroid uptake. J Nucl Med 33:237–238

Lawrence JE, Lamm SH, Braverman LE (1999) The use of perchlorate for the prevention of thyrotoxicosis in patients given iodine rich contrast agents. J Endocrinol Invest 22:405–407

Mann K, Rendl J, Busley R et al (1994) Systemic iodine absorption during endoscopic application of radiographic contrast agents for endoscopic retrograde cholangiopancreaticography. Eur J Endocrinol 130:498–501

Martin FIR, Deam DR (1996) Hyperthyroidism in elderly hospitalized patients. Clinical features and treatment outcomes. Med J Aust 164:200–203

Martin FIR, Tress BW, Colman PG et al (1993) Iodine-induced hyperthyroidism due to nonionic contrast radiography in the elderly. Am J Med 95:78–82

Martin WH, Sandler MP (2003) Thyroid imaging: In: Sandler MP, Coleman RE, Patton JE, Wackers FJT, Gottschalk A (eds) Diagnostic nuclear medicine, 4th edn. Lippincott, Williams and Wilkins, Baltimore, pp 607–651

Mönig H, Arendt T, Eggers S et al (1999) Iodine absorption in patients undergoing ERCP compared with coronary angiography. Gastrointest Endosc 50:79–81

Nolte W, Müller R, Siggelkow H et al (1996) Prophylactic application of thyrostatic drugs during excessive iodine exposure in euthyroid patients with thyroid autonomy: a randomized study. Eur J Endocrinol 134:337–341

Nygaard B, Nygaard T, Jensen LI et al (1998) Iohexol: effects on uptake of radioactive iodine in the thyroid and on thyroid function. Acad Radiol 5:409–414

Rendl J, Saller B (2001) Schilddrüse und Röntgenkontrastmittel: Pathophysiologie, Häufigkeit und Prophylaxe der jodin-duzierten Hyperthyreose. Dtsch Ärztebl 98:A402–A406

Roberts CGP, Ladenson PW (2004) Hypothyroidism. Lancet 363:793–803

Roti E, Uberti ED (2001) Iodine excess and hyperthyroidism. Thyroid 11:493–500

Saam T, Hess T, Kasperk C, Kauffmann GW, Düx M (2005) [Prevalence of latent and manifest hyperthyroidism in an iodine-deficient area: non-selected patient population admitted for CT studies with iodine-containing contrast agents] Rofo Fortschr Roentgenstr 177:1250–1254 [in German]

Stanbury JB, Ermans AE, Bourdoux P et al (1998) Iodine-induced hyperthyroidism: occurence and epidemiology. Thyroid 8:83–100

Stiedle B (1989) Iodine-induced hyperthyroidism after contrast media. Animal experimental and clinical studies. In: Tänzer V, Wend S (eds) Recent developments in nonionic contrast media. Thieme, New York, pp 6–14

Thomsen HS, Almén T, Morcos SK and members of the Contrast Media Safety Committee of the European Society of Urogenital Radiology (2002) Gadolinium-containing contrast media for radiographic examinations: a position paper. Eur Radiol 12:2600–2605

Tuttle RM, Becker DV, Hurley JR (2003) Radioiodine treatment of thyroid disease: In: Sandler MP, Coleman RE, Patton JE, Wackers FJT, Gottschalk A (eds) Diagnostic nuclear medicine, 4th edn. Lippincott, Baltimore, pp 653–670

Van der Molen AJ, Thomsen HS, Morcos SK, and members of the Contrast Media Safety Committee of the European Society of Urogenital Radiology (2004) Effect of iodinated contrast media on thyroid function in adults. Eur Radiol 14:902–907

Van Guldener C, Blom DM, Lips P et al (1998) Hyperthyre-oidie door jodiumhoudende röntgencontrastmiddelen. Ned Tijdschr Geneeskd 142: 1641–1644

Vitti P, Delange F, Pinchera A et al (2003) Europe is iodine deficient. Lancet 361:1226

Wilson GA, O'Mara RE (1997) Uptake tests, thyroid and whole body imaging with isotopes: In: Falk SA (ed) Thyroid disease: endocrinology, surgery, nuclear medicine and radiotherapy. Lippincott-Raven, Philadelpha, pp 113–133

Pulmonary Effects

19

Sameh K. Morcos

CONTENTS

19.1 Introduction   *147*

19.2 Effects of Contrast Media on Airways
Resistance   *147*

19.3 Effects of Contrast Media on Pulmonary
Circulation   *149*

19.4 Contrast Medium-Induced Pulmonary
Edema   *150*

References   *150*

Introduction

The lung is an important target organ for the effects of water-soluble radiographic contrast media. The pulmonary circulation is the first important vascular bed exposed to contrast medium following intravenous injection and during the venous return after arteriographic examinations (Morcos 2003). Several adverse pulmonary effects may follow the intravascular injection of contrast media, including bronchospasm, pulmonary arterial hypertension, and pulmonary edema (Morcos 2000, 2003). In this chapter the effects of contrast media on airways resistance and pulmonary circulation following intravascular administration are discussed.

Sameh K. Morcos
Department of Diagnostic Imaging, Northern General Hospital NHS Trust, Sheffield S5 7AU, UK

Effects of Contrast Media on Airways Resistance

The adverse respiratory reactions that have been reported with the intravascular use of contrast media include apnea, dyspnea, and bronchospasm (Morcos 2000, 2003; Littner et al. 1977, 1981; Dawson et al. 1983a; Longstaff and Henson 1985; Wilson and Davis 1988). Bronchospasm has been reported to be a contributory factor in 23% of moderate and 5% of severe adverse reactions to intravascular administration of radiographic contrast media (Morcos 2003). While symptomatic bronchospasm is rare, occurring in 0.01% of patients (Morcos 2003), subclinical bronchospasm, detected by a fall in forced expiratory volume in 1 s (FEV1), is common. It tends to be less pronounced with low-osmolar nonionic contrast media (Littner et al. 1977, 1981; Dawson et al. 1983a; Longstaff and Henson 1985). However, Wilson and Davies (1988) found that both high-osmolar ionic and low-osmolar nonionic contrast media produce a comparable fall in FEV_1 and forced vital capacity. Experimental studies in the guinea pig found that the high-osmolar ionic monomer diatrizoate, the low-osmolar nonionic monomer iopromide, and the iso-osmolar nonionic dimer iotrolan did not induce significant increase in airways resistance, and only the low-osmolar ionic dimer ioxaglate caused bronchospasm (Table 19.1) (Cipolla et al. 1995; Laude et al. 1999). Some retrospective clinical studies have also documented a higher incidence of allergy-like reactions with ioxaglate in comparison to other types of contrast media (Lasser et al. 1997; Greenberger and Patterson 1991; Laroche et al. 1998). However, there are no prospective clinical studies that have confirmed these observations. In one prospective clinical study,

Table 19.1. Summary of the different pulmonary effects of different classes of iodinated contrast media

Effect	Most marked with following categories of contrast medium	Mechanism
Bronchospasm (LITTNER et al. 1981; LONGSTAFF and HENSON 1985; CIPOLLA et al. 1995; LAUDE et al. 1999)	Low-osmolar ionic dimer High-osmolar ionic monomer	Remains unknown
Pulmonary edema (MORCOS 2003; MARE et al. 1984; SENDO et al. 2000; TOMINAGA et al. 2001; HAUGGAARD 1996; PAUL and GEORGE 2002)	Low-osmolar ionic dimer High-osmolar ionic monomer	Endothelial injury Fluid overload in cardiac patients
Increase in pulmonary vascular resistance (EMERY et al. 2001; WANG et al. 1997; DAWSON et al. 1983; LISS et al. 1996; SPITZER et al. 1999)	High-osmolar ionic monomer Low-osmolar ionic dimer Iso-osmolar nonionic dimer	Vasoconstriction Pulmonary edema Rheological effects on red blood cells
Histamine release from lung mast cells (PEACHELL and MORCOS 1998)	High-osmolar ionic monomer	Direct effect on the mast cells Complement activation
Histamine release from basophils (ASSEM et al. 1991; PEACHELL and MORCOS 1998)	High-osmolar ionic monomer Low-osmolar ionic dimer Iso-osmolar nonionic dimer	Direct effect on basophils Complement activation

ioxaglate was found to be less likely than conventional high-osmolar agents to produce coughing during pulmonary arteriography (SMITH et al. 1987).

The pathophysiology of the changes in airways resistance induced by contrast media remains obscure and could be multifactorial. The underlying mechanism may involve the release of bronchospastic mediators (such as histamine, endothelin (ET), 5-hydroxytryptamine, prostaglandins, thromboxane, and bradykinin), cholinesterase inhibition, vagal reflex, or a direct effect on the bronchi (DAWSON et al. 1983a; LAUDE et al. 1999; ASSEM et al. 1991; PEACHELL and MORCOS 1998; SZOLAR et al. 1995a, b; LASSER et al. 1971; RING and SOVAK 1981). Contrast media can cause the release of histamine, a potent bronchoconstrictor, from mast cells and basophils through a direct effect and indirectly by activating the complement system (ASSEM et al. 1991; PEACHELL and MORCOS 1998). In vitro studies showed dose-dependent histamine release from human lung mast cells and basophils in response to all types of contrast media (ASSEM et al. 1991; PEACHELL and MORCOS 1998). The high-osmolar diatrizoate induced the largest histamine release from human basophils and human lung mast cells. Ioxaglate and iotrolan caused histamine release from human basophils but not from human lung mast cells. The low-osmolar nonionic monomer iopromide was a relatively ineffective activator of histamine release from both human lung mast cells and basophils (Table 19.1) (PEACHELL and MORCOS 1998). The

importance of histamine in causing contrast media-induced bronchospasm has not been proved conclusively. Experimental studies have shown that pretreatment with antihistamine H1 receptor antagonist did not prevent contrast media-induced increase in airways resistance (CIPOLLA et al. 1995; LAUDE et al. 1999). Pretreatment with prednisolone did not offer any protection against contrast media-induced bronchospasm in spite of using the two-dose regime recommended by LASSER et al. (1987) (CIPOLLA et al. 1995; LAUDE et al. 1999; LASSER 1981, 1994, 1998). The use of corticosteroid prophylaxis in preventing contrast media reactions including bronchospasm is controversial. It has been suggested that the use of nonionic agents alone is better in preventing all categories of reactions than the use of high-osmolar ionic agents with corticosteroid prophylaxis (DAWSON and SIDHU 1993; WOLF et al. 1991).

The role of endothelin (ET) in mediating the bronchospastic effects of contrast media has also been investigated (LAUDE et al. 1999). ET is a potent smooth-muscle constrictor and produces an increase in the vascular resistance and marked bronchospasm in the lung (LAUDE et al. 1999; OLDROYD and MORCOS 2000). A pharmacologically effective dose of nonselective ET antagonist provided no protection against iodinated contrast media-induced bronchospasm in the guinea pig (LAUDE et al. 1999).

Leakage of fluids from the microcirculation into the lung tissues and bronchi may also cause an increase in airways resistance. Experimental studies in the guinea pig did not show fluid accumulation in the lungs and the bronchi in association with contrast medium-induced rise in airways resistance (LAUDE et al. 1999). Also, aerosolized β_2-adrenergic agonist treatment was able to reverse contrast medium-induced increases in airways resistance completely, suggesting that any airway narrowing resulting from edema is minimal (CIPOLLA et al. 1995; LAUDE et al. 1999).

A role for cholinesterase inhibition or the vagal reflex in mediating contrast medium-induced bronchospasm has not been confirmed. A direct effect of contrast medium on bronchial smooth muscle cells is possible, and the contribution of other bronchospastic mediators such as leucotrienes and kinins requires further investigation.

Effects of Contrast Media on Pulmonary Circulation

An increase in pulmonary artery pressure has been reported following the intravascular injection of contrast media (FRISINGER et al. 1965; MILLS et al. 1980; PECK et al. 1983; SCHRADER et al. 1987; NICOD et al. 1987; REES et al. 1988; TAJIMA et al. 1994; PITTON et al. 1996; ALMEN et al. 1980; SUNNEGARDH et al. 1990; SORENSON et al. 1994). This sudden increase in pulmonary artery pressure is thought to contribute to the morbidity and mortality associated with pulmonary angiography, particularly in patients suffering from pulmonary hypertension (SCHRADER et al. 1987; NICOD et al. 1987; REES et al. 1988; TAJIMA et al. 1994; PITTON et al. 1996). There are conflicting reports in the literature about the mechanisms responsible for these effects (PECK et al. 1983; SCHRADER et al. 1984, 1987; REES et al. 1988; ALMEN et al. 1980; SUNNEGARDH et al. 1990; SORENSON et al. 1994; KUHTZ-BUSCHBECK et al. 1997; EMERY et al. 2001).

Some studies showed that the rise in pulmonary artery pressure is secondary to an increase in pulmonary vascular resistance (PVR) (SCHRADER et al. 1984; EMERY et al. 2001), whereas others indicated that it is due to an increase in cardiac output associated with a decrease in pulmonary vascular resistance (ALMEN et al. 1980; SUNNEGARDH et al. 1990; SORENSON et al. 1994; KUHTZ-BUSCHBECK et al. 1997). In the studies that suggested a fall in the vascular resistance, the pulmonary vascular resistance

was not directly measured and was calculated from the formula *pulmonary vascular resistance = (pulmonary artery pressure – pulmonary venous pressure)/ cardiac output*. The increase in cardiac output was attributed to reduced peripheral vascular resistance of the systemic circulation caused by contrast medium-induced vasodilatation (PECK et al. 1983; SCHRADER et al. 1987; ALMEN et al. 1980; SUNNEGARDH et al. 1990; SORENSON et al. 1994; KUHTZ-BUSCHBECK et al. 1997). The fall in pulmonary vascular resistance could be due to an increase in the capacity of the pulmonary vascular bed by recruitment of closed vessels and active vasodilatation of pulmonary arteries (EMERY et al. 2001). Experimental studies have shown that contrast media can induce both dilatation and constriction of pulmonary arteries, but in systemic vascular beds they induce mainly vasodilatation except in the kidney where vasoconstriction predominates (MORCOS et al. 1998; WANG et al. 1997; MORCOS 1998).

In the isolated blood-perfused lung of the normal rat, iodinated contrast media (iotrolan, iopromide, ioxaglate, and diatrizoate) and hypertonic solutions of mannitol caused an overall rise in pulmonary artery pressure, reflecting an increase in the pulmonary vascular resistance. The maximum increase in pulmonary artery pressure was observed with the ionic dimer ioxaglate and the least increase with the nonionic monomer iopromide (EMERY et al. 2001). In isolated lungs from chronically hypoxic rats, where baseline pulmonary artery pressure and resistance are high, a slow rise in pulmonary artery pressure was observed in response to the contrast media (ioxaglate, iotrolan, and iopromide) (EMERY et al. 2001). The rise observed in pulmonary artery pressure with ioxaglate was comparable to that of iotrolan but significantly greater than that with iopromide (EMERY et al. 2001).

Surprisingly, the iso-osmolar iotrolan with the lowest vasoactivity induced a significant increase in the pulmonary vascular resistance of the isolated blood-perfused lung of both the normal and chronic hypoxic rat (EMERY et al. 2001). High viscosity and rheological effects on red blood cells of iotrolan could be responsible for the observed increase in the vascular resistance of the isolated lung preparation, which is perfused with blood (Table 19.1) (EMERY et al. 2001). The nonionic monomer iopromide had the least effect on pulmonary vascular resistance of both the normotensive and hypertensive rat lung preparation (EMERY et al. 2001). This is understandable as iopromide has low vasoactive properties including low viscosity. Its effects on the endothelium are minimal and unlikely to cause pulmonary edema leading to an increase in pulmonary vascular resistance (EMERY et al. 2001; ZHANG et al. 2000). Clinical experience has also shown the absence of major hemodynamic effects with the use of low-osmolar nonionic monomers in pulmonary angiography even in patients with pulmonary hypertension (ZUCKERMAN et al. 1996; NILSSON et al. 1998).

The increase in pulmonary vascular resistance induced by contrast media is most likely caused by a combination of active vasoconstriction of the pulmonary arteries, pulmonary edema, and possibly also by increased blood viscosity (WANG et al. 1997; DAWSON et al. 1983b; LISS et al. 1996; SPITZER et al. 1999). The increased blood viscosity could be secondary to cellular effects (increased aggregation of red blood cells with nonionic media and rigidity with high-osmolar solutions) and the high viscosity of some of the contrast agents (DAWSON et al. 1983b; LISS et al. 1996; SPITZER et al. 1999). Contrast media may also activate adhesion of leucocytes to the endothelium, causing capillary plugging and stasis of red blood cells in the small vessels precipitating an increase in vascular resistance (EMERY et al. 2001).

In summary, iodinated contrast media can induce an increase in pulmonary vascular resistance and rise in pulmonary artery pressure through direct effects on the pulmonary circulation. Nonionic monomers produce the least increase in pulmonary artery pressure. The mechanisms responsible for the rise in pulmonary artery pressure remain poorly defined.

19.4
Contrast Medium-Induced Pulmonary Edema

Contrast medium-induced pulmonary edema is often secondary to endothelial injury, leading to an increase in the permeability of the microcirculation and accumulation of fluid in the lung (MORCOS 2003).

Pulmonary edema produced by contrast media could also be responsible for the increase in the pulmonary vascular resistance and rise in pulmonary artery pressure caused by these agents. Experimental studies have shown that ioxaglate, which induced the largest increase in the pulmonary vascular resistance of the isolated rat lung preparation, is more cytotoxic

to the vascular endothelium than diatrizoate and nonionic media (see Table 19.1) (EMERY et al. 2001; ZHANG et al. 2000; BENYON et al. 1994). Ioxaglate induced greater pulmonary edema in the rat than nonionic monomeric contrast media (MARE et al. 1984; SENDO et al. 2000; TOMINAGA et al. 2001). Interestingly, in the rat nitric oxide (SENDO et al. 2000) and estrogen (TOMINAGA et al. 2001) offered some protection against ioxaglate-induced pulmonary edema.

Pulmonary edema may also occur in patients with incipient cardiac failure, when large doses of contrast medium, particularly of high-osmolar agents, are used (MORCOS 2003; FRISINGER et al. 1965). Pulmonary edema has been reported in 10–20% of cases of fatal reaction to intravenous infusion of contrast media (HAUGGAARD 1996; PAUL and GEORGE 2002). Subclinical pulmonary edema without obvious signs or symptoms of respiratory distress is thought to be common after intra-vascular contrast media administration but its true incidence is difficult to establish (MORCOS 2003).

References

Almen T, Aspelin P, Nilsson P (1980) Aortic and pulmonary arterial pressure after injection of contrast media into the right atrium of the rabbit. Acta Radiol [Suppl] 362:37–41

Assem ES, Bray K, Dawson P (1991) The release of histamine from human basophils by radiological contrast agents. Br J Radiol 56:695–712

Benyon HLC, Walport MJ, Dawson P (1994) Vascular endothelial injury by intravascular contrast agents. Invest Radiol 29 [Suppl 2]:195–197

Cipolla P, Castano M, Kirchin MA, de Haen C, Tirone P (1995) Effects of iodinated contrast media on pulmonary airway resistance in anesthetized guinea pigs. Acad Radiol 2:306–312

Dawson P, Sidhu PS (1993) Is there a role for corticosteroid prophylaxis in patients at increased risk of adverse reactions to intravascular contrast agents? Clin Radiol 48:225–226

Dawson P, Pitfield J, Britain J (1983a) Contrast media and bronchospasm: a study with iopamidol. Clin Radiol 34:227–230

Dawson P, Harrison MJ, Weisblatt E (1983b) Effects of contrast media on red cell filterability and morphology. Br J Radiol 56:707–710

Emery CJ, Fang L, Laude EA, Morcos SK (2001) Effects of radiographic contrast media on pulmonary vascular resistance of normoxic and chronically hypoxic pulmonary hypertensive rats. Br J Radiol 74:1109–1117

Frisinger G, Schaffer J, Criley M, Gartner R, Ross J (1965) Haemodynamic consequences of the injection of radiopaque material. Circulation 31:730–740

Greenberger PA, Patterson R (1991) The prevention of immediate generalized reactions to radiocontrast media in high-risk patients. J Allergy Clin Immunol 87:867–872

Hauggaard A (1996) Non-cardiogenic pulmonary oedema after intravenous administration of nonionic contrast media. Acta Radiol 37:823–825

Kuhtz-Buschbeck JP, Ehrhardt K, Kohnlein S, Radtke W, Heintzen P (1997) Gadopentetate dimeglumine and iodinated contrast media. Haemodynamic side effects after bolus injection in pigs. Invest Radiol 32:111–119

Laroche D, Aimone-Gastin, Dubois F et al (1998) Mechanisms of severe immediate reactions to iodinated contrast material. Radiology 209:183–190

Lasser EC (1981) Adverse reactions to intravascular administration of contrast media. Allergy 36:369–373

Lasser EC (1998) Pretreatment with corticosteroids to prevent reactions to IV contrast material: overview and implications. AJR Am J Roentgenol 150:257–259

Lasser EC, Walter A, Reuter SR, Lang I (1971) Histamine release by contrast media. Radiology 100:683–686

Lasser EC, Berry CC, Talner LB et al (1987) Pretreatment with corticosteroids to alleviate reactions to intravenous contrast material. N Engl J Med 317:845–849

Lasser EC, Berry CC, Mishkin MM, Williamson B, Zheutlin N, Silverman JM (1994) Pretreatment with corticosteroids to prevent adverse reactions to nonionic contrast media. AJR Am J Roentgenol 162:523–526

Lasser EC, Lyon SG, Berry CC (1997) Reports on contrast media reactions: analysis of data from reports to the US Food and Drug Administration. Radiology 203:605–610 (erratum 876)

Laude EA, Emery CJ, Suvarna SK, Morcos SK (1999) The effect of antihistamine, endothelin antagonist and corticosteroid prophylaxis on contrast media induced bronchospasm. Br J Radiol 72:1058–1063

Liss P, Nygren A, Olsson U, Ulfendahl HR, Erikson U (1996) Effects of contrast media and mannitol on renal medullary blood flow and red cell aggregation in the rat kidney. Kidney Int 49:1268–1275

Littner MR, Rosenfield AT, Ulreich S, Putman CE (1977) Evaluation of bronchospasm during excretory urography. Radiology 124:17–21

Littner MR, Ulreich S, Putman CE, Rosenfield AT, Meadows G (1981) Bronchospasm during excretory urography: lack of specificity for the methyl glucamine. AJR Am J Roentgenol 137:477–481

Longstaff AJ, Henson JHL (1985) Bronchospasm following intravenous injection of ionic and nonionic low osmolality contrast media. Clin Radiol 36:651–653

Mare K, Violante M, Zack A (1984) Contrast media induced pulmonary edema. Comparison of ionic and nonionic agents in an animal model. Invest Radiol 19:566–5699

Mills SR, Jackson BF, Older RA, Heaston DK, Moore AV (1980) The incidence, aetiologies and avoidance of complications of pulmonary angiography in a large series. Radiology 136:295–299

Morcos SK (1998) Contrast media-induced nephrotoxicity-questions and answers. Br J Radiol 71:357–365

Morcos SK (2000) Radiological contrast media. In: Dukes MNG, Aronson JK (eds) Meyler's side effects of drugs, 14th edn, chap 46.1. Elsevier Science, Amsterdam, pp 1596–1630

Morcos SK (2003) Effects of radiographic contrast media on the lung. Br J Radiol 76:290–295

Morcos SK, Dawson P, Pearson JD et al (1998) The haemodynamic effects of iodinated water soluble radiographic contrast media: a review. Eur J Radiol 29:31–46

Nicod P, Peterson K, Levine M et al (1987) Pulmonary angiography in severe chronic pulmonary hypertension. Ann Intern Med 107:565–568

Nilsson T, Carlsson A, Mare K (1998) Pulmonary angiography: a safe procedure with modern contrast media and technique. Eur Radiol 8:86–89

Oldroyd SD, Morcos SK (2000) Endothelin: what does the radiologist need to know? Br J Radiol 73:1246–125

Paul RE, George G (2002) Fatal non-cardiogenic pulmonary oedema after intravenous nonionic radiographic contrast. Lancet 359:1037–1038

Peachell P, Morcos SK (1998) Effect of radiographic contrast media on histamine release from human mast cells and basophils. Br J Radiol 71:24–30

Peck WW, Slutsky RA, Hackney DB et al (1983) Effects of contrast media on pulmonary hemodynamics: comparison of ionic and nonionic agents. Radiology 149:371–374

Pitton MB, Duber C, Mayer E, Thelen M (1996) Hemodynamic effects of nonionic contrast bolus injection and oxygen inhalation during pulmonary angiography in patients with chronic major vessel thromboembolic pulmonary hypertension. Circulation 94:2485–2491

Rees CR, Palmaz JC, Garcia O, Alvarado R, Siegle RL (1988) The hemodynamic effects of the administration of ionic and nonionic contrast material into the pulmonary arteries of a canine Model of acute pulmonary hypertension. Invest Radiol 23:184–189

Ring J, Sovak M (1981) Release of serotonin from human platelets in vitro by radiographic contrast media. Invest Radiol 16:245–248

Schrader R, Wolpers HG, Korb H et al (1984) Central venous injection of large amounts of contrast media – advantages of low osmolar contrast medium in experimentally induced pulmonary hypertension. Z Kardiol 73:434–441

Schrader R, Hellige G, Kaltenbach M, Kober G (1987) The haemodynamic side-effects of ionic and nonionic contrast media in the presence of pulmonary hypertension: experimental and clinical investigation. Eur Heart J 8:1322–1331

Sendo T, Kataoka Y, Takeda Y, Furuta W, Oishi R (2000) Nitric oxide protects against contrast media-induced pulmonary vascular permeability in rats. Invest Radiol 35:427–428

Smith DC, Lois JF, Gomes AS, Maloney MD, Yahiku PY (1987) Pulmonary angiography: comparison of cough stimulation effects of diatrizoate and ioxaglate. Radiology 162:617–618

Sorenson L, Sunnegardh O, Svanegard J, Lundquist S, Hietala SO (1994) Systemic and pulmonary haemodynamic effects of intravenous infusion of nonionic isoosmolar dimeric contrast media. An investigation in the pig of two ratio 6 contrast media. Acta Radiol 35:383–390

Spitzer S, Munster W, Sternitzky R, Bach R, Jung F (1999) Influence of iodixanol-270 and iopentol-150 on the microcirculation in man: influence of viscosity on capillary perfusion. Clin Hemorheol 20:49–55

Sunnegardh O, Hietala SO, Wierell S et al (1990) Systemic, pulmonary and renal haemodynamic effects of intravenously infused Iopental. A comparison in the pig of a new low osmolar nonionic medium with saline and iohexol. Acta Radiol 31:395–399

Szolar DH, Saeed M, Flueckiger F et al (1995a) Effects of Iopromide on vasoactive peptides and allergy-mediated substances in healthy volunteers. Invest Radiol 30:144–149

Szolar DH, Saeed M, Flueckiger F et al (1995b) Response of vasoactive peptides to a nonionic contrast media in patients undergoing pulmonary angiography. Invest Radiol 30:511–516

Tajima H, Kumazaki T, Tajima N, Murakami R, Gemma K (1994) Effect of iohexol on pulmonary arterial pressure at pulmonary angiography in patients with pulmonary hypertension. Radiat Med 12:197–199

Tominaga K, Kataoka Y, Sendo T, Furuta W, Niizeki M, Oishi AR (2001) Contrast media-induced pulmonary vascular hyperpermeability is aggravated in a rat climacterium model. Invest Radiol 36:131–135

Wang YX, Emery CJ, Laude E, Morcos SK (1997) Effects of radiocontrast media on the tension of isolated small pulmonary arteries. Br J Radiol 70:1229–1238

Wilson ARM, Davis P (1988) Ventilatory function during urography: a comparison of iopamidol and sodium iosalamate. Clin Radiol 39:490–493

Wolf GL, Mishkin MM, Roux SG et al (1991) Comparison of the rates of adverse drug reactions. Ionic agents, ionic agents combined with steroids and nonionic agents. Invest Radiol 26:404–410

Zhang H, Holt CM, Malik N, Shepherd L, Morcos SK (2000) Effects of radiographic contrast media on proliferation and apoptosis of human vascular endothelial cells. Br J Radiol 73:1034–1041

Zuckerman DA, Sterling KM, Oser RF (1996) Safety of pulmonary angiography in the 1990s. J Vasc Interv Radiol 7:199–205

MRContrast Media

Non-Tissue Specific Extracellular MR Contrast Media

Chelates and Stability

Chelates and Stability

Sameh K. Morcos

CONTENTS

20.1
Introduction

Extracellular gadolinium-based MRI contrast media are all chelates containing Gd ions (Gd^{3+}). Free gadolinium is highly toxic and can cause splenic degeneration, central lobular necrosis of the liver, enzyme inhibition, calcium channel blocking and a variety of haematological abnormalities (Dawson 1999; Desreux and Gilsoul 1999). Therefore, it is crucially important that Gd^{3+} should be strongly attached to a chelate to avoid its toxic effects.

There are seven extracellular gadolinium-based contrast agents currently available for clinical use (Table 20.1) (Idee et al. 2006; Morcos 2007). The configuration of the molecule is either linear or cyclic and they are available as ionic or nonionic preparations. There are differences in the chemical stability of these agents and in their liability to release

Sameh K. Morcos
Department of Diagnostic Imaging, Northern General
Hospital, Sheffield Teaching Hospitals NHS Trust,
Sheffield S5 7AU, UK

free gadolinium ions. Recently, there is increasing evidence that the instability of Gd-contrast agents could be an important factor in the pathogenesis of the serious complication of nephrogenic systemic fibrosis (NSF) (Morcos 2007).

In this chapter the chemical structure of Gd-contrast agents is discussed, highlighting the important features that determine the stability of the molecules. Methods to assess the stability of these agents are presented. The relevance of the stability of Gd-contrast agents to the development of NSF is addressed.

20.2
Chemistry

The chemical principles involved in the production of Gd-chelates are presented in a simplified manner but with the intention of not compromising scientific accuracy. The gadolinium ion has nine coordination sites. *Coordination sites represent the number of atoms or ligands directly bonded to the metal centre such as Gd^{3+}. A **ligand** is a molecule or atom that is bonded directly to a metal centre. The bonding between the metal centre (Gd^{3+}) and the ligands is through **valent bonds** in which shared electron pairs are donated to the metal ion by the ligand.* In an ionic linear molecule such as Gd-DTPA (Magnevist, Bayer Schering Pharma AG, Berlin, Germany), Gd^{3+} is coordinated with five carboxyl groups and three amino nitrogen atoms. The remaining vacant site is coordinated with a water molecule which is important in enhancing the signal by the contrast agent in T1 weighted MR imaging (Dawson 1999; Desreux and Gilsoul 1999; Morcos 2007; Rofsky et al. 2008). The three negatively charged carboxyl groups neutralise the three positive charges of the Gd ion and the remaining two carboxyl groups are neutralised by

Table 20.1. Stability measurements of clinically available extracellular Gd-contrast agents (Morcos 2007)

Extracellular Gd-CM	Type	Thermodynamic stability constant	Conditional stability	Amount of excess chelate (mg ml⁻¹)	Kinetic stability (dissociation half life at pH 1.0)
Gadoversetamide, Gd-DTPA-BMEA (OptiMark, Tyco, USA)	Nonionic linear	16.6	15	28.4	Not available
Gadodiamide, Gd-DTPA-BMA (Omniscan, GE, USA)	Nonionic linear	16.9	14.9	12	35 s
Gadobutrol, Gd-BT-DO3A (Gadovist, Schering, Berlin)	Nonionic cyclic	21.8	Not available	Not available	24 h
Gadoteridol, Gd-HP-DO3A (ProHance, Bracco, Italy)	Nonionic cyclic	23.8	17.1	0.23	3 h
Gadopentetate Gd-DTPA (Magnevist, Schering, Berlin)	Ionic linear	22.1	18.1	0.4	10 min
Gadobenate, Gd-BOPTA, (Multihance, Bracco, Italy)	Ionic linear	22.6	18.4	None	Not available
Gadoterate, Gd-DOTA (Dotarem, Guerbet, France)	Ionic cyclic	25.8	18.8	None	>1 month

two meglumine cations (Dawson 1999). In a nonionic linear molecule such as gadodiamide (Omniscan, GE Healthcare, Chalfont St. Giles, UK) or gadoversetamide (OptiMark, Covidien, St Louis, USA), the number of carboxyl groups is reduced to three because each of the other two carboxyl groups has been replaced by a nonionic methyl amide (Dawson 1999). Although both amide carbonyl atoms are directly coordinated to Gd³⁺, the binding is weaker in comparison to that with carboxyl groups. This weakens the grip of the nonionic chelate on the Gd³⁺ and decreases the stability of the complex (Dawson 1999; Desreux and Gilsoul 1999; Morcos 2007).

The other feature that influences the binding between the Gd³⁺ and the chelate is whether the configuration of the molecule is cyclic or linear. The macrocyclic molecule offers better protection and binding of Gd³⁺ by virtue of being a preorganised rigid ring of almost optimal size to cage the Gd ion. In contrast, the linear structure which is a flexible open chain provides weaker protection of the Gd ion (Idee et al. 2006; Morcos 2007). All the macrocyclic agents available for clinical use, whether ionic or nonionic, are derived from a 12-membered macrocyclic polyaminocarboxylate ring (Brücher and Sherry 2001). The number and identity of the side chains affect the stability of these agents and a minimum of three carboxylate side groups is necessary to form reasonably stable Gd-complexes (Fig. 20.1).

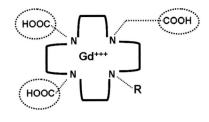

Gd-DOTA   (Dotarem)   **R= COOH**
Gd-HP-DO3A   (ProHance) **R= Hydroxy**
Gd-BT-DO3A   (Gadovist) **R= Dihydroxypropyl**

Fig. 20.1. The chemical structure of macrocyclic Gd-contrast agents. All the macrocyclic agents available for clinical use have three carboxylate side groups (COOH). The difference between these agents is related to the fourth side chain (R)

Because of charge neutralisation in the complexation process, lanthanides prefer carboxylate donor atoms rather than etherial or alcoholic oxygens (Tweedle 1992; Kumar 1997). The negatively charged carboxylate oxygens are more powerful donor atoms than are uncharged hydroxyl oxygen atoms (Tweedle 1992). Using the ionic macrocyclic complex Gd-DOTA (Dotarem, Guerbet, Paris, France) which has four carboxylate side groups as a reference, when one carboxylate group is replaced with a hydroxy-propyl group [Gd-DOTA to Gd-HP-DO3A (ProHance, Bracco, Milan, Italy)], the stability and binding constants decrease (BRÜCHER and SHERRY 2001; TWEEDLE 1992). The replacement of the sterically uncrowded hydroxypropyl group of Gd-HP-DO3A with the bulky 2,3-dihydroxy-(1-hydroxymethyl)-propyl group to form Gd-BT-DO3A (Gadovist, Bayer Schering Pharma AG, Berlin, Germany) results in further destabilization of the complex. The bulky side chain destabilizes binding interaction between Gd^{3+} and each of the three car-boxylate side arms (KUMAR 1997). The bulky chain is also more acidic than the hydroxypropyl group and weakens the binding with Gd^{3+}. Lanthanides such as Gd^{3+} behave like typical "hard" acids and interact preferentially with hard bases rather than with softer bases (BRÜCHER and SHERRY 2001; KUMAR 1997). Therefore, increasing the acidity of the side chain decreases the stability of the Gd-chelate (BRÜCHER and SHERRY 2001; KUMAR 1997). According to these chemical principles, the stability of the three available macrocyclic agents follows the order of DOTA > HP-DO3A > BT-DO3A (MORCOS 2007). However, it is fair to state that all macrocyclic agents available for clinical use are quite stable in comparison to the linear gadolinium chelates. For the Gd^{3+} to break free from a macrocy-clic chelate, it must simultaneously break 5–6 coor-dination sites. On the other hand, Gd^{3+} can break free easily from the linear chelate as the separation occurs sequentially (GIBBY et al. 2004).

20.3

In Vitro Measurements to Assess Stability

The following measurements are used to assess the stability of the chelate molecules:

the thermodynamic stability constant (measured under very alkaline conditions (pH ~ 11), because at this pH there are no competing hydrogen ions for the chelate and a theoretical maximum stability for the chelate is obtained), *the conditional stability constant* (measured at physiological pH of 7.4) and *the kinetic stability* (dissociation half life under very acidic condi-tions (pH 1)) (GIBBY et al. 2004; ROFSKY et al. 2008). The details of how to obtain these measurements are beyond the scope of this chapter. The higher the value of these measurements, the higher is the stability of the molecule (IDEE et al. 2006; MORCOS 2007).

The amount of excess chelate in the Gd-contrast agent preparations is another marker of the stability of these agents. A large amount of excess chelate is

Table 20.2. Dissociation half life ($T\frac{1}{2}$) of Gd-contrast agents under the same laboratory conditions (PORT et al. 2008)

Gd-contrast agents	$T\frac{1}{2}$, pH 1.2	$T\frac{1}{2}$, pH 1	$T\frac{1}{2}$, pH 1
Temp	37°	37°	25°
Dotarem (Guerbet, France)	85 h	23 h	338 h
Gadovist ((Bayer Schering Pharma AG, Germany),	18 h	7 h	43 h
ProHance (Bracco, Italy)	4 h	1.6 h	3.9 h
All linear chelates	ND	ND	<5 s

present in Gd-contrast agents of low stability (GREEN and KRESTIN 2006). The excess chelate is included in the preparation to ensure the absence of free Gd^{3+} in solution. The addition of excess chelate to gadodi-amide (nonionic linear chelate) dramatically reduces the acute toxicity of non-formulated preparations (no excess chelate) by a factor of 2.5 as demonstrated by acute toxicity studies (intravenous LD_{50}) (IDEE et al. 2006).

As expected from the chemical structure, the stabi-lity measurements confirm the superior stability of the ionic macrocyclic chelate and the low stability of the nonionic linear chelates (MORCOS 2007). The former has the highest stability values and the longest dissociation half life and no excess chelate is required in the commercial preparation (Table 20.1). In contrast, the nonionic linear chelates have a short dissociation half life, the lowest stability values, and the highest amount of excess chelate (Table 20.1) (MORCOS 2007). A recent study evaluating the disso-ciation half life ($T\frac{1}{2}$) of Gd-contrast agents under the same laboratory conditions confirmed that the ionic macrocyclic chelate has the highest kinetic stability followed by the nonionic macrocyclic chelates (PORT et al. 2008). The linear chelates had the lowest kinetic stability in this study (Table 20.2).

20.4

In Vivo Measurements to Assess Stability

There are several factors in vivo such as endogenous ions, enzymes and other biological elements that may work simultaneously to dissociate the Gd-chelate with unpredictable effects. Therefore, it has been suggested that ex-vivo data are not reliable to predict the behaviour of Gd-contrast agents in vivo as the conditions under which these measurements are obtained are different from those occurring in vivo (TWEEDLE 2007). However, dissociation half life under acidic conditions has been accepted as a reliable ex-vivo measurement that can predict the stability of these agents in vivo (WEDEKING et al. 1992).

Retention of Gd in tissues has been used to assess the stability of Gd-CM in vivo. Once the Gd cation is dissociated from the chelate, it is immediately carried away by endogenous anions such as citrates and phosphates and is deposited in the body tissues. Once within the tissues, Gd can persist for long periods of time. On the other hand, virtually all the injected Gd chelate would have been eliminated from the body by 5 days after administration. Therefore, most of the Gd detected in the body 3–8 days after administration of a Gd-contrast agent is likely to have been released from the original chelate (GIBBY et al. 2004). Thus, the higher the retention of Gd in tissues, the lower is the stability of the Gd-contrast agent.

Animal studies in vivo in rats and mice with normal renal function showed that Gd retention in tissues 2 weeks after injection of the nonionic linear chelate gadodiamide was three times greater than that observed with the ionic linear chelate Gd-DTPA. Gd retention in tissues was minimal with the tested macrocyclic agents Gd-DOTA and Gd-HP-DO3A, and the least retention was observed with the nonionic macrocyclic agent Gd-HP-DO3A (WEDEKING et al. 1992; TWEEDLE et al. 1995). Clinical studies have also showed that gadodiamide leaves 2–4 times more Gd^{3+} in the bone than Gd-HP-DO3A in patients with normal renal function (WHITE et al. 2006).

In summary, in vivo data have confirmed the ex vivo measurements, which indicate that the least stable agents are the nonionic linear chelates. However, in vivo data did not identify any difference in stability between the ionic and nonionic macrocyclic agents, although in vitro data suggest that the ionic macrocyclic agent Gd-DOTA is the most stable Gd-contrast agent. Further studies in vivo using suitable animal models of chronic renal impairment are required to elucidate whether the differences in the stability of these agents are important in vivo under biological conditions similar to those of patients with marked reduction in renal function.

Transmetallation

Transmetallation of Gd-CM leads to release of free gadolinium by replacement of the Gd^{3+} within the chelate molecule by body cations such as iron, copper, zinc and calcium (LAURENT et al. 2001). Only zinc can displace a significant amount of Gd^{3+}, because its concentration in the blood is relatively high (55–125 µmol L^{-1}) whereas copper is present in very small amounts (1–10 µmol L^{-1}) and calcium ions have low affinity to organic ligands (LAURENT et al. 2001). Iron ions are tightly bound by the storage proteins ferritin and haemosiderin and are not available for transmetallation with Gd^{3+} (CACHERIS et al. 1990). Transmetallation between Gd^{3+} and zinc results in the formation of zinc chelate, which is excreted in urine. The released Gd^{3+} becomes attached to endogenous anions such as phosphate, citrate, hydroxide or carbonate, which deposit in the tissues as insoluble compounds (Fig. 20.2) (GIBBY et al. 2004). In vivo (COROT et al. 1998), in vitro (LAURENT et al. 2001, 2006) and human studies (KIMURA et al. 2005; PUTTAGUNTA et al. 1996) have shown that linear chelates, particularly the nonionic ones, cause a large increase in zinc excretion in urine. The nonionic linear chelate gadodiamide induced a decrease of 32% of plasma zinc after a single injection in healthy

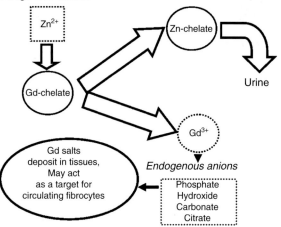

Fig. 20.2. A diagram of the process of transmetallation between Gd^{3+} and endogenous cations such as zinc (Zn^{2+}). The zinc replaces the Gd of the chelate and is eliminated from the body in urine as zinc chelate. The Gd^{3+} combines with endogenous anions and deposits in tissues

volunteers (PUTTAGUNTA et al. 1996). This is thought to be secondary to transmetallation and the presence of excess chelate in the gadodiamide preparation. In patients undergoing contrast enhanced MRI examination, gadodiamide caused a large increase in zinc in the urine excretion that was almost three times greater than the zinc excretion induced by the ionic linear molecule Gd-DTPA (KIMURA et al. 2005). On the other hand, the ionic macrocyclic Gd-DOTA had no effect on zinc excretion (KIMURA et al. 2005). Ex-vivo studies have also confirmed that all macrocyclic Gd-contrast agents are insensitive to transmetallation by zinc ions in comparison to the open-chain complexes (LAURENT et al. 2001, 2006).

It is interesting that animal studies in rats and monkeys showed that repeated administration of high doses (3–5 mmol/kg) of nonionic linear Gd chelates (gadoversetamide and gadodiamide) for 28 days produced skin ulceration and testicular atrophy (IDEE et al. 2006). These lesions are similar to those described with zinc deficiency (PRASAD 2003). Much higher cumulative doses were required to produce similar lesions with the ionic agents Gd-DTPA and Gd-DOTA (IDEE et al. 2006).

20.6
Stability and Nephrogenic Systemic Fibrosis

Gd-contrast agents are eliminated from the body through the kidneys and their biological half life in patients with normal renal function is 1.5 h. In patients with advanced renal impairment elimination, half life can be prolonged to 30 h or more (THOMSEN et al. 2006). Patients on haemodialysis would require three consecutive dialysis sessions over 6 days to remove 97% of the administered dose of Gd-contrast agents from the body. Continuous ambulatory peritoneal dialysis for 20 days eliminates 69% of the injected dose of Gd-contrast agents (MORCOS et al. 2002). Transmetallation is likely to occur when the Gd-chelate remains in the body for a long period, as, for example, in patients with end stage renal disease including those on dialysis (MORCOS 2007). Transmetallation of Gd-contrast agents leads to release of free gadolinium, which is deposited in the tissues as phosphates, carbonate, hydroxide or citrate complexes. It is postulated that the gadolinium salts are engulfed by local macrophages, leading to the release of a variety of cytokines, particularly transforming growth factor beta

(TGF-ß), which is a potent fibrogenic cytokine (DOUTHWAITE et al. 1999; PERAZELLA 2007). The cytokines would attract circulating fibrocytes, which would leave the circulation and deposit in the dermis and other organs containing Gd. The fibrocytes could then mature into fibroblasts, leading to fibrotic changes and deposition of collagen in the affected tissues (PERAZELLA 2007).

20.7
Conclusion

The chemical structure of Gd-contrast agents determines their stability. The least stable Gd-contrast agents are the nonionic linear chelates and the most stable is the ionic macrocyclic chelate. However, based on in vivo data, all macrocyclic agents seem to have similar high stability. Furthermore, no cases of NSF have been reported so far following the exclusive administration of any of the macrocyclic agents. The stability of the Gd chelate is likely to be an important factor in the pathogenesis of NSF in patients with end-stage renal disease (ESRD).

References

Brücher E, Sherry AD (2001) Stability and toxicity of contrast agents. In: Merbach AE, Toth E (eds) The chemistry of contrast agents in medical magnetic resonance imaging. Wiley, Chichester, Chapter 6, pp 249–257

Cacheris WP, Quay SC, Rocklage SM (1990) The relationship between thermodynamics and the toxicity of gadolinium complexes. Magn Reson Imag 8:467–481

Corot C, Idee JM, Hentsch AM, Santus R, Mallet C, Goulas V, Bonnemain B, Meyer D (1998) Structure-activity relationship of macrocyclic and linear gadolinium chelates: investigation of transmetallation effect on the zinc-dependent metallopeptidase angiotensin-converting enzyme. J Magn Reson Imag 8:695–702

Dawson P (1999) Gadolinium chelates: chemistry. In: Dawson P, Cosgrove DO, Grainger RG (eds) Textbook of contrast media. Isis Medical Media, Oxford, Chapter 22, pp 291–296

Desreux JF, Gilsoul D (1999) Chemical synthesis of paramagnetic complexes. In: Thomsen HS, Muller RN, Mattrey (eds) Trends in contrast media. Springer, Heidelberg, Chapter 15, pp 161–169

Douthwaite JA, Johnson TS, Haylor JL, Watson P, El Nahas AM (1999) Effects of transforming growth factor-beta1 on renal extracellular matrix components and their regulating proteins. J Am Soc Nephrol 10:2109–2119

Gibby WA, Gibby KA, Gibby WA (2004) Comparison of Gd DTPA-BMA (Omniscan) versus Gd-Hp-DO3A (ProHance) retention in human bone tissue by inductive coupled plasma atomic emission spectroscopy. Invest Radiol 39:138–142

Green RWF, Krestin GP (2006) Non-tissue specific extra cellular MR contrast media. In: Thomsen (ed) Contrast media. Safety issues and ESUR guidelines. Springer, Heidelberg, Chapter 16, pp 107–112

Idee J-M, Port M, Raynal I, Schaefer, Greneur SL, Corot C (2006) Clinical and biological consequences of transmetallation induced by contrast agents for magnetic resonance imaging: a review. Fundam Clin Pharmacol 20:563–576

Kimura J, Ishguchi T, Matsuda J, Ohno R, Nakamura A, Kamei S, Ohno K, Kawamura T, Murata K (2005) Human comparative study of zinc and copper excretion via urine after administration of magnetic resonance imaging contrast agents. Radiation Med 23:322–326

Kumar K (1997) Macrocyclic polyamino carboxylate complexes of Gd (III) as magnetic resonance imaging contrast agents. J Alloys Compounds 249:163–172

Laurent S, Elst LV, Copoix F, Muller RN (2001) Stability of MRI paramagnetic contrast media, a proton relaxometric protocol for transmetallation assessment. Invest Radiol 36:115–122

Laurent S, Elst LV, Copoix F, Muller RN (2006) Comparative study of the physicochemical properties of six clinical low molecular weight gadolinium contrast agents. Contrast Media Mol Imaging1:128–137

Morcos SK (2007) Nephrogenic systemic fibrosis following the administration of extracellular gadolinium based contrast agents: Is the stability of the contrast agent molecule an important factor in the pathogenesis of this condition? Br J Radiol 80:73–76

Morcos SK, Thomsen HS, Webb JAW, Members of the Contrast Media Safety Committee of the European Society of Urogenital Radiology (ESUR) (2002) Dialysis and contrast media. European Radiology 12:3026–3030

Perezella MA (2007) Nephrogenic systemic fibrosis, kidney disease and gadolinium: is there a link? Clin J Am Soc Nephrol 2:200–2002

Prasad AS (2003) Zinc deficiency. BMJ 326:409–410

Port M, Idée JM, Medina C, Robic C, Sabatou M, Corot C (2008) Efficiency, thermodynamic and kinetic stability of marketed gadolinium chelates and their possible clinical consequences: a critical review. Biometals 21:469–490

Puttagunta NR, Gibby WA, Smith GT (1996) Human in vivo comparative study of zinc and copper transmetallation after administration of magnetic resonance imaging contrast agents. Invest Radiol 12:739–742

Rofsky NM, Sherry AD, Lenkinski RE (2008) Nephrogenic systemic fibrosis: a chemical prespective. Radiology 247:608–612

Thomsen HS, Morcos SK, Dawson P (2006) Is there a causal relation between the administration gadolinium based contrast media and the development of nephrogenic systemic fibrosis (NSF)? Clin Radiol 61:905–906

Tweedle MF (1992) Physicochemical properties of gadoteridol and other magnetic resonance contrast agents. Invest Radiol 27:S2–S6

Tweedle MF, Wedeking P, Kumar K (1995) Biodistribution of radiolabeled formulated gadopentetate, gadoteridol, gadoterate and gadodiamide in mice and rats. Invest Radiol 30:372–380

Tweedle MF (2007) Stability of gadolinium chelates (letter to the Editor). Br J Radiol 80:583–584

Wedeking P, Kumar K, Tweedle MF (1992) Dissociation of gadolinium chelates in mice: relationship to chemical characteristics. Magn Reson Imaging 10:641–648

White GW, Gibby WA, Tweedle MF (2006) Comparison of Gd (DTPA-BMA) (Omniscan) versus Gd(HP-DO3A) (ProHance) relative to gadolinium retention in human bone tissue by inductively coupled plasma mass spectroscopy. Invest Radiol 41:272–278

Diagnostic Efficacy

AART J. VAN DER MOLEN

CONTENTS

21.1
Introduction

After the invention of MRI by Lauterbur and others in the early 1970s, it was believed that the multiple variable image acquisition parameters would produce sufficient intrinsic image contrast to make contrast agents unnecessary. However, in the late 1970s and early 1980s, experiments with a number of paramagnetic compounds led to the first MR images using gadopentetate dimeglumine by Schering AG and the University of California at San Francisco, which were shown at the Society for Magnetic

AART J. VAN DER MOLEN
Department of Radiology, C-2S, Leiden University Medical Center, PO Box 9600, 2300 RC Leiden, The Netherlands

Resonance in Medicine meeting in 1983. It took until the beginning of 1988 before gadopentetate dimeglumine (Gd-DTPA, Magnevist®, Bayer Schering Pharma, Germany) was introduced to the market, and within a short time contrast-enhanced MRI as a routine procedure became a clinical reality (DE HAËN 2001).

Since the introduction of gadopentetate dimeglumine, a number of other extracellular Gd-based contrast agents have been introduced. These agents together with their most important physicochemical data have been summarized in Table 21.1.

21.2
Terminology and Populations

In this era of evidence-based medicine, it is important to understand the terminology used. The terms efficacy, effectiveness, and efficiency all refer to different concepts (HAYNES 1999). Efficacy ("Can it work?") refers to the extent that contrast media do more good than harm under ideal conditions. With optimized clinical trial conditions, the effects are usually studied in selected populations in which confounding factors such as concomitant medications, interventions, etc. are limited as much as possible.

Effectiveness ("Does it work in practice?") refers to the extent that contrast media do more good than harm under everyday conditions in routine clinical practice. The criteria for trials studying effectiveness are much more relaxed, and concomitant medications and interventions, etc are permitted. While efficacy trials are designed to study causal relationships, effectiveness trials study management of disease. Ineffectiveness of a specific intervention such as the use of contrast media may therefore not only relate to its efficacy, but also to other factors such as the particular clinical setting, provider compliance, patient adherence, reimbursement, etc.

Table 21.1. Physicochemical characteristics of extracellular Gadolinium-based contrast agents

Name	Brand name	Ligand	Structure	Ionicity	Osmolality (mOsm kg⁻¹)	Viscosity 37°C (mPa s)	T1 relaxivity in blood, 1.5 T (L mmol⁻¹ s⁻¹)	T2 relaxivity in blood, 1.5 T (L mmol⁻¹ s⁻¹)	Renal excretion (T½; h)
Gadopentetate	Magnevist	DTPA	Linear	Ionic	1960	2.9	4.3	4.4	1.6
Gadoterate	Dotarem	DOTA	Macrocyclic	Ionic	1350	2.0	4.2	6.7	1.6
Gadodiamide	Omniscan	DTPA-BMA	Linear	Nonionic	789	1.4	4.6	6.9	1.3
Gadoteridol	ProHance	HP-DO3A	Macrocyclic	Nonionic	630	1.3	4.4	5.5	1.6
Gadoversetamide	OptiMARK	DTPA-BMEA	Linear	Nonionic	1110	2.0	5.2	6.0	1.7
Gadobutrol	Gadovist	BT-DO3A	Macrocyclic	Nonionic	1390	4.9	5.3	5.4	1.5
Gadobenate[a]	MultiHance	BOPTA	Linear	Ionic	1970	5.4	6.7	8.9	1.2–2

[a] Also liver-specific – 4–5% is excreted via the hepatocytes

Finally, efficiency ("Is it worth it?") measures the effect of an intervention in relation to the resources it consumes. Trials of efficiency are commonly referred to as cost-effectiveness trials.

21.3
Efficacy in Single Dose Administration

The value of using extracellular Gd-contrast agents in neurological, spine, cardiac, abdominal, and vascular imaging has been described in many clinical studies in the literature. Most of the specific quantitative efficacy data reviewed in this chapter comes from the clinical trials necessary for registration of these agents. In the first section, only studies that deal with one specific agent are described.

21.3.1
Standard (0.5M) Concentration Agents

Specific efficacy data were published for *gadopentetate dimeglumine* in the late 1980s and early 1990s, especially for brain and spine applications. First results using T1-weighted (T1w) spin echo sequences showed enhancement that made small posterior fossa tumors more conspicuous (STACK et al. 1988). In the brain, use of gadolinium revealed many lesions not shown by unenhanced imaging (HESSELINK et al. 1988; RUSSELL et al. 1989), and the diagnosis was changed in up to 37% of patients (RUNGE et al. 1988; RUSSELL et al. 1989). In the spine, the use of contrast medium was especially helpful for intradural tumors (STIMAC et al. 1988), providing additional information in almost all cases and changing the diagnosis in 30% of patients (SZE et al. 1990). Gadopentetate administration in infants and children also led to improved tumor detection and lesion conspicuity (BIRD et al. 1988; ELSTER and RIESER 1989; ELDEVIK and BRUNBERG 1994). As a result of the immature renal function in infants, the imaging time window is significantly prolonged (ELSTER 1990). In infants and children, Gd-contrast agents should be used selectively based on the findings of the clinical examination and unenhanced imaging (ELSTER and RIESER 1989; ELDEVIK and BRUNBERG 1994). In MR angiography, a review of more than 4,000 patients showed good efficacy of gadopentetate in doses of 0.1–0.3 mmol kg^{-1} (GOYEN and DEBATIN 2004).

In brain imaging, the use of *gadoterate meglumine* (Gd-DOTA, Dotarem®, Guerbet, Paris, France) improved the definition of pathologic lesions and so improved sensitivity and specificity (PARIZEL et al. 1989). In vascular imaging, it produced better definition between mural thrombus and slow flow in time-of-flight MRA (LAISSY et al. 1995). In children, gadoterate use was helpful for diagnosing tumors in the brain and spine (LIPSKI et al. 1990).

Use of the nonionic, linear agent *gadodiamide* (Gd-DTPA-BMA, Omniscan®, GE Healthcare, Chalfont St. Giles, UK) improved lesion detection and delineation, which facilitated diagnosis in the brain or head and neck in the majority of patients (KAPLAN et al. 1991; SZE et al. 1991, ASLANIAN et al. 1996; EKHOLM et al. 1996, 2001). In large, multicenter studies it was shown that its use could change diagnosis in 17.0–28.6% of patients (SZE et al. 1991, ASLANIAN et al. 1996). In children, efficacy was similar, and in infants efficacy was good (MARTI-BONMATI et al. 2000). In older children, postcontrast imaging yielded additional diagnostic information in 65–82% of cases (LUNDBY et al. 1996; HANQUINET et al. 1996).

After *gadoteridol* (Gd-HP-DO3A, ProHance®, Bracco, Milan, Italy), additional diagnostic information was obtained in the majority of patients, making a change in diagnosis possible in 29.4% of cranial, 33.5% of spinal, and 35.1% of head and neck studies (RUNGE et al. 1990, 1991a,b, 1992; ZOARSKI et al. 1993). In children, the benefit was even greater in brain compared to spinal imaging, with a modified brain diagnosis in 48% and a modified spinal diagnosis in 20% (BALL et al. 1993). Efficacy was not reduced by using higher doses (CARVLIN et al. 1992). Early studies using enhanced time-of-flight intracranial MRA showed a more limited benefit, with additional findings only changing the diagnosis in 8% of patients (MCLACHLAN et al. 1994).

The experience with *gadoversetamide* (Gd-DTPA-BMEA, OptiMark®, Covidien, USA) is limited. Like the other agents, administration in adults and children resulted in increased diagnostic confidence and better delineation of brain pathology (GROSSMANN et al. 1998; LOWE et al. 2006).

21.3.2
High (1.0M) Concentration and Protein-Binding Agents

While all the agents already discussed are available in a 0.5M concentration, *gadobutrol* (Gd-BT-DO3A, Gadovist®, Bayer Schering Pharma, Berlin, Germany) was introduced to the market in a 1.0M concentration to improve the gadolinium flux during contrast agent injection for newer applications such as MR perfusion imaging and contrast-enhanced MR angiography.

In routine brain imaging it was found that a 0.1 mmol kg^{-1} dose (i.e., half the volume of the other agents) was sufficient (LEMKE et al. 1997), but in brain perfusion studies better results could be achieved with a 0.3 mmol kg^{-1} dose (BENNER et al. 2000). Compared to gadobutrol in a 0.5 M formulation, the 1.0 M concentration showed a sharper contrast peak and improved quality and superior contrast in the relative Cerebral Blood Flow and Mean Transit Time parameter maps (TOMBACH et al. 2003). In multiple studies, the use of gadobutrol for contrast-enhanced MRA produced high sensitivity (92–96% for aortoiliac or total body MRA) and a high specificity (89–97% for aortoiliac or total body MRA). There was excellent interobserver agreement and comparable performance for therapy planning using intraarterial DSA (SCHÄFER, 2003; HENTSCH, 2003; HERBORN, 2004; MOHRS, 2004).

Gadobenate dimeglumine (Gd-BOPTA, Multi-Hance®, Bracco, Milan, Italy) was initially developed for liver imaging. It has a slightly higher R1- and R2-relaxivity in vitro, but due to protein binding the relaxivity in blood is almost 50% higher than gadopentetate (Table 21.1). The beneficial effect of this increased relaxivity was soon investigated in other applications such as brain imaging, perfusion MR, and MR angiography. Using gadobenate in brain studies improved the detection and delineation of lesions and increased diag-nostic confidence (SCHNEIDER et al. 2001; BALERIAUX et al. 2002). In brain perfusion, the increased R2-relaxivity allowed good T2* perfusion MRI and post-processed maps, even with a dose of 0.1 mmol kg^{-1} (COTTON 2006).

Contrast-enhanced MR angiography produces a significant gain in diagnostic quality over unenhanced MRA. Diagnostic quality in multiple vascular beds is better at 0.1 mmol kg^{-1} than at lower doses (SCHNEIDER et al. 2007). A further dose increase has no clinically relevant benefit (KROENCKE et al. 2002; WIKSTROM et al. 2003). In the run-off vessels, MRA enhanced with gadobenate led to improved sensitivity and specificity for clinically relevant (>50%) stenoses compared to time-of-flight MRA (THURNHER et al. 2007). For the diagnosis of internal carotid artery stenosis, 3D contrast-enhanced MRA correlated better with 3D rotational angiography than did intra-arterial (2D) DSA (ANZALONE et al. 2005).

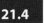

21.4
Efficacy in Triple vs. Single Dose Administration

For a number of agents, higher dose or dose accumulation studies have been performed to improve efficacy. Doses up to 0.3 mmol kg^{-1} have been studied in the brain for diagnosing metastases and for MR angiography.

In the brain, *gadopentetate* in 0.3 mmol kg^{-1} doses was associated with an improved contrast to noise ratio (CNR) and better visual assessment ratings (HAUSTEIN et al. 1993). It was shown that the number of metastases detected increased significantly by 15% and 43%, respectively, when 0.2 and 0.3 mmol kg^{-1} were administered (VAN DIJK et al. 1997). However, triple doses showed no additional benefit when the single-dose study was negative, but were helpful MRI findings where equivocal or when a single dose study showed a solitary lesion (SZE et al. 1998). More recent studies of MR angiography showed no benefit of higher doses for vessel enhancement, but vessel contrast improved. In large vessels like the abdominal arteries (HEVERHAGEN et al. 2007) or the carotids (JOURDAN et al. 2007), a dose of 0.1 mmol kg^{-1} is deemed sufficient.

A high dose of *gadodiamide* resulted in better delineation of pathologic structures and tumor size in the brain, with increasing contrast agent dose (DEMAEREL et al. 1994). In peripheral MRA, high doses improved sensitivity, specificity, and the depiction of collateral circulation was similar to intra-arterial DSA (KRAUSE et al. 2005).

With *gadoteridol*, brain lesions were also shown better at higher dose with improved lesion detection (RUNGE et al. 1992; YUH et al. 1992, 1994, 1995). In a preliminary study it was shown that additional information from high dose gadoteridol led to a potential modification in the treatment of 35% of patients, which was likely to be cost-effective (YUH et al. 1992; MAYR et al. 1994).

High doses of *gadobutrol* can be administered with relatively smaller volumes or lower injection rates. The added benefit from triple dose imaging was less than that between standard dose imaging and unenhanced MRI. Nevertheless, the added information from triple dose examinations could change treatment in up to 20% of patients (LEMKE et al. 1997; VOGL et al. 1995). Application of Magnetization Transfer combined with a single dose may be equivalent to triple dose imaging (KNAUTH et al. 1996).

Because of its improved T1-relaxivity, *gadobenate* improved reader confidence and lesion conspicuity. There was only improvement in the number of detected lesions up to a dose of 0.2 mmol kg^{-1}, but not beyond that (SCHNEIDER et al. 2001). Results were similar if the first dose of 0.1 mmol kg^{-1} was split into two lower doses of 0.05 mmol kg^{-1} each (BALERIAUX et al. 2002).

21.5

Comparative Efficacy of Agents

21.5.1
Standard (0.5M) Concentration Agents

Most of the newer agents have been compared with the older ones, especially with gadopentetate and to a lesser extent with gadoterate.

Gadoterate was compared to gadopentetate in two studies. No differences in efficacy were found by BRUGERIES et al. (1994). Interestingly, the authors concluded that "the greater stability of gadoterate theoretically might reduce biological interactions in man." Similar results were obtained in a large central nervous system study by OUDKERK et al. (1995), who found that additional findings changed treatment in 17.0% of gadoterate and 17.3% of gadopentetate patients, respectively.

Multiple studies have compared the efficacy of *gadodiamide* to gadopentetate and/or gadoterate in CNS applications and none showed any significant differences in efficacy (MYHR et al. 1992, BALERIAUX et al. 1993; VALK et al. 1993; AKESON et al. 1995). In a double-blind randomized MR angiography study with intra-arterial DSA as reference standard, SCHÄFER et al. (2006) found no substantial differences between Gd-DTPA-BMA and Gd-DTPA in sensitivity and specificity for detecting stenosis.

Gadoteridol and *gadoversetamide* have been compared with gadopentetate in liver and brain imaging. Multiple readers found no significant difference between the agents at either site (GRECO et al. 2001; RUBIN et al. 1999; GROSSMAN et al. 2000).

21.5.2
High (1.0M) Concentration and Protein-Binding Agents

Agents with special characteristics may have a special role. In particular, gadobenate with its higher relaxivity in plasma due to protein binding has been extensively tested.

Gadobutrol for contrast-enhanced pulmonary perfusion MRI performed best at 0.1 mmol kg^{-1}, but did not lead to increased signal-to-noise ratio (SNR) compared to gadopentetate in the low-dose range (0.025–0.100 mmol kg^{-1}) (FINK et al. 2004). In multiple MR angiography studies in volunteers and patients improved signal-to-noise and contrast-to-noise of gadobutrol 1 M compared to equimolar doses of gadopentetate 0.5 M was shown, with a high sensitivity and specificity for diagnosis of aorto-iliac stenosis (GOYEN et al. 2001, 2003). In a recent large multicenter study on focal renal lesions 0.1 mmol kg^{-1} gadobutrol 1 M was diagnostically equivalent to an equimolar dose of gadopentetate 0.5 M (TOMBACH et al. 2008).

MRI of the brain with normal dose *gadobenate* may be a valid alternative to using high doses of the other agents. Comparative cross-over studies with equal doses of gadopentetate or gadoterate have repeatedly shown improved percentage contrast enhancement, higher sensitivity for lesion detection, increased lesion-to-brain contrast, and reader preference for gadobenate in both intra-axial and extra-axial CNS tumors (COLOSIMO et al. 2001, 2004; ESSIG et al. 2006b; KNOPP et al. 2004; MARAVILLA et al. 2006; KUHN et al. 2007). In a multicenter study comparing multiple doses of gadobenate and gadodiamide, both agents had similar efficacy, but at a slightly lower dose for gadobenate (RUNGE et al. 2001, 2002).

Another application in which the higher relaxivity may be beneficial is MR angiography of the aorto-iliac and run-off vessels. Higher signal-to-noise and contrast-to-noise ratios with higher diagnostic image quality in the smaller femoro-tibial vessels was demonstrated with gadobenate compared to gadopentetate (VON TENGG-KOBLIGK et al. 2003; KNOPP et al. 2003). However, when gadoterate was the comparative agent, sensitivity and specificity was equal between agents. Most of the benefit is probably in showing vessels below the knee, where the number of nonassessable vessel segments was lower for gadobenate (WYTTENBACH et al. 2003). In the renal arteries and lower aorta, efficacy was not reduced when single dose (0.1 mmol kg^{-1}) gadobenate was compared to double-dose (0.2 mmol kg^{-1}) gadopentetate (PROKOP et al. 2005; SOULEZ et al. 2008).

21.5.3
High (1.0M) Concentration vs. Protein-Binding Agents

Finally, some studies have directly compared both methods of achieving higher signal intensities, that is, higher concentration agents (gadobutrol) and protein-binding agents (gadobenate). In brain perfusion MRI, susceptibility effects for a single dose were not significantly different between the agents, for quantitative parameters and parametric maps, either at 1.5 T (ESSIG et al. 2002) or at 3 T (THILMANN et al. 2005). Double doses of the two agents produced better overall image quality but no clinical benefit over single dose examinations. (THILMANN et al. 2005; ESSIG et al. 2006a).

In MR angiography, both diluted and undiluted gadobutrol and gadobenate resulted in significantly higher signal-to-noise than gadopentetate, but there was no difference between the higher signal-to-noise ratio agents (HERBORN et al. 2003).

<table>
<tr><td>**21.6**</td></tr>
</table>

Summary and Conclusions

Since the introduction of the first gadolinium-based contrast agent in 1988, it has become clear that these agents significantly improve the diagnostic efficacy of MRI. Studies on single agents have shown that, when compared to unenhanced sequences, all agents help to improve the detection and delineation of lesions and this can alter diagnosis in up to 40% of patients.

Doubling or tripling the standard dose of 0.1 mmol kg^{-1} body weight may be beneficial for selected indications (e.g., brain perfusion, equivocal single dose study in MRI for brain metastasis, small vessel MR angiography). A more limited number of studies have compared the various agents. These studies do *not* show clinically significant differences in diagnostic efficacy between the various extracellular Gd-CA. Agents with higher concentration or protein binding may be relatively more suitable for particular applications (e.g., perfusion MRI). The higher relaxivity agents may be used in somewhat lower doses than the extracellular agents.

References

Akeson P, Jonsson E, Haugen I, Holtås S (1995) Contrast-enhanced MRI of the central nervous system: comparison between gadodiamide injection and gadolinium-DTPA. Neuroradiology 37:229–233

Anzalone N, Scomazzoni F, Castellano R et al. (2005) Carotid artery stenosis: intraindividual correlations of 3D time-of-flight MR angiography, contrast-enhanced MR angiography, conventional DSA, and rotational angiography for detection and grading. Radiology 236:204–213

Aslanian V, Lemaignen H, Bunouf P, Svaland MG, Borseth A, Lundby B (1996) Evaluation of the clinical safety of gadodiamide injection, a new nonionic MRI contrast medium for the central nervous system: a European perspective. Neuroradiology 38:537–541

Balériaux D, Matos C, De Greef D (1993) Gadodiamide injection as a contrast medium for MRI of the central nervous system: a comparison with gadolinium-DOTA. Neuroradiology 35:490–494

Balériaux D, Colosimo C, Ruscalleda J et al. (2002) Magnetic resonance imaging of metastatic disease to the brain with gadobenate dimeglumine. Neuroradiology 44:191–203

Ball WS Jr, Nadel SN, Zimmerman RA et al. (1993) Phase III multicenter clinical investigation to determine the safety and efficacy of gadoteridol in children suspected of having neurologic disease. Radiology 186:769–774

Benner T, Reimer P, Erb G et al. (2000) Cerebral MR perfusion imaging: first clinical application of a 1 M gadolinium chelate (Gadovist 1.0) in a double-blinded randomized dose-finding study. J Magn Reson Imaging 12:371–380

Bird CR, Drayer BP, Medina M, Rekate HL, Flom RA, Hodak JA (1988) Gd-DTPA-enhanced MR imaging in pediatric patients after brain tumor resection. Radiology 169:123–126

Brugières P, Gaston A, Degryse HR et al. (1994) Randomised double blind trial of the safety and efficacy of two gadolinium complexes (Gd-DTPA and Gd-DOTA). Neuroradiology 36:27–30

Carvlin MJ, De Simone DN, Meeks MJ (1992) Phase II clinical trial of gadoteridol injection, a low-osmolal magnetic resonance imaging contrast agent. Invest Radiol 27 (Suppl 1): S16–S21

Colosimo C, Ruscalleda J, Korves M et al. (2001) Detection of intracranial metastases: a multicenter, intrapatient comparison of gadobenate dimeglumine-enhanced MRI with routinely used contrast agents at equal dosage. Invest Radiol 36:72–81

Colosimo C, Knopp MV, Barreau X et al. (2004) A comparison of Gd-BOPTA and Gd-DOTA for contrast-enhanced MRI of intracranial tumours. Neuroradiology 46:655–665

Cotton F (2006) Diffusion-perfusion in intra-axial brain tumors with high relaxivity contrast agents. Neuroradiology 48 (Suppl 1):34–40

De Haën C (2001) Conception of the first magnetic resonance imaging contrast agents: a brief history. Top Magn Reson Imaging 12:221–230

Demaerel P, Marchal G, Wilms G et al. (1994) Gadodiamide injection at 0.1 and 0.3 mmol/kg body weight: a phase III double-blind, parallel, randomised clinical investigation of known or suspected central nervous system lesions at 1.5T. Neuroradiology 36:355–359

Ekholm SE, Jonsson E, Sandvik L et al. (1996) Tolerance and efficacy of Omniscan (gadodiamide injection) in MR imaging of the central nervous system. Acta Radiol 37:223–228

Ekholm SE, Björk-Eriksson T, Western A et al. (2001) MRI staging using gadodiamide for soft-tissue tumors of the head and neck region. Results from a phase II trial and a 5-year clinical follow-up. Eur J Radiol 39:168–175

Eldevik OP, Brunberg JA (1994) Gadopentetate dimeglumine-enhanced MR of the brain: clinical utility and safety in patients younger than two years of age. AJNR Am J Neuroradiol 15:1001–1008

Elster AD (1990) Cranial MR imaging with Gd-DTPA in neonates and young infants: preliminary experience. Radiology 176:225–230

Elster AD, Rieser GD (1989) Gd-DTPA-enhanced cranial MR imaging in children: initial clinical experience and recommendations for its use. AJR Am J Roentgenol 153:1265–1268

Essig M, Hartmann M, Lodemann KP et al. (2001) Comparison of contrast behavior of gadobenate-dimeglumine and Gd-DTPA in intra-axial brain tumors. A double-blind randomized intraindividual cross-over study [in German]. Radiologe 41:1063–1071

Essig M, Lodemann KP, LeHuu M, Schönberg SO, Hübener M, Van Kaick G (2002) Comparison of MultiHance and Gadovist for cerebral MR perfusion imaging in healthy volunteers [in German]. Radiologe 42:909–915

Essig M, Lodemann KP, Le-Huu M, Brüning R, Kirchin M, Reith W (2006a) Intraindividual comparison of gadobenate dimeglumine and gadobutrol for cerebral magnetic resonance perfusion imaging at 1.5 T. Invest Radiol 41:256–263

Essig M, Tartaro A, Tartaglione T, Pirovano G, Kirchin MA, Spinazzi A (2006b) Enhancing lesions of the brain: intraindividual crossover comparison of contrast enhancement after gadobenate dimeglumine versus established gadolinium comparators. Acad Radiol 13:744–751

Fink C, Puderbach M, Ley S et al. (2004) Contrast-enhanced three-dimensional pulmonary perfusion magnetic resonance imaging: intraindividual comparison of 1.0 M gadobutrol and 0.5 M Gd-DTPA at three dose levels. Invest Radiol 39:143–148

Goyen M, Debatin JF (2004) Gadopentetate dimeglumine-enhanced three-dimensional MR-angiography: dosing, safety, and efficacy. J Magn Reson Imaging 19:261–273

Goyen M, Lauenstein TC, Herborn CU, Debatin JF, Bosk S, Ruehm SG (2001) 0.5 M Gd chelate (Magnevist) versus 1.0 M Gd chelate (Gadovist): dose-independent effect on image quality of pelvic three-dimensional MR-angiography. J Magn Reson Imaging 14:602–607

Goyen M, Herborn CU, Vogt FM et al. (2003) Using a 1 M Gd-chelate (gadobutrol) for total-body three-dimensional MR angiography: preliminary experience. J Magn Reson Imaging 17:565–571

Greco A, Parker JR, Ratcliffe CG, Kirchin MA, McNamara MT (2001) Phase III, randomized, double-blind, cross-over comparison of gadoteridol and gadopentetate dimeglumine in magnetic resonance imaging of patients with intracranial lesions. Australas Radiol 45:457–463

Grossman RI, Kuhn MJ, Maravilla K et al. (1998) Multicenter evaluation of the safety, tolerance, and efficacy of OptiMARK in magnetic resonance imaging of the brain and spine. Acad Radiol 5 (Suppl 1):S154–S155; discussion S156

Grossman RI, Rubin DL, Hunter G et al. (2000) Magnetic resonance imaging in patients with central nervous system pathology: a comparison of OptiMARK (Gd-DTPA-BMEA) and Magnevist (Gd-DTPA). Invest Radiol 35:412–419

Hanquinet S, Christophe C, Greef DD, Gordon P, Perlmutter N (1996) Clinical evaluation of gadodiamide injection in paediatric MR imaging. Pediatr Radiol 26:806–810

Haustein J, Laniado M, Niendorf HP et al. (1993) Triple-dose versus standard-dose gadopentetate dimeglumine: a randomized study in 199 patients. Radiology 186:855–860

Haynes B (1999) Can it work? Does it work? Is it worth it? The testing of healthcare interventions is evolving. BMJ 319:652–653

Hentsch A, Aschauer MA, Balzer JO et al. (2003) Gadobutrol-enhanced moving-table magnetic resonance angiography in patients with peripheral vascular disease: a prospective, multi-centre blinded comparison with digital subtraction angiography. Eur Radiol 13:2103–2114

Herborn CU, Lauenstein TC, Ruehm SG, Bosk S, Debatin JF, Goyen M (2003) Intra-individual comparison of gadopentetate dimeglumine, gadobenate dimeglumine, and gadobutrol for pelvic 3D magnetic resonance angiography. Invest Radiol 38:27–33

Herborn CU, Goyen M, Quick HH et al. (2004) Whole-body 3D MR angiography of patients with peripheral arterial occlusive disease. AJR Am J Roentgenol 182:1427–1434

Hesselink JR, Healy ME, Press GA, Brahme FJ (1988) Benefits of Gd-DTPA for MR imaging of intracranial abnormalities. J Comput Assist Tomogr 12:266–274

Heverhagen JT, Reitz I, Pavlicova M, Levine AL, Klose KJ, Wagner HJ (2007) The impact of the dosage of intravenous gadolinium-chelates on the vascular signal intensity in MR angiography. Eur Radiol 17:626–637

Jourdan C, Heverhagen JT, Knopp MV (2007) Dose comparison of single- vs. double-dose in contrast-enhanced magnetic resonance angiography of the carotid arteries: Intraindividual cross-over blinded trial using Gd-DTPA. J Magn Reson Imaging 25:557–563

Kaplan GD, Aisen AM, Aravapalli SR (1991) Preliminary clinical trial of gadodiamide injection: a new nonionic gadolinium contrast agent for MR imaging. J Magn Reson Imaging 1:57–62

Knauth M, Forsting M, Hartmann M, Heiland S, Balzer T, Sartor K (1996) MR enhancement of brain lesions: increased contrast dose compared with magnetization transfer. AJNR Am J Neuroradiol 17:1853–1859

Knopp MV, Giesel FL, von Tengg-Kobligk H et al. (2003) Contrast-enhanced MR angiography of the run-off vasculature: intraindividual comparison of gadobenate dimeglumine with gadopentetate dimeglumine. J Magn Reson Imaging 17:694–702

Knopp MV, Runge VM, Essig M et al. (2004) Primary and secondary brain tumors at MR imaging: bicentric intraindividual crossover comparison of gadobenate dimeglumine and gadopentetate dimeglumine. Radiology 230:55–64

Krause U, Kroencke T, Spielhaupter E et al. (2005) Contrast-enhanced magnetic resonance angiography of the lower extremities: standard-dose vs. high-dose gadodiamide injection. J Magn Reson Imaging 21:449–454

Kroencke TJ, Wasser MN, Pattynama PM et al. (2002) Gadobenate dimeglumine-enhanced MR angiography of the abdominal aorta and renal arteries. AJR Am J Roentgenol 179:1573–1582

Kuhn MJ, Picozzi P, Maldjian JA et al. (2007) Evaluation of intra-axial enhancing brain tumors on magnetic resonance imaging: intraindividual crossover comparison of gadobenate dimeglumine and gadopentetate dimeglumine for visualization and assessment, and implications for surgical intervention. J Neurosurg 106:557–566

Laissy JP, Soyer P, Tebboune D, Tiah D, Hvass U, Menu Y (1995) Abdominal aortic aneurysms: assessment with gadolinium-enhanced time-of-flight coronal MR angiography (MRA). Eur J Radiol 20:1–8

Lemke AJ, Sander B, Balzer T, Geens V, Hosten N, Felix R (1997) Safety and use of gadobutrol in patients with brain tumors (phase III trial) [in German]. RöFo 167:591–598

Lipski S, Baraton J, Mamou Mani T, Tavière V, Brunelle F, Lallemand D (1990) Utilization of gadolinium DOTA in the diagnosis of tumors of the central nervous system of the child. Diagn Interv Radiol 2:163–167

Lowe LH, Kearns GL, Wible JH Jr (2006) The safety and efficacy of neuroimaging with gadoversetamide injection in pediatric patients. Curr Med Res Opin 22:2515–2524

Lundby B, Gordon P, Hugo F (1996) MRI in children given gadodiamide injection: safety and efficacy in CNS and body indications. Eur J Radiol 23:190–196

Maravilla KR, Maldjian JA, Schmalfuss IM et al. (2006) Contrast enhancement of central nervous system lesions: multicenter intraindividual crossover comparative study of two MR contrast agents. Radiology 240:389–400

Martí-Bonmatí L, Vega T, Benito C et al. (2000) Safety and efficacy of Omniscan (gadodiamide injection) at 0.1 mmol/kg for MRI in infants younger than 6 months of age: phase III open multicenter study. Invest Radiol 35:141–147

Mayr NA, Yuh WT, Muhonen MG et al. (1994) Cost-effectiveness of high-dose MR contrast studies in the evaluation of brain metastases. AJNR Am J Neuroradiol 15:1053–1061

McLachlan SJ, Francisco JC, Pernicone JR, Hasso AN (1994) Efficacy evaluation of gadoteridol for MR angiography of intracranial vascular lesions. J Magn Reson Imaging 4:405–411

Mohrs OK, Oberholzer K, Krummenauer F et al. (2004) Comparison of contrast-enhanced MR angiography of the aortoiliac vessels using a 1.0 molar contrast agent at 1.0 T with intra-arterial digital subtraction angiography [in German]. RöFo 176:985–991

Myhr G, Rinck PA, Børseth A (1992) Gadodiamide injection and gadopentetate dimeglumine. A double-blind study in MR imaging of the CNS. Acta Radiol 33:405–409

Oudkerk M, Sijens PE, Van Beek EJ, Kuijpers TJ (1995) Safety and efficacy of Dotarem (Gd-DOTA) versus Magnevist (Gd-DTPA) in magnetic resonance imaging of the central nervous system. Invest Radiol 30:75–78

Parizel PM, Degryse HR, Gheuens J et al. (1989) Gadolinium-DOTA enhanced MR imaging of intracranial lesions. J Comput Assist Tomogr 13:378–385

Prokop M, Schneider G, Vanzulli A et al. (2005) Contrast-enhanced MR Angiography of the renal arteries: blinded multicenter crossover comparison of gadobenate dimeglumine andgadopentetate dimeglumine. Radiology 234:399–408

Rubin DL, Desser TS, Semelka R et al. (1999). A multicenter, randomized, double-blind study to evaluate the safety, tolerability, and efficacy of OptiMARK (gadoversetamide injection) compared with Magnevist (gadopentetate dimeglumine) in patients with liver pathology: results of a Phase III clinical trial. J Magn Reson Imaging 9:240–250

Runge VM, Schaible TF, Goldstein HA et al. (1988) Gd-DTPA. Clinical efficacy. Radiographics 8:147–159

Runge VM, Gelblum DY, Pacetti ML, Carolan F, Heard G (1990) Gd-HP-DO3A in clinical MR imaging of the brain. Radiology 177:393–400

Runge VM, Bradley WG, Brant-Zawadzki MN et al. (1991a) Clinical safety and efficacy of gadoteridol: a study in 411 patients with suspected intracranial and spinal disease. Radiology 181:701–709

Runge VM, Dean B, Lee C, Carolan F, Heard G (1991b) Phase III clinical evaluation of Gd-HP-DO3A in head and spine disease. J Magn Reson Imaging 1:47–56

Runge VM, Kirsch JE, Burke VJ, Price AC, Nelson KL, Thomas GS et al. (1992) High-dose gadoteridol in MR imaging of intracranial neoplasms. J Magn Reson Imaging 2:9–18

Runge VM, Armstrong MR, Barr RG et al. (2001) A clinical comparison of the safety and efficacy of MultiHance (gadobenate dimeglumine) and Omniscan (gadodiamide) in magnetic resonance imaging in patients with central nervous system pathology. Invest Radiol 36:65–71

Runge VM, Parker JR, Donovan M (2002) Double-blind, efficacy evaluation of gadobenate dimeglumine, a gadolinium chelate with enhanced relaxivity, in malignant lesions of the brain. Invest Radiol 37:269–280

Russell EJ, Schaible TF, Dillon W et al. (1989) Multicenter double-blind placebo-controlled study of gadopentetate dimeglumine as an MR contrast agent: evaluation in patients with cerebral lesions. AJR Am J Roentgenol 152:813–823

Schäfer FK, Schäfer PJ, Jahnke T et al. (2003) First clinical results in a study of contrast enhanced magnetic resonance angiography with the 1.0 molar gadobutrol in peripheral arterial occlusive disease – comparison to intra-arterial DSA [in German]. RöFo 175:556–564

Schäfer FK, Schäfer PJ, Altjohann C et al. (2007) A multicenter, site-independent, blinded study to compare the diagnostic accuracy of contrast-enhanced magnetic resonance angiography using 1.0M gadobutrol (Gadovist) to intra-arterial digital subtraction angiography in body arteries. Eur J Radiol 61:315–323

Schäfer PJ, Boudghene FP, Brambs HJ et al. (2006) Abdominal and iliac arterial stenoses: comparative double-blinded randomized study of diagnostic accuracy of 3D MR angiography with gadodiamide or gadopentetate dimeglumine. Radiology 238:827–840

Schneider G, Kirchin MA, Pirovano G, et al (2001) Gadobenate dimeglumine-enhanced magnetic resonance imaging of intracranial metastases: effect of dose on lesion detection and delineation. J Magn Reson Imaging 14: 525–539

Schneider G, Ballarati C, Grazioli L et al. (2007) Gadobenate dimeglumine-enhanced MR angiography: Diagnostic performance of four doses for detection and grading of carotid, renal, and aorto-iliac stenoses compared to digital subtraction angiography. J Magn Reson Imaging 26: 1020–1032

Soulez G, Pasowicz M, Benea G, et al. (2008) Renal artery stenosis evaluation: diagnostic performance of gadobenate dimeglumine-enhanced MR Angiography-comparison with DSA. Radiology 247:273–285

Stack JP, Antoun NM, Jenkins JP, Metcalfe R, Isherwood I (1988) Gadolinium-DTPA as a contrast agent in magnetic resonance imaging of the brain. Neuroradiology 30: 145–154

Stimac GK, Porter BA, Olson DO, Gerlach R, Genton M (1988) Gadolinium-DTPA-enhanced MR imaging of spinal neoplasms: preliminary investigation and comparison with unenhanced spin-echo and STIR sequences. AJR Am J Roentgenol 151:1185–1192

Sze G, Johnson C, Kawamura Y et al. (1990) Comparison of single- and triple-dose contrast MR contrast agent: evaluation in patients with spinal tumors. AJNR Am J Neuroradiol 11:967–974

Sze G, Brant-Zawadzki M, Haughton VM et al. (1991) Multicenter study of gadodiamide injection as a contrast agent in MR imaging of the brain and spine. Radiology 181:693–699

Sze G, Stimac GK, Bartlett C et al. (1998) Multicenter study of gadopentetate dimeglumine as an material in the MR screening of brain metastases. AJNR Am J Neuroradiol 19:821–828

Thilmann O, Larsson EM, Björkman-Burtscher IM, Ståhlberg F, Wirestam R (2005) Comparison of contrast agents with high molarity and with weak protein binding in cerebral perfusion imaging at 3 T. J Magn Reson Imaging 22:597–604

Thurnher S, Miller S, Schneider G et al. (2007) Diagnostic performance of gadobenate dimeglumine enhanced MR angiography of the iliofemoral and calf arteries: a large-scale multicenter trial. AJR Am J Roentgenol 189:1223–1237

Tombach B, Benner T, Reimer P et al. (2003) Do highly concentrated gadolinium chelates improve MR brain perfusion imaging? Intraindividually controlled randomized crossover concentration comparison study of 0.5 versus 1.0 mol/L gadobutrol. Radiology 226:880–888

Tombach B, Bohndorf K, Brodtrager W, et al. (2008) Comparison of 1.0 M gadobutrol and 0.5 M gadopentate dimeglumine-enhanced MRI in 471 patients with known or suspected renal lesions: results of a multicenter, single-blind, interindividual, randomized clinical phase III trial. Eur Radiol 18:2610–2619

Valk J, Algra PR, Hazenberg CJ, Slooff WB, Svaland MG (1993) A double-blind, comparative study of gadodiamide injection and gadopentetate dimeglumine in MRI of the central nervous system. Neuroradiology 35:173–177

Van Dijk P, Sijens PE, Schmitz PI, Oudkerk M (1997) Gd-enhanced MR imaging of brain metastases: contrast as a function of dose and lesion size. Magn Reson Imaging 15:535–541

Vogl TJ, Friebe CE, Balzer T et al. (1995) Diagnosis of cerebral metastasis with standard dose gadobutrol vs. a high dose protocol. Intraindividual evaluation of a phase II high dose study [in German]. Radiologe 35:508–516

Von Tengg-Kobligk H, Floemer F, Knopp MV (2003) Multiphasic MR angiography as an intra-individual comparison between the contrast agents Gd-DTPA, Gd-BOPTA, and Gd-BT-DO3A [in German]. Radiologe 43:171–178

Wikström J, Wasser MN, Pattynama PM et al. (2003) Gadobenate dimeglumine-enhanced magnetic resonance angiography of the pelvic arteries. Invest Radiol 38:504–515

Wyttenbach R, Gianella S, Alerci M, Braghetti A, Cozzi L, Gallino A (2003) Prospective blinded evaluation of Gd-DOTA- versus Gd-BOPTA-enhanced peripheral MR angiography, as compared with digital subtraction angiography. Radiology 227:261–269

Yuh WT, Engelken JD, Muhonen MG, Mayr NA, Fisher DJ, Ehrhardt JC (1992) Experience with high-dose gadolinium MR imaging in the evaluation of brain metastases. AJNR Am J Neuroradiol 13:335–345

Yuh WT, Fisher DJ, Runge VM, et al (1994) Phase III multicenter trial of high-dose gadoteridol in MR evaluation of brain metastases. AJNR Am J Neuroradiol 15:1037–1051

Yuh WT, Tali ET, Nguyen HD, Simonson TM, Mayr NA, Fisher DJ (1995) The effect of contrast dose, imaging time, and lesion size in the MR detection of intracerebral metastasis. AJNR Am J Neuroradiol 16:373–380; Erratum in: AJNR Am J Neuroradiol 16:1384

Zoarski GH, Lufkin RB, Bradley WG Jr et al. (1993) Multicenter trial of gadoteridol, a nonionic gadolinium chelate, in patients with suspected head and neck pathology. AJNR Am J Neuroradiol 14:955–961

Radiography with Gadolinium Contrast Agents

22

Henrik S. Thomsen

CONTENTS

22.1
Introduction

At the kV (~70) used for digital angiography, the attenuation of X-rays by gadolinium is approximately the same as for iodine and at the kV (~120) used for CT, the attenuation of X-rays by gadolinium is approximately double that of iodine, so theoretically gadolinium could therefore replace iodine as a radiographic contrast agent.

Henrik S. Thomsen
Department of Diagnostic Sciences, Faculty of Health Sciences, University of Copenhagen, DK-2200 Copenhagen N, Denmark
and
Department of Diagnostic Radiology,
Copenhagen University Hospital Herlev, 2730 Herlev, Denmark

It has been suggested that patients with significant renal impairment and/or previous severe reactions to iodinated contrast media should receive gadolinium-based MRI contrast agents instead of the traditional iodinated radiographic contrast agents (Albrecht and Dawson 2000; Bittner et al. 1997; Engelbrecht et al. 1996). Another possible indication suggested for using gadolinium based contrast agents rather than iodinated agents is before thyroid treatment with radioactive iodine to avoid interference by iodinated agents with the therapeutic iodine uptake.

Gadolinium based contrast agents are in general known to be safe and not nephrotoxic in the usual MRI doses of up to 0.3 mmol kg^{-1} body weight (BW) However, the dose requirement for a satisfactory diagnostic study differs between MR and X-ray examination because different properties of the gadolinium are being used in the two modalities. The use of gadolinium-based contrast agents in radiographic examinations is contentious and the risks are poorly understood (Thomsen et al. 2002; Thomsen 2003).

22.2
Molar Concentrations of Gadolinium and Iodinated Contrast Agents

The first four marketed gadolinium contrast media (gadopentate dimeglumine, gadoterate, gadodiamide, gadoteridol) are available in a concentration of 0.5 mmol ml^{-1}. Gadobenate dimeglumine is also available in this concentration but unlike the other four agents, it is also excreted via the liver (4%) (Chap. 25). Gadobutrol has been introduced in a concentration of 1 mmol ml^{-1}. For all the six agents there is one Gd-atom in each molecule, so the molar concentration of the agent and of gadolinium is the same. Traditionally, iodine radiographic contrast media are marketed based on the mg of iodine per ml. The concentration of 300 mg I ml^{-1} is equal to 2.38 mmol I ml^{-1}. Since there are three iodine atoms per molecule, the molar concentration of the agent is only 0.8 mmol ml^{-1}.

The commonly used dose for body CT is 150 ml of a 300 mg I ml^{-1} (2.38 mmol I ml^{-1}) solution. For body CT, a patient weighing 70 kg would receive 120 mmol of the iodinated agent molecule (0.8 mmol ml^{-1} × 150 ml) and 360 mmol of iodine (2.38 mmol ml^{-1} × 150 ml). The standard dose for contrast-enhanced MR examination is 0.2 ml kg^{-1} BW of a 0.5 mmol ml^{-1} gadolinium-based contrast agent. For MR examination, the same 70 kg patient would receive 7 mmol of the gadolinium based agent molecule and 7 mmol of gadolinium [0.5 mmol ml^{-1} × 14 ml (0.2 ml kg^{-1} BW × 70 kg BW)]. Thus, the number of iodinated contrast agent molecules administered for CT would be almost 17 times that of gadolinium containing molecules for MR, and the number of iodine atoms administered would be 51 times that of gadolinium. For a patient weighing 50 kg, the difference is even larger [~24 times (molecule) and ~72 times (atom)], whereas for a patient weighing 100 kg it is less [~12 times (molecule) and ~ 36 times (atom)].

22.3

Attenuation of X-Rays by Iodine and Gadolinium

Iodine has the atomic number 53 and an atomic weight of 127, whereas gadolinium has the atomic number 64 and an atomic weight of 157. Attenuation increases with the atomic number of the atom but decreases with the energy (keV) of the X-ray photons, except at the K-edges. At photon energies between the K-edge of iodine [33 kilo electron Volt (keV)] and that of gadolinium (52 keV), iodine attenuates approximately twice as many X-ray photons as gadolinium does. At all other photon energies, the opposite prevails (NYMAN et al. 2002). For CT, the maximal X-ray photon energy is between 120–140 keV and the most common photon energies in the spectrum are between 60–70 keV. This is above the K-edge of gadolinium, so the attenuation by gadolinium in this situation is about twice that of iodine; but since there are three iodine atoms per contrast medium molecule, the iodinated contrast agent molecule attenuates 1.5 times more radiation than the gadolinium-based contrast molecule does. For common radiographic examinations, the maximal X-ray photon energy is

between 70–90 keV and the most common photon energies in the spectrum are above and below the K-edge of gadolinium (50 keV). Because of the range of photon energies, attenuation is approximately the same for iodine and gadolinium atoms. Hence, the attenuation by the iodinated contrast agent molecule is three times that of the gadolinium based contrast molecule (NYMAN et al. 2002).

It should theoretically be possible to obtain radiographic images of diagnostic quality with gadolinium-based contrast agents, but the image quality will generally be inferior to that achieved with iodinated contrast agents. This can be explained by the difference in molar concentrations between gadolinium- and iodine-based contrast agents. A 0.5 mmol ml^{-1} concentration of iodinated contrast agent contains 63 mgI ml^{-1}. Assuming that a 0.5 mmol ml^{-1} concentration of gadolinium based contrast agent attenuates to the same extent as a 0.5 mmol ml^{-1} concentration of the iodinated agent, a patient receiving these equi-attenuating concentrations receives only 1/3 of the contrast medium molecules with the iodinated agent that would be necessary with the gadolinium based agent. Considering the molar concentration of an iodinated contrast agent at 300 mgI ml^{-1}, the attenuation of this preparation is almost five times that of gadolinium preparations of the same volume. Thus, the volume of gadolinium preparation required to obtain "comparable" attenuation is five times that of the iodine preparation.

22.4

Pharmacokinetics

The gadolinium chelates have pharmacokinetics similar to those of iodinated radiographic contrast agents with the exception of gadobenate dimeglumine which is also excreted by the liver in small amounts (Chap. 25). Gadobenate dimeglumine is however mainly used for non liver specific indications similar to the five other "extracellular" gadolinium chelates (Chap. 21). Both gadolinium and iodinated agents are distributed in the extracellular space and excreted by glomerular filtration. Thus, the T½ is almost the same, and both types of agents can be used to measure the glomerular filtration rate. In patients with normal kidney function about 98% of these agents are excreted within 24 h of injection. However, in patients with severe renal impairment, excretion of gadolinium and iodinated agents differs. Nearly no gadolinium is found in the feces in patients with renal insufficiency, whereas up to 6% of the injected iodine has been recovered in the feces of such patients (JOFFE et al. 1998). No free gadolinium is found in the blood several days after injection of gadolinium chelates in patients with end-stage renal failure despite the slow excretion (JOFFE et al. 1998; NORMANN et al. 2000).

22.5
Toxicity (LD$_{50}$)

Acute intravenous LD$_{50}$ of contrast media in mice is expressed as mmol iodine or gadolinium per kg BW. For the five gadolinium-based contrast agents, dimeglumine gadopentate, gadobenate dimeglumine, gadoterate, gadoteridol and gadodiamide, the figures are 6, 8, 8, 18 and 20 mmol gadolinium kg^{-1}, respectively. According to IDÉE et al (2006)the determination with regard to gadodiamide is based on two subsequent injections 30 min. apart. The LD$_{50}$ for the conventional high osmolality iodinated contrast agent diatrizoate is about 50 mmol iodine kg^{-1}. The LD$_{50}$ of low osmolality nonionic monomers, e.g. iopromide, is much higher, about 150 mmol iodine per kg) (WEINMANN et al. 1990; WEINMANN 1999). These LD$_{50}$ values suggest that, comparing attenuating atoms, the acute intravenous toxicity of the gadolinium-based contrast media is 6–25 times that of the nonionic iodinated monomers.

22.6
Incidence of General Reactions to Gadolinium Based Contrast Agents

General adverse reactions similar to those observed with iodinated contrast media may be seen following injection of gadolinium based contrast agents, but the frequency is lower with the incidence of moderate and severe reactions well below 1% (NIENDORF et al. 1991; THOMSEN 1997). However, the number of patients exposed to unapproved dosages (above 0.3 mmol kg^{-1} BW) is still too small to draw any conclusion about the safety of these higher doses. In the few published studies, varying doses of gadolinium-based agents (20–440 ml) have been used and the number of patients has been small.

22.7
Clinical Studies

PRINCE et al. (1996) studied 64 patients undergoing MR examination with a gadolinium-based agent and a radiographic examination with an iodinated contrast medium. They concluded that high-dose gadolinium chelates are significantly less nephrotoxic than iodinated agents, since eleven of the 64 patients had a significant increase in serum creatinine after intravenous or intraarterial administration of iodine-based contrast media whereas none had increased serum creatinine levels after intravenous administration of a gadolinium-based contrast agent. However, the molar doses and concentrations of the iodine and gadolinium atoms were not comparable. Although the exact dose of the iodinated contrast agent used for each patient could not be verified, between 30 and 60 g I was administered. For the MR examinations between 0.2 and 0.4 mmol kg^{-1} BW were used. Assuming that all patients were standard (~70 kg), the dose of iodine atoms was approximately 17 times higher than that of gadolinium atoms. Thus, the doses were not comparable and had equi-attenuating doses been used, the results might have been different.

Over recent years, gadolinium-based contrast agents have been used for examinations such as CT, intravenous urography and digital subtraction angiography of various parts of the body (e.g. liver, renal and peripheral arteries). ALBRECHT and DAWSON (2000) studied 15 patients receiving 0.3 mmol kg^{-1} BW gadopentate dimeglumine; five had abdominal CT, five abdominal DSA and five had intravenous urography. No side-effects were reported, but generally the image quality was inferior to that obtained subsequently with standard doses of iodinated contrast media (50–150 ml of a 300 or 350 mgI ml^{-1} solution). The authors suggested that higher doses including more concentrated solutions of gadolinium-based contrast media might be useful (ALBRECHT and DAWSON 2000).

Gadolinium-based contrast media have also been used for endoscopic retrograde cholangiography, cystography, urethrocystography, and retrograde pyelography and during percutaneous nephrostomy and biliary tract drainage with resultant adequate image quality and no side-effects (VELMAS and MARKKOLA 1998). COCHE et al. (2001) reported successful detection of pulmonary embolism using gadolinium-enhanced helical CT (0.4 mmol kg^{-1} gadodiamide), without any problems, in a 77-year-old woman with previous allergy-like reaction to iodinated contrast medium and renal insufficiency (serum creatinine of 200 µmol ml^{-1}). A total of 14 patients with abnormal S-creatinine levels underwent digital subtraction vena cavography with a gadolinium-based contrast agent (maximum 0.4 mmol kg^{-1} BW) for filter placement, thrombolysis or diagnosis. Three of the 14 patients had a significant increase in serum creatinine (>44 µmol ml^{-1}), but there were other concurrent causes, which might account for the deterioration of renal function (KAUFMANN et al. 1999). It was concluded that gadolinium-based contrast agents were suitable for digital subtraction venography in patients with renal insufficiency.

In an azotemic patient with suspected renal artery stenosis, a total of 40 ml (0.5 mmol ml^{-1}) undiluted dimeglumine gadopentate was injected arterially (MATCHETT et al. 1996). The serum creatinine increased from 290 µmol l^{-1} to 390 µmol l^{-1}, but this might have been attributable to a myocardial infarction which the patient developed 3 days after the procedure. Acute renal failure was described following lower extremity arteriography with 80 ml of 0.5 mmol ml^{-1} (0.44 mmol kg^{-1} BW) of gadoteridol in an insulin-dependent diabetic patient with nephropathy (GEMERY et al. 1998). S-creatinine transiently increased from 350 to 820 µmol ml^{-1} and the deterioration was considered most likely due to the contrast agent.

A total of 31 patients with azotemia or previous severe adverse reaction to iodinated contrast media underwent digital subtraction angiography with between 20 and 60 ml of 0.5 mmol ml^{-1} gadopentate (HAMMER et al. 1999). In nine cases, CO_2 was also used and in eight cases between 6 and 40 ml of iohexol 350 mgI ml^{-1} (mean 17.8 ml) were used. In no patient did S-creatinine increase more than 44 µmol l^{-1} within 48 h. SPINOSA et al. (1998) studied 13 renal transplant patients with suspected vascular causes of renal insufficiency and/or accelerated hypertension with both CO_2 and a gadolinium-based contrast agent (16–60 ml gadodiamide). Digital subtraction angiography was considered adequate in all patients. In two patients renal failure progressed (>44 µmol l^{-1} within 48 h), but concurrent causes of the renal dysfunction were also present; one had received 20 and the other had received 60 ml of gadodiamide. During peripheral arteriography SPINOSA et al. (1999) found that gadodiamide with an osmolality of 789 mOsm per kilogram of water was less painful than gadopentate dimeglumine with an osmolality of greater than 1,800 mOsm per kilogram of water. No effects on

renal function were found. Later SPINOSA et al. (2000) reported one of 18 azotemic patients (6%) whose renal function deteriorated after undergoing CO_2 angiography supplemented with 0.5 mmol ml^{-1} gadodiamide (20–100 ml; mean volume 55 ml; 0.13–.04 mmol kg^{-1}). The affected patient received 70 ml gadodiamide (0.3 mmol kg^{-1} BW)

Injections of 80–440 ml of gadodiamide during arteriography have also been reported (GEMMETE et al. 2001). A S-creatinine increase of 53 µmol ml^{-1} or more occurred in eight of 20 patients (40%) with a preprocedural S-Cr of 115–548 µmol ml^{-1}. In three of the eight patients, the creatinine values did not return to baseline value. Following peripheral gadolinium arteriography, angioplasty and stent placement, a patient with renal insufficiency (340 ìmol l^{-1}) developed acute renal failure and acute pancreatitis (SCHENKER et al. 2001). Acute pancreatitis has been seen both after intraarterial (GEMERY et al. 1998) and intravenous (TERZI and SOKMEN 1999) injection of a gadolinium-based contrast agent.

22.8
Experimental Nephrotoxicity

Intravenous injection (9 ml kg^{-1}) of gadopentate (0.1 mol ml^{-1}), iohexol (300 mgI ml^{-1}), metrizoate (300 mgI ml^{-1}) and normal saline in rabbits produced nephrotoxicity of the same order for all three contrast agents (LEANDER et al. 1992). The molar concentration and dose of iodine atoms was 24 times higher than the molar concentration and dose of gadolinium atoms. Thus, the iodinated agents might have had a lower nephrotoxic effect than the gadolinium media if the two agents had been compared in equiattenuating doses and concentrations. Rat studies where high equimolar doses (4.59 mmol kg^{-1} BW) of gadolinium (gadopentate and gadodiamide) and iodinated (diatrizoate and iohexol) contrast agents were injected intravenously showed no significant deterioration in the function of normal and diseased kidneys (THOMSEN et al. 1994, 1995). There was a significant correlation between albuminuria and the osmolality of the contrast medium; gadopentate caused the highest excretion of albumin and gadodiamide and iohexol the least. However, the degree of albuminuria does not correlate with the nephrotoxic potential of a contrast medium. In these studies the dose of iodine atoms was three times the dose of gadolinium atoms.

In an ischemic rat model, intra-aortic injections of 1.5 ml (0.5 mmol ml^{-1}) gadopentate (0.75 mmol Gd atoms) and 2.6 ml 370 mgI ml^{-1} diatrizoate (7.6 mmol iodine atoms) caused a significant decrease in creatinine clearance of similar magnitude, 50 and 67%, respectively (Deray et al. 1990; Brillet et al. 1994). Gadoterate [1.5 ml (0.5 mmol l^{-1})] alone caused no decrease in renal function in this model. The dose of iodine was ten times higher than the dose of gadolinium and the two different doses produced a similar significant decrease in creatinine clearance. Whether the iodinated contrast medium would produce less decrease in creatinine clearance than the gadolinium medium if equimolar doses had been given remains speculative.

In an experimental model of renal ischemia in pigs, 0.5 molar gadopentate dimeglumine (3 ml kg^{-1} BW) caused severe impairment of renal function; the low-osmolar gadodiamide caused less deterioration in renal function, and the low-osmolar iohexol (3 ml of 190 mgI ml^{-1} per kg BW) caused even less (Elmståhl et al. 2004). Three ml per kg BW of iohexol (70 mg iodine ml^{-1}), which for angiography is equi-attenuating with 0.4 M gadopentate dimeglumine, caused no change in renal function. Iodine based contrast agents showed a better renal tolerance and radiodensity than did gadolinium based contrast agents during arteriography in ischemic porcine kidneys (Elmståhl et al. 2008). An in vitro study using the isolated perfused rat kidney showed that a large dose of gadopentate dimeglumine (0.3 mmol kg^{-1} BW) did not cause significant reduction in renal function (Brown et al. 1993). However, an equimolar dose per kg BW of iodine atoms in a 70 kg man would be 10 ml at concentration of 265 mg iodine ml^{-1}.

22.9
MR Examinations and Nephrotoxicity

Sam et al. (2003) reported that in 3.5% of 195 patients with abnormal pre-examination creatinine clearance levels, acute renal failure (anuria) developed after gadolinium-based contrast medium administration. For MR angiography the incidence was 1.9% and for digital subtraction angiography 9.5%. Dialysis was required in three of the seven patients who developed acute renal failure. The average creatinine clearance in the whole group was 38.2 ± 1.6 ml min^{-1} 1.73 m^{-2} and in the seven patients who developed

contrast medium induced nephropathy it was 32.5 ± 7.8 ml min^{-1} 1.73 m^{-2}. The doses of gadolinium-DTPA ranged from 0.31 to 0.41 mmol kg^{-1} for MR angiography and 0.27 to 0.42 mmol kg^{-1} for digital subtraction angiography. Contrast medium induced nephropathy occurred after a moderate (0.14 mmol kg^{-1}) – approved – dose of a gadolinium-based contrast medium in a patient with moderate to severe diabetic nephropathy and chronic heart failure (Thomsen 2004). Akgun (2006) reported acute tubular necrosis in a renal biopsy following exposure to a gadolinium based contrast agent. In diabetic patients with multiple risk factors it may be appropriate to take the same precautions before enhanced MR examinations as before enhanced radiographic examinations. The possibility remains that for CT aortography, iodine based contrast media of equal attenuation to gadolinium based contrast agents may have less risk of causing contrast medium induced nephropathy (Nyman et al. 2008).

22.10
Conclusion

Nephrotoxicity of gadolinium-based contrast agents when used for radiographic studies, CT and MRI has now been described in both man and animals. Use of high doses (>0.3 mmol kg^{-1} BW) of the gadolinium agents in patients with impaired renal function is contraindicated. Patients with reduced renal function are also at risk of developing nephrogenic systemic fibrosis after less stable gadolinium agents (see Chap. 24)

Several reports have shown the usefulness of gadolinium-based agents in radiographic examinations including CT when iodinated contrast agents were contraindicated for a variety of reasons. The major drawback when using gadolinium-based contrast agents for CT or radiography is that commercially available contrast media have only one gadolinium atom per molecule and a low molar concentration. In comparison, iodinated monomers for radiographic examinations contain three iodine atoms per molecule and have a molar concentration five times that of gadolinium in the four gadolinium-based contrast agents (dimeglumine gadopentate, gadobenate dimeglumine, gadoteridol, gadodiamide, gadoterate). Hence, image quality is generally inferior when gadolinium-based contrast media are used for radiography. Gadolinium-based contrast media should not be used for radiographic examinations (Chap. 29).

References

Akgun H, Gonlusen G, Cartwright J, Suki WN, Truong LD (2006) Are gadolinium based contrast media nephrotoxic? A renal biopsy study. Arch Pathol Lab Med 130:1354–1357

Albrecht T, Dawson P (2000) Gadolinium-DTPA as X-ray contrast medium in clinical studies. Br J Radiol 73:878–882

Bittner CA, Goodwin SC, Lu D, McNamara TO, Joseph T (1997) Gadolinium-based contrast agents for angiographic use as a safe radiocontrast in patients with impaired renal function. J Vasc Interv Radiol [Suppl] 8:178

Brillet G, Dubois M, Beaufils H, Bourboze R, Deray G (1994) Renal tolerance of gadolinium-DOTA and gadolinium-DTPA in rats. Invest Radiol 29:352–354

Brown PWG, Haylor JL, Morcos SK, El Nahas AM (1993) The functional effects of gadolinium-DTPA on the isolated perfused rat kidney. Eur J Radiol 16:85–89

Coche EE, Hammer FD, Gofette PP (2001) Demonstration of pulmonary embolism with dynamic gadolinium-enhanced spiral CT. Eur Radiol 11:2306–2309

Deray G, Dubois M, Martinez F, Baumelou B, Beaufils H, Bourboze R, Baumelou A, Jacobs C (1990) Renal effects of radiocontrast agents in rats: A new model of acute renal failure. Am J Nephrol 10:507–513

Elmståhl B, Nyman U, Leander P et al (2004) Gadolinium contrast media are more nephrotoxic than low dose iodine medium employing doses with equal X-ray attenuation in renal arteriography: an experimental study in pigs. Acad Radiol 11:1219–1228

Elmståhl B, Nyman U, Leander P, Golman K, Chai CM, Grant D, Doughty R, Pehrson R, Björk J, Almén T (2008) Iodixanol 320 results in better renal tolerance and radiodensity than do gadolinium-based contrast media: arteriography in ischemic porcine kidneys. Radiology 247:88–97

Engelbrecht V, Koch JA, Rassek M, Mödder U (1996) Gadodiamide and gadolinium-DTPA as intravenous media in computed tomography. Röfo Fortschr Geb Rontgenstr Neuen Bildgeb Verfahr 165:24–28

Gemery J, Idelson B, Reid S et al (1998) Acute renal failure after arteriography with a gadolinium-based contrast agent. AJR Am J Roentgenol 171:1277–1278

Gemmete JJ, Forauer AR, Kazanjian S, Dasika N, Williams DM, Cho K (2001) Safety of large volume gadolinium angiography. J Vasc Interv Radiol 12(part 2):S28

Hammer FD, Gofette PP, Maliase J, Mathurin P (1999) Gadolinium dimeglumine: an alternative contrast agent for digital subtraction angiography. Eur Radiol 9:128–136

Idée J-M, Port M, Raynal I, Schaefer, Le Greneur S, Corot C (2006) Clinical and biological consequences of transmetallation induced by contrast agents for magnetic resonance imaging: a review. Fundam Clin Pharmacol 20:563–576

Joffe P, Thomsen HS, Meusel M (1998) The pharmacokinetics of gadodiamide injection in patients with severe renal insufficiency treated conservatively or undergoing hemodialysis or continuous ambulatory peritoneal dialysis. Acad Radiol 5:491–502

Kaufmann JA, Geller SC, Bazari H, Waltman AC (1999) Gadolinium-based contrast agents as an alternative at vena cavography in patients with renal insufficiency – early experiences. Radiology 212:280–284

Leander P, Allard P, Caillé JM, Golman K (1992) Early effect of gadopentate and iodinated contrast media on rabbit kidneys. Invest Radiol 27:922–926

Matchett WJ, McFarland DR, Rusell DK, Sailors DM, Moursi MM (1996) Azotemia: gadopentate dimeglumine as contrast agent at digital subtraction angiography. Radiology 201:569–571

Niendorf HP, Gifford LM, Haustein J, Cornelius I, Alhassan A, Clauss W (1991) Tolerance data of Gd-DTPA: a review. Eur J Radiol 13:15–20

Normann PT, Joffe P, Martinsen I, Thomsen HS (2000) Identification and quantification of gadodiamide in serum, peritoneal dialysate and faeces from end-stage renal patients dosed with gadodiamide injection by inductively coupled plasma-atomic emission spectroscopy and comparative analysis by high-performance liquid chromatography. J Pharma Biomed Anal 22:939–947

Nyman U, Elmståhl B, Leander P, Nilsson M, Golman K, Almén T (2002) Are gadolinium-based contrast media really safer than iodinated contrast media for digital subtraction angiography in patients with azotemia? Radiology 223:311–318

Nyman U, Elmståhl B, Leander P, Almén T (2008). Iodine contrast media doses equal-attenuating with gadolinium chelates at CT-aortography may have less risk of contrast-induced nephropathy and no risk of nephrogenic systemic fibrosis in azotaemic patients! Eur Radiol 18(9):2013–2014

Prince MR, Arnoldus C, Frisoli JK (1996) Nephrotoxicity of high-dose gadolinium compared with iodinated contrast. JMRI 1:162–166

Sam AD II, Morasch MD, Collins J, Song G, Chen R, Pereles FS (2003) Safety of gadolinium contrast angiography in patients with chronic renal insufficiency. J Vasc Surg 38:313–318

Schenker MP, Solomon JA, Roberts DA (2001) Gadolinium arteriography complicated by acute pancreatitis and acute renal failure. J Vasc Interv Radiol 12:393

Spinosa DJ, Matsumo AH, Angle JF, Hagspiel KD, Iassacs R (1998) Gadolinium based contrast and carbon dioxide angiography to evaluate transplants for vascular causes of renal insufficiency and accelerated hypertension. J Vasc Interv Radiol 9:909–916

Spinosa DJ, Matsumoto AH, Hagspiel KD, Angle JF, Hartwell GD (1999) Gadolinium-based contrast agents in angiography and interventional radiology. AJR Am J Roentgenol 173:1403–1409

Spinosa DJ, Angle JF, Hagspiel KD, Kern JA, Hartwell GD, Matsumoto AH (2000) Lower extremity arteriography with use of iodinated contrast material or gadodiamide to supplement CO2 angiography in patients with renal insufficiency. JVIR 11:35–43

Terzi C, Sokmen S (1999) Acute pancreatitis induced by magnetic-resonance-imaging contrast agent. Lancet 354:1789–1790

Thomsen HS (1997) Frequency of acute adverse events to a nonionic low-osmolar contrast medium: the effect of verbal interview. Pharmacol Toxicol 80:108–110

Thomsen HS (2003) ESUR Guidelines in contrast media. Am J Roentgenol 181:1461–1471

Thomsen HS (2004) Gadolinium-based contrast media may be nephrotoxic even at approved doses. Eur Radiol 14:1654–1656

Thomsen HS, Dorph S, Larsen S et al (1994) Urine profiles and kidney histology after intravenous injection of ionic and nonionic radiologic and magnetic resonance contrast media in normal rats. Acad Radiol 1:128–135

Thomsen HS, Dorph S, Larsen S et al (1995) Urine profiles and kidney histology after intravenous injection of ionic and nonionic radiologic and magnetic resonance contrast media in rats with cisplatin nephropathy. Acad Radiol 2:675–682

Thomsen HS, Almén T, Morcos SK, Members of Contrast Media Safety Committee of European Society of Urogenital Radiology (2002) Gadolinium-containing contrast media for radiographic examinations: a position paper. Eur Radiol 12:2600–2605

Velmas T, Markkola T (1998) Gd-DTPA as an alternative contrast agent in conventional and interventional radiology. Acta Radiol 39:223–226

Weinmann HJ (1999) Gadolinium chelates: physico-chemical properties, formulation and toxicology. In: Dawson P, Cosgrove DO, Grainger RG (eds) Textbook of contrast media. Isis Medical Media, Oxford, p 228

Weinmann JH, Press WR, Gries H (1990) Tolerance of extracellular contrast agents for magnetic resonance imaging. Invest Radiol 25:S49–S50

MR Contrast Media

Gadolinium-Based Contrast Agents

Acute Adverse Reactions

Gertraud Heinz-Peer

23.1
Introduction

For many years, gadolinium based contrast agents have been considered quite safe, with minimal associated risk. However, gadolinium based contrast agents are not inert drugs. They may cause acute non-renal adverse reactions (e.g. anaphylactoid reactions), acute renal adverse reactions (e.g. contrast induced nephropathy), delayed adverse reactions (nephrogenic systemic fibrosis), problems at the site of injection (e.g. local necrosis) and laboratory abnormalities. The use of contrast enhanced MRI has increased over the past decade, as a variety of new applications have been described and put into clinical practice. Consequently, the number of administrations of gadolinium based contrast agents have also increased considerably. This chapter focuses on acute adverse reactions to gadolinium contrast agents which are similar to reactions which occur

Gertraud Heinz-Peer
Medical University of Vienna, Department of Radiology,
Währinger Gürtel 18-20 1090 Vienna, Austria

after iodine based contrast media. Delayed adverse reactions, extravasation and laboratory abnormalities are covered in Chaps 24, 15 and 14, respectively.

23.2
Acute Non-Renal Adverse Reactions

Because of differences in study design and definitions of adverse reactions used, it is difficult to draw definite conclusions about the incidence of adverse effects following gadolinium contrast media. In European and Japanese studies, gadopentetate dimeglumine had low adverse incidence rates (0.63%), whereas in the USA, with legally imposed differences in registration and documentation of adverse events, the incidence was 7.6% (Niendorf et al. 1991a). Nonetheless, it appears that safety profiles of gadopentetate dimeglumine, gadoterate meglumine, gadoteridol, gadodiamide, gadobenate dimeglumine and gadoversetamide are comparable (Kirchin and Runge 2003; Shellock and Kanal 1999). In general, the total incidence rate of adverse events appears to be less than 5% and the incidence of a single adverse event is below 1% (Niendorf et al. 1991a, b; Thomsen 1997). Dillman et al. (2007) reported in a retrospective study that there were 54 (0.07%) acute allergy-like reactions in 78,353 intravenous administrations of gadolinium based contrast agents over 6 years. One patient experienced three acute allergy-like reactions during the period. 74% of the reactions were considered mild. In another study Murphy et al. (1996) described a 0.1% frequency of allergy-like reactions to gadolinium based contrast agents among 21,000 patients over an almost 5-year period. A retrospective survey involving 53 institutions showed that 241 allergy-like reactions (0.03%) occurred after 825,535 injections (MURPHY et al. 1999). However retrospective studies may underestimate the actual rate. In particular, mild reactions may be underestimated whereas the rate of severe reactions is more likely to be correct. A recent post marketing surveillance study (HERBORN et al. 2007) of 24,308 patients who received gadoterate meglumine intravenously for a variety of diagnostic examinations reported that the incidence of adverse events was 0.4%; most of them were rated as minor, such as a feeling of warmth or altered taste. LI et al. (2006) reported a reaction frequency of 0.2% in 9,528 patients.

The most common reported adverse events with gadolinium based contrast agents are headache, nausea, vomiting, hives and altered taste (KIRCHIN and RUNGE 2003; RUNGE 2000; SHELLOCK and KANAL 1999). Treatment for adverse reactions is the same as for iodine based contrast agents (Chap. 8). Anaphylactoid reactions to gadolinium based contrast agents do occur, but their incidence is very low. The first documented anaphylactoid reaction to gadopentetate dimeglumine was observed not in clinical trials but some time after approval (RUNGE 2000). The true incidence of such reactions for Gd chelates is not known, but appears to be between 1:100,000 and 1:500,000 (SHELLOCK and KANAL 1999).

There are large differences in the incidence of adverse events in studies of various gadolinium agents (GREENEN and KRESTIN 2006). For gadopentetate dimeglumine the incidence of doubtful to highly probable related adverse events varied between 0.77–18%. The figures were 0–18.8% for gadodiamide, 0.97–14.1% for gadoterate meglumine and 0–22% for gadobenate dimeglumine. Interestingly, the study with the largest patient population ($n = 1,038$) showed lowest incidence rate of adverse events (OUDKERK et al. 1995). In none of the studies was there a significant difference in adverse events between agents.

In a descriptive study of moderate to severe reactions after either gadopentetate dimeglumine or gadoterate meglumine in approximately 30,000 patients over a 10-year time period, three moderate to severe reactions occurred, all after gadoterate meglumine (DE RIDDER et al. 2001). In a study of 56 patients with multiple sclerosis, who received monthly MRI examinations with gadopentetate dimeglumine 0.1 mmol kg^{-1} for research purposes, no significant effects on routine haematology, serum chemistry, renal and liver function and serum iron profiles were found. Patients had received between three and 53 doses of gadopentetate dimeglumine. It was concluded that repeated monthly administration of gadopentetate dimeglumine at the standard dose is safe (TRESLEY et al. 1997). However, the long term effects have not yet been studied.

During phase I–III studies with gadoversetamide, no significant differences in adverse event rates for doses between 0.1 and 0.4 mmol kg^{-1} were noted (BROWN et al. 2002). In another study with gadoversetamide, patients received 0.1, 0.3, or 0.5 mmol kg^{-1}. The incidence of adverse events increased significantly with increasing dose (SWAN et al. 1999a). In a phase III clinical trial, 38 patients received the standard gadodiamide dose and 40 received a triple dose. Five patients from the standard dose group and two from the triple dose group reported adverse events, none of which were judged to be related to the contrast medium (DEMAEREL et al. 1994). In a double blind multicenter study with single versus triple dose gadodiamide, no adverse events possibly related to gadodiamide administration were recorded (THURNHER et al. 2001). In a phase III study in 199 patients with suspected CNS pathology, patients either received 0.1 or 0.3 mmol kg^{-1} gadopentetate dimeglumine (HAUSTEIN et al. 1993). A total of 15 adverse events in 12 patients were encountered, eight in the 0.1 mmol kg^{-1} group and seven in the 0.3 mmol kg^{-1} group.

Although acute allergy-like reactions occurred more frequently in adults than in children, and in females than male patients, these differences were not statistically significant (DILLMAN et al. 2007).

Gadobutrol produced adverse reactions are considered to be possibly drug related in 4.6% of patients (BALZER et al. 2003). Gadobutrol is contra-indicated in patients with uncorrected hypokalemia. Furthermore, special care is needed in patients with a family history of congenital long QT syndrome, previous arrhythmias after taking drugs that prolong cardiac repolarisation or who are taking class III antiarrhythmic drugs. Recommendations are based on the assumption that gadobutrol in a high dose (≥ 4 times maximal dose) can block potassium channels, resulting in prolonged QT interval and accelerated ventricular rhythm.

Potential factors that may increase an individual's risk of an acute allergy-like reaction include a history of previous allergy-like reaction to intravenous-administered contrast media (either gadolinium- or iodine-containing) and prior allergic reaction to a substance other than contrast media. The risk of adverse reactions to gadopentetate dimeglumine was 3.7 times higher in patients with a prior history of reaction to iodinated contrast media (NIENDORF et al. 1991b). The number of published studies is too small to draw any conclusions about safety of higher unapproved dosages. One of the reasons for the lower prevalence of adverse reactions to gadolinium based than iodine-based contrast agents may be the much lower dose of the agent used for MRI than for radiography, i.e. the molar dose for enhanced MRI of the brain is on average 8 times lower than that for CT of the brain. DILLMAN et al. (2008) recently reported that allergy-like reactions to gadolinium based contrast agents could occur despite premedication with corticosteroids and antihistamines. 2/3 of the reactions were mild. All patients had a history of allergy-like reactions to either a gadolinium or iodine based contrast agent.

Currently there is no evidence of any advantage of premedication before administration of gadolinium based contrast agents, even in patients who have reacted earlier to contrast agents. Prompt recognition and treatment is crucial and invaluable in blunting an adverse response of a patient to gadolinium based contrast agents and may prevent a reaction from becoming severe or even life-threatening.

23.3
Acute Renal Adverse Reactions (Contrast Induced Nephropathy)

In most patients with moderate to severe impaired renal function, gadopentetate dimeglumine, gadoterate meglumine, gadodiamide, gadobenate dimeglumine, gadoteridol, gadobutrol and gadoversetamide do not significantly affect serum creatinine levels (BELLIN et al. 1992; HAUSTEIN et al. 1992; JOFFE et al. 1998; SWAN et al. 1999a, b; TOMBACH et al. 2001; YOSHIKAWA and DAVIES 1997). However, contrast medium induced nephropathy may occur after gadolinium based contrast media, just as after iodinated contrast media (Chaps. 9 and 22).

Nephrotoxicity of the gadolinium based contrast agents has now been documented in both man and animals. Use of high doses ($>0.3 \, \mathrm{mmol \, kg^{-1} \, bw}$) of gadolinium based contrast agents in patients with impaired renal function is clearly contraindicated (THOMSEN et al. 2002). In 2003, SAM et al. reported that in 3.5% of 195 patients with abnormal creatinine clearance levels, acute renal failure developed after gadolinium based contrast agents. For MR angiography the incidence was 1.9% and for digital subtraction

angiography 9.5%. Dialysis was required in 40% of the patients developing acute renal failure. Doses of gadolinium-DTPA ranged from 0.31 to 0.41 mmol $\mathrm{kg^{-1}}$ for MR angiography and from 0.27 to 0.42 mmol $\mathrm{kg^{-1}}$ for digital subtraction angiography. Contrast medium induced nephropathy has even been reported after an intravenous injection of 0.14 mmol $\mathrm{l^{-1}}$ of a gadolinium based contrast agent (THOMSEN 2004). In an experimental study investigating whether gadolinium based contrast agents were less nephrotoxic than iodine based contrast agents in X-ray arteriography of a kidney made temporarily ischemic by arterial balloon occlusion, ELMSTÅHL et al. (2004) found that 0.5 M gadolinium based contrast agents were more nephrotoxic than both equal-attenuating (70 mg I ml^{-1}) and equimolar (190 mg I ml^{-1}) concentrations of iodine media. Using the same ischemic porcine model, they found in 2007 that the histomorphological changes caused by gadolinium based contrast agents were similar to those caused by iodine media (ELMSTÅHL et al. 2007). Vacuolization appeared to be independent of osmolality and viscosity of the contrast medium, and did not seem to be an indicator of renal impairment.

In a retrospective study that included 473 patients with stage 3 and 4 renal failure who received 0.2 ml kg^{-1} of gadolinium based contrast medium, ERGUN et al. (2006) found that risk factors for acute renal failure after gadolinium based contrast agents included diabetic nephropathy and low glomerular filtration rate. In addition, BRIGUORI et al. (2006) showed in a prospective study that using gadolinium based contrast agents did not appear to reduce the rate of contrast induced nephropathy, as compared to iodine based contrast agents in patients with chronic renal insufficiency.

The risk of contrast medium induced nephropathy is very low when MR-approved doses ($<0.3 \, \mathrm{mmol \, kg^{-1}}$) of gadolinium based contrast agents are used. In comparison, the risk of NSF is much higher when less stable agents are used (Chap. 24).

23.4
Conclusion

Clinical trials and experience have shown that in general, gadolinium based contrast agents produce relatively few acute reactions. However, acute reactions may occur. Allergy-like reactions occur after less than 1% of gadolinium based contrast agent administrations. Reactions are the same as those seen after iodine based contrast agents. In most cases they are mild, but a few severe anaphylactoid reactions have been reported. Allergy-like reactions may occur despite pretreatment with corticosteroid and antihistamine. Therefore, one must always be prepared to treat an adverse reaction after administration of gadolinium based contrast agents. Management is similar to that of reactions to iodine based contrast agents. Appropriate knowledge, training and preparation are essential to ensure prompt effective treatment. Premedication before administering gadolinium based contrast agents is not generally indicated.

Acute renal adverse reactions may occur after administration of gadolinium based contrast agents in approved doses (<0.3 mmol Kg^{-1} bw), but these occur very infrequently. Above 0.3 mmol kg^{-1} bw, the risk is much higher in patients with reduced renal function. Gadolinium based contrast agents should not be used in these patients in doses greater than 0.3 mmol kg^{-1} bw.

References

Balzer JO, Loewe C, Davis K et al (2003) Safety of contrast-enhanced MR angiography employing gadobutrol 1.0 M as contrast material. Eur Radiol 13:2067–2074

Bellin MF, Deray G, Assogba U et al (1992) Gd-DOTA: evaluation of its renal tolerance in patients with chronic renal failure. Magn Reson Imaging 10:115–118

Briguori C, Colombo A, Airoldi F, Melzi G et al (2006) Gadolinium-based contrast agents and nephrotoxicity in patients undergoing coronary artery procedures. Catheter Cardiovasc Interv 67:175–180

Brown JJ, Kristy RM, Stevens GR et al (2002) The OptiMARK clinical development program: summary of safety data. J Magn Reson Imaging 15:446–455

Demaerel P, Marchal G, Wilms G et al (1994) Gadodiamide injection at 0.1 and 0.3 mmol/kg body weight: a phase III double-blind, parallel, randomised clinical investigation of known or suspected central nervous system lesions at 1.5T. Neuroradiology 36:355–359

De Ridder F, de Maeseneer M, Stadnik T et al (2001) Severe adverse reactions with contrast agents for magnetic resonance: clinical experience in 30000 MR examinations. JBR-BTR 84:150–152

Dillman JR, Ellis JH, Cohan RH, Strouse PJ, Jan SC (2007) Frequency and severity of acute allergic-like reactions to gadolinium-containing IV contrast media in children and adults. Am J Roentgenol 189:1533–1538

Dillman JR, Ellis JH, Cohan RH, Strouse PJ, Jan SC (2008) Allergic-like breakthrough reactions to gadolinium contrast agents after corticosteroid and antihistamine premedication. Am J Roentgenol 190:187–190

Elmståhl B, Leander P, Grant D et al (2007) Histomorphological changes after renal X-ray arteriography using iodine and gadolinium contrast media in an ischemic porcine model. Acta Radiol 23:1–11

Elmståhl B, Nyman U, Leander P, Chai CM, Frennby B, Almen T (2004) Gadolinium contrast media are more nephrotoxic than a low-osmolar iodine medium employing doses with equal X-ray attenuation in renal arteriography: an experimental study in pigs. Acad Radiol 11:1219–1228

Ergun I, Keven K, Uruc I et al (2006) The safety of gadolinium in patients with stage 3 and 4 renal failure. Nephrol Dial Transplant 21:697–700

Greenen RWF, Krestin GP (2006) Non-tissue specific extracellular MR contrast media. In: Thomsen HS (ed). Contrast media: Safety issues and ESUR Guidelines. Springer, Heidelberg, pp 107–120

Herborn CU, Honold E, Wolf M et al (2007) Clinical safety and diagnostic value of the gadolinium chelate gadoterate meglumine (Gd-DOTA). Invest Radiol 42:58–62

Haustein J, Laniado M, Niendorf HP et al (1993) Triple-dose versus standard-dose gadopentetate dimeglumine: a randomized study in 199 patients. Radiology 186:855–860

Joffe P, Thomsen HS, Meusel M (1998) Pharmacokinetics of gadodiamide injection in patients with severe renal insufficiency and patients undergoing hemodialysis or continuous ambulatory peritoneal dialysis. Acad Radiol 5:491–502

Kirchin MA, Runge VM (2003) Contrast agents for magnetic resonance imaging. Safety update. Top Magn Reson Imaging 14:426–435

Li A, Wong CS, Wong MK, Lee CM, Au Yeung MC (2006) Acute adverse reactions to magnetic resonance contrast media: gadolinium chelates. Br J Radiol 79:368–371

Murphy KJ, Brunberg JA, Cohen RH (1996) Adverse reactions to gadolinium contrast media: a review of 36 cases. Am J Roentgenol 167:847–849

Murphy KPJ, Szopinski KT, Cohan RH, Mermillod B, Ellis JH (1999) Occurrence of adverse reactions to gadolinium-based contrast material and management of patients at increased risk: a survey of the American Society of Neuroradiology Fellowship Directors. Acad Radiol 6:656–664

Niendorf HP, Dinger JC, Haustein J et al (1991a) Tolerance data of Gd-DTPA: a review. Eur J Radiol 13:15–20

Niendorf HP, Haustein J, Cornelius I, Alhassan A, Clauss W (1991b). Safety of gadolinium-DTPA: extended clinical experience. Magn Reson Med 22:222–228

Oudkerk M, Sijens PE, van Beek EJR et al (1995) Safety and efficacy of Gadoterate meglumine (Gd-DOTA) versus Magnevist (Gd-DTPA) in magnetic resonance imaging of the central nervous system. Invest Radiol 30:75–78

Runge VM (2000) Safety of approved MR contrast media for intravenous injection. J Magn Reson Imaging 12:205–213

Sam II AD, Morasch MD, Collins J, Song G, Chen R, Pereles FS (2003) Safety of gadolinium contrast angiography in patients with chronic renal insufficiency. J Vasc Surg 38:313–318

Shellock FG, Kanal E (1999) Safety of magnetic resonance imaging contrast agents. J Magn Reson Imaging 10:477–484

Swan SK, Baker JF, Free R, Tucker RM et al (1999a) Pharmacokinetics, safety, and tolerability of gadoversetamide injection (OptiMARK) in subjects with central nervous system or liver pathology and varying degrees of renal function. J Magn Reson Imaging 9:317–321

Swan SK, Lambrecht LJ, Townsend R, Davies et al (1999b) Safety and pharmacokinetic profile of gadobenate dimeglumine in subjects with renal impairment. Invest Radiol 34:443–448

Thomsen HS (1997) Frequency of acute adverse events to a nonionic lowosmolar contrast medium: the effect of verbal interview. Pharmacol Toxicol 80:108–110

Thomsen HS (2004) Gadolinium-based contrast media may be nephrotoxic even at approved doses (case report). Eur Radiol 14:1654–1656

Thomsen HS, Almén T, Morcos SK, Members of Contrast Media Safety Committee of European Society of Urogenital Radiology (2002) Gadolinium-containing contrast media for radiographic examinations: a position paper. Eur Radiol 12:2600--2605

Thurnher SA, Capelastagui A, del Olmo FH et al (2001) Safety and effectiveness of single- versus triple-dose gadodiamide injection-enhanced MR angiography of the abdomen: a phase III double-blind multicenter study. Radiology 219:137–146

Tombach B, Bremer C, Reimer P et al (2001) Renal tolerance of a neutral gadolinium chelate (gadobutrol) in patients with chronic renal failure: results of a randomized study. Radiology 218:651–657

Tresley RM, Stone LA, Fields N et al (1997) Clinical safety of serial monthly administrations of gadopentetate dimeglumine in patients with multiple sclerosis: implications for natural history and early-phase treatment trials. Neurology 48:832–835

Yoshikawa K, Davies A (1997) Safety of ProHance in special populations. Eur Radiol 7(Suppl 5):S246–S250

Delayed Reactions: Nephrogenic Systemic Fibrosis 24

Henrik S. Thomsen

CONTENTS

Henrik S. Thomsen
Department of Diagnostic Sciences, Faculty of Health Sciences, University of Copenhagen, DK-2200 Copenhagen N, Denmark
and
Department of Diagnostic Radiology,
Copenhagen University Hospital Herlev, 2730 Herlev, Denmark

24.1
Introduction

Since early 2006, evidence has accumulated that some gadolinium-based contrast agents, particularly gadodiamide (Omniscan®, GE Healthcare, Chalfont St. Giles, UK), may cause a potentially devastating or even fatal scleroderma-like, fibrosing condition called nephrogenic systemic fibrosis (NSF) in patients with renal failure (Thomsen 2006; Thomsen et al. 2007a). Some months later it was shown that gadopentetate dimeglumine (Magnevist®, Bayer Schering, Berlin, Germany) may also trigger NSF, but not with the same frequency as gadodiamide (Wertman et al. 2008). This development shocked the radiological community because for many years it was believed that gadolinium-based contrast agents were very safe. However, over the past few years there have been rapid developments in MR techniques and in the use of gadolinium-based contrast agents, which could not have been foreseen when most agents were developed and underwent early testing (phase I to III trials).

24.2
Clinical Features of Nephrogenic Systemic Fibrosis

NSF was first described in San Diego, California, USA in 1997 as an idiopathic skin condition characterized by thickening and hardening of the skin of the extremities and sometimes the trunk, with an increase in the number of dermal fibroblast-like cells associated with collagen remodeling and mucin deposition. However, it took another 3 years before the observation was reported in the peer-reviewed literature (Cowper et al. 2000). Observations from four medical centers were included in the report.

NSF affects all ages and races. The typical patient has end-stage renal disease (ESRD) (Thomsen et al. 2007a; Cowper et al. 2008). Most reported patients are on regular hemodialysis treatment, but there are centers where most patients were not on hemodialysis.

The first signs of NSF may be seen within hours of exposure to gadolinium-based contrast agents, but may occur as late as 3 months after exposure (MARCKMANN et al. 2008). It has even been claimed that NSF may occur several years after exposure to a gadolinium-based contrast agent. During the latent period, gadolinium may have accumulated in a tissue other than skin, for example, bone. TWEEDLE et al. (1995) studied [153]Gd release from four different gadolinium-based contrast agents in mice and rats and found that gadolinium was retained in liver and bone. Transmetallation, in which gadolinium exchanges with cations that occur naturally in the body, starts immediately after the agent has entered the blood (Chap. 20).

In most patients the condition begins with sub-acute swelling of the distal extremities followed in subsequent weeks by severe skin induration and sometimes extends to involve the thighs, forearms, and lower abdomen (COWPER et al. 2008; MARCKMANN et al. 2008). The skin induration may be aggressive and associated with constant pain, muscle restlessness, and loss of skin flexibility. In some cases, NSF leads to serious physical disability, including becoming wheelchair bound. For many patients, the skin thickening inhibits flexion and extension of joints, resulting in contractures. Severely affected patients may be unable to walk or fully extend the upper and lower limb joints. Complaints of muscle weakness are common, and deep bone pain in the hips and ribs has been described. Radiography may show soft tissue calcification. There is great variability. NSF severity may be graded from 0 to 4: 0 – no symptoms, 1 – mild physical, cosmetic, or neuropathic symptoms not causing any kind of disability, 2 – moderate physical and/or neuropathic symptoms limiting physical performance to some extent, 3 – severe symptoms limiting daily physical activities (walking, bathing, shopping, etc), and 4 – severely disabling symptoms causing dependence on aid or devices for common, daily activities (MARCKMANN et al. 2008). MARCKMANN et al. (2008) reported that approximately 50% of their patients had developed severe or "disabling" stage 3 and 4 NSF.

NSF was initially observed in and thought to affect the skin only, so it was called nephrogenic fibrosing dermopathy (NFD), but it is now known that it may involve organs such as the liver, lungs, muscles, and heart. Involvement of internal organs may explain the suspected increased mortality of NSF patients. In up to 50% of patients the disease is progressive and severe. NSF may contribute to death by causing scarring of organs (which impairs normal function), by restricting effective ventilation, or by restricting

movement leading to falls, which may cause fractures or hemorrhage. Other patients have died as a result of renal disease or transplant surgery. In one study it was shown that 18-month mortality was increased significantly compared to patients without NSF (40% vs. 16%, respectively), with an adjusted hazard ratio of 2.9 (95% CI(1.3–6.5), $p = 0.008$) (TODD et al. 2007). SWAMINATHAN et al. (2008) showed that of 32 patients with nephrogenic systemic fibrosis, 10 died at a median of 112 days after diagnosis. At autopsy (3 patients) there were appreciable amounts of gadolinium, iron, and aluminum, as measured by indirectly coupled plasma-mass spectrometry and confirmed by X-ray fluorescence, in the heart, blood vessels, and skin. In this high-risk group, it is difficult to differentiate deaths caused by complications of the underlying disease and its treatment from those due to NSF.

24.2.1
Pathophysiology

In patients with advanced chronic kidney disease, the elimination half-life of gadolinium-based contrast agents can be prolonged to 30 h or more (MORCOS et al. 2002). Release of free Gd^{3+} from gadolinium-based contrast agents by transmetallation and spontaneous dissociation is likely to occur if the contrast agent remains in the body for a long time, as, for example, in patients with end-stage renal disease, including those on dialysis (MORCOS 2007). Three consecutive hemodialysis sessions over 6 days would be required to clear 97% of the dose of gadolinium-based contrast agents from the body. Only 69% of the dose would be removed after 20 days of continuous ambulatory peritoneal dialysis (MORCOS et al. 2002). It seems reasonable to suggest that free Gd^{3+} ions become attached to endogenous anions particularly phosphate and form insoluble salts that deposit in tissues. These insoluble molecules will then be engulfed by local macrophages, which in turn will release a range of cytokines, including TGFb1, which attract circulating fibrocytes and initiate the process of fibrosis (MORCOS 2007; PARAZELLA 2007). There is evidence that tissue fibrosis in NSF is caused by circulating fibrocytes recruited from the circulation, rather than by proliferation of resident dendritic cells. In addition, hybridization studies have showed a marked increase in TGF b-1 mRNA levels in the skin and fascia of patients with NSF (COWPER 2007; COWPER et al. 2008).

24.2.2
Validation of NSF Cases

Because NSF may mimic other skin lesions that occur in patients with end-stage renal failure (see Tables 24.1 and 24.2), the diagnosis of NSF should never be made without histological evaluation by an experienced dermatopathologist (COWPER 2007) as well as a careful inspection of the skin by an experienced dermatologist or nephrologist. Some cases reported outside the peer-reviewed literature as NSF, for example, to the health authorities, have turned out after investigation not to be NSF.

Correlation of the disease with exposure to drugs or contrast media requires adequate documentation of patient exposure. Not all radiology departments have to date had adequate registration systems for the dose and name of the contrast medium used. Sometimes nicknames are used independent of the product administered or a brand-name continues to be used even though a new product has been introduced. Also the patient's weight is often not recorded. The lack of complete records has caused problems in retrospective studies to detect unsuspected NSF cases. In the future it is very important that a record is always kept of the type and amount of each injection of gadolinium-based contrast agent given and that all

new cases of NSF are reported to the appropriate National Regulatory Authority. Interestingly, no National Medicines Agency had any record of NSF before the first 20 cases of gadodiamide-induced NSF were submitted to them in 30 March 2006 (STENVER 2008) or almost 1 year after the first thoughts about a correlation were submitted for publication (GROBNER 2006). In Denmark, one case was reported in 2004 under another diagnosis; review of the histopathologic specimen in 2006 showed that the correct diagnosis was NSF and this probably was the cause of the patient's death (MARCKMANN 2008). The authorities only need four simple facts: (1) initials, birth date, and sex of the patient, (2) the adverse event, (3) name of the drug, and (4) name of the reporting person, including occupation. However, this limited information requires validation before the case can be confirmed as being NSF associated with use of a gadolinium-based contrast agent.

Validation becomes even more difficult when several gadolinium products have been used in a short period of time. Thus if two different gadolinium-based contrast agents have been injected, for example, within 8 weeks of each other or longer, it may be impossible to determine with certainty which agent triggered the development of NSF and the situation is described as "confounded." In this situation, the agent

Table 24.1. Skin lesions that may mimic nephrogenic systemic fibrosis on clinical examination (adapted from COWPER (2007))

Scleromyxedema
Eosinophilic fasciitis
Eosinophilia–myalgia syndrome
Toxic oil syndrome
Sclerodermoid graft-versus-host disease
Fibrosis (induced by drugs, silica, or organic solvents)
Fibroblastic rheumatism
Borrelliosis
B2-microglobulin amyloidosis
Systemic sclerosis/morphea
Sclerodermia of Buschke
Amyloidosis
Carcinoid syndrome
Porphyria cutanea tarda
Calciphylaxis
Lipodermatosclerosis

Table 24.2. Histopathologic differential diagnosis for nephrogenic systemic fibrosis (adapted from COWPER (2007))

Scleromyxedema
Eosinophilic fasciitis
Eosinophilia–myalgia syndrome
Toxic oil syndrome
Sclerodermoid graft-versus-host disease
Fibroblastic rheumatism
B2-microglobulin amyloidosis
Systemic sclerosis/morphea
Sclerodermia of Buschke
Amyloidosis
Carcinoid syndrome
Porphyria cutanea tarda
Calciphylaxis
Lipodermatosclerosis
Dermatofibrosarcoma protuberans
Melanoma (spindle-cell variant)
Granuloma annulare

that is most likely to be responsible is the one that has triggered NSF in other unconfounded situations.

24.2.3
Cofactors in the Development of NSF

Time has shown that two factors are important for the development of NSF: (1) reduced renal function and (2) exposure to one of the less stable gadolinium-based contrast agents. However, NSF does not develop in all at-risk patients after exposure to the less stable gadolinium-based contrast agents (Thomsen et al. 2007a). Therefore, many investigators have been looking for cofactors that may destabilize these agents.

Several cofactors have been suggested: high doses of erythropoietin (EPO), metabolic acidosis, iron and ferritin, chronic inflammation, hypercoagulability, thrombotic events, recent vascular surgery, recent renal transplant failure, recent surgery, anion gap, or increased phosphate. However, no universal cofactor apart from renal failure has been identified. Marckmann et al. (2007) could not identify any exposure/event other than gadodiamide common to more than a minority of the patients who developed NSF. The Center for Disease Control and Prevention found that only exposure to gadolinium-based contrast agents during the preceding 6 months or preceding year remained statistically significant in their case–control study of 19 NSF cases (Center for Disease and Prevention 2007). Thirty-six percent of the patients in the four American University Study were outpatients (Wertman et al. 2008). The authors concluded that NSF is also seen in patients who have renal compromise but a relatively stable medical condition, in which acute concurrent events may be absent or undetected. The majority of 19 patients in the study by Marckmann et al. (2007) belonged to this group.

Our current knowledge suggests that there may be several cofactors that increase the risk of NSF after some gadolinium-based contrast agents. However, some of the factors may have been listed just by chance because enhanced MRI was performed when the particular factors were present. For example, in some departments enhanced MRI is done as part of the evaluation of thromboembolic symptoms, post surgical complications, etc., whereas in other departments MRI is not used in these situations. Therefore, one institution may report that NSF occurs more frequently in patients with particular conditions but

others cannot confirm it because they use enhanced MRI differently.

24.2.4
Prevalence

In several studies based on pathologic or nephrologic registers, the prevalence of NSF after exposure to gadodiamide has been reported to be between 3 and 7% in patients with reduced renal function (Thomsen and Marckmann 2008). In patients with CKD 5 (GFR less than $15\,ml\,min^{-1}\,1.73\,m^{-2}$), who have been contacted and examined, it may be as much as 18% (Rydahl et al. 2008); all those with suspicious lesions had a skin biopsy. The prevalence was higher after two injections (or more) (36%) than after a single injection (12%), indicating a cumulative effect (Rydahl et al. 2008). Todd et al. (2007) reported that 30% of patients on dialysis had developed NSF based on a systematic examination of the patients in five dialysis centers; biopsies were only taken in a few patients. In the peer-reviewed literature only one center has reported a large number (>10) of NSF cases after gadopentetate dimeglumine (Todd et al. 2007), whereas many centers, including our own, have reported more than 10 cases after gadodiamide (Thomsen and Marckmann 2008). This difference is not just a reflection of the market share of the two products, because gadopentetate dimeglumine has been administered to as many as 4–5 times the number of patients who have had gadodiamide. In the Four American University Study, the overall incidence was 0.039% after gadodiamide and 0.003% after gadopentetate dimeglumine (Wertman et al. 2008). The benchmark incidence of NSF was one in 2,913 patients who underwent gadodiamide-enhanced MRI and one in 44,224 patients who underwent gadopentetate dimeglumine-enhanced MRI ($p < 0.001$). The study was based on patient records from databases of dermatology, pathology, internal medicine, nephrology, transplant surgery, and radiology departments and not systematic examination of patients with reduced renal function exposed to a gadolinium-based contrast agent.

Thirty-two months after the first paper (Grobner 2006) indicating a link between gadolinium-based contrast agents and development of NSF, no case of NSF after exposure to a macrocyclic agent or to the high-relaxivity agents has been published in the peer-reviewed literature. When all three of the macrocyclic agents are taken together, macrocyclic agents have been used in nearly the same number of patients as the nonionic linear agents.

24.2.5
Registries

Many registries have collected data about NSF cases and this leads to confusion. The International Center for Nephrogenic Fibrosing Dermopathy Research (ICNFDR, http://www.icnfdr.org) has collected cases of NSF submitted to them since 2000. A case can only be registered if the head of the registry, Dr. Shawn Cowper, has evaluated the histologic specimen and agrees with the diagnosis of NSF. Since 8 June 2006, the FDA has encouraged reporting of American cases through Med-Watch. The cases are not validated and many do not fulfill the aforementioned criteria or the criteria for being included in the International Registry. Nonetheless, the figures are quoted frequently. The same applies to the reports submitted to National Regulatory Authorities in the various European countries, all of which rely on the vendor to collect the validating data. Both the Contrast Media Committees of American College of Radiology and the European Society of Urogenital Radiology have asked their members to report cases, but these again are not validated. Also the vendors have a registry, which should be identical to that of the National Regulatory Authorities. Finally, there is the peer-reviewed literature, which provides the most reliable information, but suffers from delays in the collection of data and the publication process. By 1 February 2008, 190 cases (confirmed by biopsy *and* clinical examination) had been reported in the peer-reviewed literature: 157 had had gadodiamide, 8 had gadopentetate, 3 had gadoversetamide, and in 5 no exposure could be verified. In 18, the agent could not be identified and 4 received several agents (Broome 2008).

24.3

Patients at Risk for NSF

Patients at higher risk are those with CKD 4 and 5 (GFR < 30 ml min^{-1}), those on hemo- or peritoneal dialysis and patients with reduced renal function who have had or are awaiting liver transplantation (Thomsen et al. 2007a; Thomsen 2007). Patients at lower risk are those with CKD 3 (GFR 30–59 ml min^{-1}) and children under 1 year, because of their immature renal function. To date, no cases where the patient had normal renal function, CKD 1 and 2 (GFR > 60 ml min^{-1} 1.73 m^{-2}), have been reported in the literature. Patients with acute renal failure are at particular risk as the reduced renal function may be overlooked by a single determination of their estimated glomerular filtration rate (eGFR). If they receive a less stable gadolinium agent when they have low renal function and then develop NSF, NSF does not disappear when the renal function improves (Kalb et al. 2008).

24.3.1
Determination of Glomerular Filtration Rate

Accurate determination of the glomerular filtration rate is not easy. The most precise method measures inulin clearance and isotope methods give similar results (Blaufox et al. 1996). However, both methods are cumbersome and impractical for daily use (Thomsen et al. 2005). Measurement of serum creatinine is not satisfactory because more than 25% of older patients have normal serum creatinine levels but reduced glomerular filtration rates. A single determination of the glomerular filtration rate does not exclude acute renal insufficiency

Renal function can also be estimated using specially derived predictive equations that use not only serum creatinine but also characteristics such as weight, height, race, and gender. The most accurate results are obtained with the Cockroft–Gault equation (Cockroft and Gault 1976), whereas the most precise formula is the Modification of Diet in Renal Disease (MDRD) study equation (Levey et al. 1999, 2000, 2007). Unfortunately, the predictive capabilities of these formulae are suboptimal (Bostom et al. 2002). In addition, they are not useful for patients with a glomerular filtration rate above 60 ml min^{-1} (Stevens et al. 2006). Different methods also can result in very different values for glomerular filtration rate (Stevens et al. 2006; Band et al. 2007; Eken and Kilicaslan 2007). For example, a 43-year-old 70 kg male patient with a creatinine level of 264 μmol l^{-1} has a glomerular filtration level of 32 ml min^{-1} if it is calculated by the Cockroft–Gault equation. The same patient will have a glomerular filtration level calculated by the MDRD equation of 33 ml min^{-1} if he is Afro–American and 27 ml min^{-1} if he is Caucasian. Thus, it would have been illegal to use one of the less stable agents in a Caucasian if the glomerular filtration rate had been estimated by the MDRD equation, but not if it had been estimated by the Cockcroft–Gault equation. The situation is further complicated in Asians, because their glomerular filtration rates are lower, but appropriate equations have not been established.

24.3.2
What to Do

In practice, it is easier to use one of the more stable gadolinium agents, for which eGFR measurement before administration may not be mandatory. No differences in diagnostic efficacy have been demonstrated between the six extracellular agents (Chap. 21).

If departments continue to use two agents, other problems arise (Wertman et al. 2008):

- A suitable agent must be chosen for each individual patient.
- Patients with reduced renal function must be identified. Serum creatinine should be measured within 7 days of contrast medium administration in patients with previously elevated serum creatinine or who have a history suggesting the possibility of elevated serum creatinine, namely (1) renal disease, (2) renal surgery, (3) proteinuria, (4) diabetes mellitus, (5) hypertension, (6) gout, and/or (7) recent nephrotoxic drugs (Thomsen et al. 2005).
- Some at-risk patients may be missed because of operator or laboratory error.
- The possibility that NSF is only one of potentially several diseases related to the presence of gadolinium in the body is not accounted for.
- The possibility remains that there will be greater retention of gadolinium in the body with potential late sequelae if the less stable agents are used.

There are several conditions where alternative imaging is diagnostically inferior and cannot replace enhanced MRI. The risk of the NSF is low if the nonionic linear chelates are avoided, and if the most stable agents are used in the smallest dose consistent with a diagnostic result in at-risk patients. Despite the American College of Radiology recommendation that hemodialysis should be used in at-risk patients (Kanal et al. 2007), initiating dialysis should be considered with care, since the morbidity of hemodialysis in a patient not already adjusted to hemodialysis is higher than the risk of NSF after

exposure to a macrocyclic gadolinium agent. The risk of complications (procedural, allergy-like reactions, contrast-induced nephropathy, radiation) following conventional or CT arteriography with iodinated contrast medium must also be weighed carefully against performing MR using a stable gadolinium agent. In most cases there is no better alternative to enhanced MRI (Diego 2008; Thomsen et al. 2007b).

24.4
Why did it take so long?

It took nearly 9 years from the diagnosis of the first NSF case to the recognition that the disease was associated with exposure to the less stable gadolinium-based contrast agents. There are many good reasons for this. Uremic patients are exposed to many drugs and the drugs change during the progress of their disease. Generally contrast agents, in particular MR agents, have been considered safe inert drugs. NSF is a delayed reaction that mainly occurs weeks (or years) after the patient has received the contrast medium. It does not occur in all CKD 5 patients (GFR less than $15\,\mathrm{ml\,min^{-1}\,1.73\,m^{-2}}$ and/or dialysis) and to date has only been reported in the peer-reviewed literature after administration of the less stable gadolinium-based contrast agents. Most patients have not been exposed to nonionic linear agents, which are the least stable (Chap. 20). Access to MRI has increased considerably since the beginning of the century and new techniques such as step-wise angiography based on a single contrast medium injection are now available. Until recently, most physicians did not know about NSF. Mild changes, for example, on the legs, may have gone undiagnosed and only severe changes that have led to significant disability have been noticed. With all these circumstances, it is not surprising that it took a time for the connection to be recognized.

24.5
Legal Aspects

In the US, the Food and Drug Administration in 2007 required that an identical black box warning be placed on package-insert for all approved gadolinium-based contrast agents. The European Medicines Agency concluded that the agents have different risks. In their public assessment report (European Medicines Agency 2007) of 26 June 2007, the European Agency wrote *"Are all Gd-based CA associated with the same risk of NSF? No. Current evidence suggests that the risk of developing NSF is related to the physicochemical and pharmacokinetic properties of Gd-based CA. The physicochemical properties affect the release of toxic Gd³⁺ from the chelate complex, and the pharmacokinetic properties influence how long the agent remains in the body."* Today in Europe, gadodiamide (Omniscan®, GE Healthcare, Chalfont St. Giles, UK), gadopentetate dimeglumine (Magnevist®, Bayer Schering, Berlin, Germany), and gadoversetamide (OptiMARK®, Covidien, St. Louis, USA) are contraindicated in patients with a glomerular filtration rate less than $30\,\text{ml min}^{-1}\,1.73\,\text{m}^{-2}$, including those on dialysis (CKD 4 and 5). The European recommendation is that these agents should be only used with caution in patients with moderately reduced kidney function ($30\text{–}60\,\text{ml min}^{-1}\,1.73\,\text{m}^{-2}$ (CKD 3)).

24.6

Experimental Data

A rat model of NSF in which there were repeated injections over a 20 day period of $2.5\,\text{mmol kg}^{-1}$ of gadolinium-based contrast agents was reported by Siebert et al. (2008a). $2.5\,\text{mmol kg}^{-1}$ is a high dose for human beings, but not for rats (see below). Skin lesions consistent with human NSF were observed as early as 8 days after starting nonformulated gadodiamide exposure and 20 days after starting formulated gadodiamide and caldiamide (Omniscan) solution, but not when Gd-DTPA (Magnevist) was given. The highest Gd³⁺ concentrations in the skin and the most advanced skin lesions were found in animals that received low stability gadolinium-based contrast agents. These data are strongly supportive of a link between the release of Gd³⁺ secondary to low stability of chelates and the development of NSF-like skin lesions. In this study the rats had normal renal function and the biological half life of the gadolinium-based contrast agents would be approximately 20 min, one-sixth of that in man. Nonetheless, NSF-like skin lesions developed, suggesting that some dissociation of the gadolinium-based contrast agent and release of free Gd³⁺ occurs even in the presence of normal renal function. It is reasonable to conclude from Siebert et al. (2008b)'s findings that multiple injec-

tions of low stability gadolinium based contrast agents in the absence of renal impairment can lead to gradual accumulation of Gd³⁺ in tissues until it reaches a threshold level that triggers the fibrotic process. A previous study in humans has shown that Gd³⁺ deposition in bone occurs in patients with normal renal function. In this study, the Gd³⁺ retention in bone with gadodiamide (Omniscan) was 2–4 times more than with gadoteridol (ProHance, Bracco, Italy, a nonionic macrocyclic Gd-CA) (White et al. 2006). From these studies it is tempting to postulate that multiple administrations of large doses of low stability gadolinium-based contrast agents may cause heavy metal intoxication even in patients with normal renal function.

Serum from NSF patients has recently been shown to stimulate fibroblast hyaluron synthesis by up to sevenfold and collagen by up to 2.4-fold compared to control fibroblast cultures incubated with serum derived from healthy volunteers and dialysis patients not suffering from NSF. Fibroblasts exposed to Gd-DTPA–BMA (1.0 mM) for up to 7 days showed significant stimulation of proliferation but no response to incubation with GdCl₃. The authors suggested that Gd³⁺ may not be responsible for the cell growth. Omniscan (Gd-DTPA–BMA) has also induced the expression of α-smooth muscle actin staining, suggesting induction of a myofibroblast phenotype (Edward et al. 2008). Additional studies comparing various gadolinium-based contrast agents are required to elicit whether there is a difference in their effect on fibroblasts.

24.7

Gadolinium and Patients with Normal Renal Function

Gadolinium has been demonstrated in the skin (High et al. 2007; Abraham et al. 2008) of patients with NSF and in the bone of patients who had received a gadolinium-based contrast agent but did not develop NSF (White et al. 2006). The bone accumulation was about four times greater after a linear chelate agent than after a nonionic cyclic agent in patients with normal renal function (White et al. 2006). The rates of dissociation of gadolinium from macrocyclic ligands are several orders of magnitude slower that their dissociation from linear systems (Rosky et al. 2008). The amount of gadolinium in the skin of patients with NSF seems to increase up to 3 years after the last exposure to a gadolinium-based contrast agent (Abraham et al. 2008). Where does it come from? Bone has a slow turnover. The long-term implications of gadolinium deposition in bone, which is likely to occur more commonly in pediatric patients because of the more active bone creation in this population, have yet to be determined (Wertman et al. 2008). Another risk group could be patients who undergo multiple enhanced MRI examinations, for example, women with an increased risk of breast cancer who may follow recommendations to undergo annual enhanced MRI. After each examination some gadolinium will accumulate in the bone and it will stay there for many years (Abraham and Thakral 2008). What will happen when the gadolinium is released from bone, for example, when osteoporosis increases bone turnover? The release of an overload of gadolinium might cause classic toxicity symptoms, not NSF. Free gadolinium may produce liver necrosis, obstruct calcium ion passage through muscle cells, and interfere with intracellular enzymes and cell membranes by the process of transmetallation, a phenomenon whereby Gd^{3+} replaces endogenous metals such as zinc and copper. The safety of multiple injections of gadolinium-based contrast agents has never been studied; the phase I–III studies that led to approval by the health authorities included only a single injection in man and in most cases at a dose of $0.1\,mmol\,kg^{-1}$ body weight. Since then there has been a major revolution in the use of enhanced MRI. The chance of having several enhanced MRI examinations within a shorter period is much higher now than 15 years ago when there were only 1,000–2,000 MRI units world-wide and each had a lower throughput. The phase I–III studies did not foresee these changes and can therefore not be used to document safety of these products as they are now used. One product could easily be safe in the 1993 environment, but not 15 years later.

Another risk group could be patients with diabetes mellitus; after approximately 10 years, 50% may develop diabetic nephropathy, but these patients cannot be identified when they have normal renal function. If some gadolinium remains in the body from a MR-examination when the patient had normal function, it is possible that this patient will develop more severe NSF after enhanced MRI with a less stable agent when their GFR becomes severely reduced (CKD 5). Marckmann et al. (2007) showed that, independent of renal function, patients with severe NSF had had a higher life-time dose of the gadolinium-based agent than those developing nonsevere NSF.

A lot of detailed and careful research is vital before we can be sure that there will not be new problems in 10–20 years because of retention of the heavy metal gadolinium in the body for long periods of time.

24.8
Conclusion

NSF is an important delayed adverse reaction to some gadolinium-based contrast agents, which occurs in patients with impaired renal function (Thomsen 2006). The recognition of this reaction to agents previously considered to be very safe emphasizes the need to have a good clinical indication for all enhanced MRI examinations, to choose an agent that leaves the smallest amount of gadolinium in the body (stable agents and high relaxivity agents), and to keep complete records of the type and dose of agent given.

Research into the etiology of NSF has drawn attention to the retention of gadolinium in the body tissues long after an enhanced MR examination and the safety implications of this are as yet unclear.

References

Abraham JL, Thakral C (2008) Tissue distribution and kinetics of gadolinium and nephrogenic systemic fibrosis. Eur J Radiol 66:200–207

Abraham JL, Thakral C, Skov L et al (2008) Dermal inorganic gadolinium concentrations: evidence for in vivo transmetallation and long-term persistence in nephrogenic systemic fibrosis. Br J Dermatol 158:273–280

Band RA, Gaieski DF, Mills AM et al (2007) Discordance between serum creatinine and creatinine clearance for identification of ED patients with abdominal pain at risk for contrast induced nephropathy. Am J Emerg Med 25:268–272

Blaufox MD, Aurell M, Bubeck B et al (1996) Report of the Radionuclide in Nephrourology Committee on renal clearance. J Nucl Med 37:1883–1890

Bostom AG, Kronenberg F, Ritz E (2002) Predictive performance of renal function equations for patients with chronic kidney disease and normal serum creatinine levels. J Am Soc Nephrol 13:2140–2144

Broome DR (2008) Nephrogenic Systemic Fibrosis Associated with Gadolinium Based Contrast Agents: A Summary of the Medical Literature Reporting. Eur J Radiol 6:230–234

Center for Disease Control and Prevention (CDC) (2007) Nephrogenic fibrosing dermopathy associated with exposure to gadolinium-containing contrast agents – St. Louis, Missouri, 2002–2006. MMWR Morb Mortal Wkly Rep 56:137–141

Cockroft DW, Gault MH (1976) Prediction of creatinine clearance from serum creatinine. Nephron 16:31–41

Cowper SE (2007) Nephrogenic systemic fibrosis. Adv Dermatol 23:131–154

Cowper SE, Robin HS, Steinberg SM et al (2000) Scleromyxoedema-like cutaneous disease in renal dialysis patients. Lancet 356:1000–1001

Cowper SE, Rabach M, Girardi M (2008) Clinical and Histological Findings in Nephrogenic Systemic Fibrosis. Eur J Radiol 66:200–207

Diego DR (2008) Nephrogenic System Fibrosis: A Radiologist's Practical Perspective. Eur J Radiol 66:220–224

Edward M, Quinn JA, Mukherjee S (2008) Gadodiamide contrast agent 'activates' fibroblasts: a possible cause of nephrogenic systemic fibrosis. J Pathol 214:584–593

Eken C, Kilicaslan I (2007) Differences between various glomerular filtration rate calculation methods in predicting patients at risk for contrast-induced nephropathy. Am J Emerg Med 25:487 (Correspondence)

European Medicines Agency (2007), Public Assessment Report, June 26th 2007. www.esur.org. Accessed 22 July 2008

Grobner T (2006) Gadolinium: a specific trigger for the development of nephrogenic fibrosing dermopathy and nephrogenic systemic fibrosis? Nephrol Dial Transplant 21:1104–1108

High W, Ayers RA, Chandler J, Zito G, Cowper SE (2007) Gadolinium is detectable within the tissue of patients with nephrogenic systemic fibrosis. J Am Acad Dermatol 56:27–30

Kalb RE, Helm TN, Sperry H, Thrakral C, Abraham JL, Kanal E (2008) Gadolinium-induced nephrogenic systemic fibrosis in a patient with an acute and transient kidney injury. Br J Dermatol 8:607–610

Kanal E, Barkovich AJ, Bell C et al (2007) ACR Blue Ribbon Panel on MR Safety. ACR guidance document for safe MR practices: 2007. Am J Roentgenol 188:1447–1474

Levey AS, Bosch JP, Lewis JB, Greene T, Rogers N, Roth D (1999) A more accurate method to estimate glomerular filtration rate from serum creatinine: a new prediction equation. Ann Intern Med 130:461–470

Levey AS, Greene T, Kusek J, Beck GA (2000) A simplified equation to predict glomerular filtration rate from serum creatinine. J Am Soc Nephrol 11:155A

Levey AS, Coresh J, Greene T et al (2007) Expressing the modification of diet in renal disease study equation for estimating glomerular filtration rate with standardized serum creatinine values. Clin Chem 53:766–772

Marckmann P (2008) An epidemic outbreak of nephrogenic systemic fibrosis in a Danish hospital. Eur J Radiol 66(2):187–190

Marckmann P, Skov L, Rossen K, Heaf JG, Thomsen HS (2007) Case-control study of gadodiamide-related nephrogenic systemic fibrosis. Nephrol Dial Transplant 22:3174–3178

Marckmann P, Skov L, Rossen K, Thomsen HS (2008) Clinical manifestations of gadodiamide-related nephrogenic systemic fibrosis. Clin Nephrol 69:161–168

Morcos SK (2007) Nephrogenic systemic fibrosis following the administration of extracellular gadolinium based contrast agents: is the stability of the contrast agent molecule an important factor in the pathogenesis of this condition? Br J Radiol 80:73–76

Morcos SK, Thomsen HS, Webb JAW, Contrast media safety committee of the European Society of Urogenital Radiology (ESUR) (2002) Dialysis and contrast media. Eur Radiol 12:3026–3030

Parazella MA (2007) Nephrogenic systemic fibrosis, kidney disease, and gadolinium: is there a link? Clin J Am Soc Nephrol 2:200–2002

Rosky NM, Sherry AD, Lenkinski RE (2008) Nephrogenic systemic fibrosis: A chemical perspective. Radiology 247:608–612

Rydahl C, Thomsen HS, Marckman P (2008) High prevalence of nephrogenic systemic fibrosis in chronic renal failure patients exposed to gadodiamide, a Gadolinium(Gd)-containing magnetic resonance contrast agent. Invest Radiol 43:141–144

Sieber MA, Pietsch H, Walter J et al (2008a) A preclinical study to investigate the development of nephrogenic systemic fibrosis: a possible role for gadolinium based contrast media. Invest Radiol 43:65–75

Sieber MA, Lengsfeld P, Walter J et al (2008b) Gadolinium based contrast agents and their potential role in the pathogenesis of nephrogenic systemic fibrosis: the role of excess ligand. J Magn Reson Imaging 27:955–962

Stenver DI (2008) Pharmacovigilance: What to do if you see an adverse reaction and the consequences. Eur J Radiol 66:184–186

Stevens LA, Coresh J, Greene T, Levey AS (2006) Assessing kidney function – measured and estimated glomerular filtration rate. N Engl J Med 354:2473–2483

Swaminathan S, High WA, Ranville et al (2008) Cardiac and vascular metal deposition with high mortatlity in nephrogenic systemic fibrosis. Kidney Int 73:1413–1418

Thomsen HS (2006) Nephrogenic systemic fibrosis: A serious late adverse reaction to gadodiamide. Eur Radiol 16: 2619–2621

Thomsen HS (2007) ESUR guideline: gadolinium-based contrast media and nephrogenic systemic fibrosis. Eur Radiol 17:2692–2696

Thomsen HS, Marckmann P (2008) Extracellular Gd-CA: Differences in prevalences of NSF. Eur J Radiol 66: 180–183

Thomsen HS, Morcos SK, Members of Contrast Media Safety Committee of European Society of Urogenital Radiology (ESUR) (2005) In which patients should serum-creatinine be measured before contrast medium administration? Eur Radiol 15:749–754

Thomsen HS, Marckmann P, Logager VB (2007a) Nephrogenic systemic fibrosis (NSF): a late adverse reaction to some of the gadolinium based contrast agents. Cancer Imag 7:130–137

Thomsen HS, Marckmann P, Logager VB (2007b) Enhanced Computed Tomography or Magnetic Resonance Imaging: A choice between contrast medium-induced nephropathy and nephrogenic systemic fibrosis? Acta Radiol 48: 593–596

Todd DJ, Kagan A, Chibnik LB, Kay J (2007) Cutaneous changes of nephrogenic systemic fibrosis. Predictor of early mortality and association with gadolinium exposure. Arthritis Rheumat 56:3433–3441

Tweedle MF, Wedeking P, Kumar K (1995) Biodistribution of radiolabeled, formulated gadopentetate, gadoteridol, gadoterate, and gadodiamide in mice and rats. Invest Radiol 30:372–380

Wertman R, Altun E, Martin DR (2008) Risk of nephrogenic systemic fibrosis: evaluation of gadolinium chelate contrast agents at four American universities. Radiology 248:799–806

White GW, Gibby WA, Tweedle MF (2006) Comparison of Gd (DTPA-BMA) (Omniscan) versus GD(HP-DO3A) (Prohance) relative to gadolinium retention in human bone tissue by inductively coupled plasma mass spectroscopy. Invest Radiol 41:272–278

MR Contrast Media

Organ-Specific MR Contrast Agents

Gadolinium-Based Contrast Agents

Marie-France Bellin

CONTENTS

25.1
Introduction

Although nonspecific extracellular gadolinium (Gd) chelates dominate the MR contrast agent market, organ-specific contrast agents (Gd-based and non-Gd-based) have tissue-specific properties that permit targeted MRI of organs such as the liver and lymph nodes or MR angiography. Gadolinium-based organ-specific contrast agents (Table 25.1) are increasingly used to detect and characterize liver lesions better (Bellin et al. 1994, 2003; Bluemke et al. 2005; Kirchin and Runge 2003; Kopp et al. 1997; Marti-Bonmati et al. 2003; Ros et al. 1995; Spinazzi et al. 1999) and to improve the efficacy of MR angiography (Rapp et al. 2005; Goyen et al. 2005; Nikolaou et al. 2006). Although

Marie-France Bellin
Université Paris-Sud 11, AP-HP, Service de Radiologie,
Hôpital Paul Brousse, 12–14 avenue Paul Vaillant Couturier,
94804 Villejuif Cedex, France

there are theoretical safety concerns, these MR contrast agents have been shown to be safe and well-tolerated in clinical use.

25.2
Hepatobiliary Gadolinium Chelates

Hepatobiliary gadolinium chelates include gadobenate dimeglumine (Gd–BOPTA), which is currently approved in Europe for MRI of the central nervous system (CNS) and liver, and gadoxetic acid disodium (Gd–EOB–DTPA), which is approved for hepatic MRI in some European countries and the United States of America. They are paramagnetic compounds that are taken up by functioning hepatocytes and excreted in bile. Gadobenate dimeglumine and gadoxetic acid disodium are eliminated by both the renal and hepatobiliary routes. Hepatic uptake accounts for 2–4% of the injected dose of gadobenate (kidney pathway: 96–98%) and 50% of the injected dose of gadoxetic acid disodium (kidney pathway: 50%).

25.2.1
Gadobenate Dimeglumine

The ionic, linear agent *gadobenate dimeglumine* (Gd–BOPTA, MultiHance®, Bracco, Italy) was initially developed for liver imaging. It has only slightly greater R1- and R2-relaxivity than gadopentetate in vitro, but its relaxivity in plasma is almost twice that of gadopentetate because of protein binding. The beneficial effect of this increased relaxivity was soon explored in other routine applications such as brain imaging, perfusion MR, and MR angiography. Unlike other available gadolinium-based agents that are

Table 25.1. Overview of the various organ-specific gadolinium chelates that are commercially available

Organ specific MR agents	Target cell	Main effect on signal intensity		Short names (trade names)	Main route of elimination
		T1	T2		
Hepatobiliary gadolinium chelates	Hepatocytes	↑	~	Gd-BOPTA[a] (MultiHance®)	Renal (96–98%) and biliary (2–4%)
				Gd-EOB-DTPA (Primovist®)	Renal (50%) and biliary (50%)
MR angiography	Vascular bed Blood pool agent	↑↑	~	Gadofosveset (Vasovist®)	Renal (91%) and biliary (9%)

[a]Also extracellular agent

excreted exclusively by glomerular filtration by the kidneys, Gd–BOPTA is eliminated by both the renal and hepatobiliary pathways (KIRCHIN et al. 1998, 2001; SPINAZZI et al. 1999). Hepatic uptake accounts for 2–4% of the injected dose. In addition, this agent has a capacity for weak and transient protein binding (CAVAGNA et al. 1997), making it potentially suitable for MR angiography with an in vivo T_1 relaxivity approaching twice that of the conventional gadolinium chelates. The approved dose for hepatic imaging is 0.05 mmol kg^{-1} (0.1 ml kg^{-1} of a 0.5 M solution) and for CNS imaging 0.1 mmol kg^{-1} (0.2 ml kg^{-1} of a 0.5 M solution). Gadobenate dimeglumine should be administered undiluted followed by a bolus of 0.9% sodium chloride solution. It is currently approved in the United States and Canada for MR imaging of the central nervous system (CNS) and related tissues and in Europe and various countries in Asia and Australasia for MR imaging of the CNS and liver.

Gadobenate dimeglumine behaves as a conventional extracellular contrast agent in the first minutes following administration and can be used for dynamic bolus imaging. It then behaves as a liver-specific agent in a later, delayed phase, 40–120 min after administration. As it is taken up specifically by normally functioning hepatocytes through a complex interplay of various carrier systems, it produces a marked and long-lasting enhancement of the normal liver parenchyma. As most tumor nodules are devoid of functional hepatocytes, they do not take up the agent and thus appear hypointense on enhanced MR images (HAMM et al. 1999; KIRCHIN et al. 2001). Numerous clinical trials have shown that Gd–BOPTA increases sensitivity and specificity and thus increases detection and characterization of liver tumors

(CAUDANA et al. 1996; GRAZIOLI et al. 2000; HAMM et al. 1999; KIRCHIN et al. 1998; MANFREDI et al. 1998, 1999; PETERSTEIN et al. 2000; ROSATI et al. 1994; VOGL et al. 1997).

Four exhaustive reviews have been published (HAMM et al. 1999; KIRCHIN et al. 2001; ROSATI et al. 1994; SHELLOCK et al. 2006), including extended clinical experience from phase I studies to post-marketing surveillance. They reported a low incidence of serious events and confirmed the excellent safety profile of Gd–BOPTA. Between July 1990 and September 2000, 2,891 subjects participated in 65 clinical trials, including 2,540 subjects (2,430 adults and 110 children) who received Gd–BOPTA. One thousand nine hundred and eighty-six (78.2%) subjects received a single injection and 554 subjects received two or more injections. For adult patients and volunteers, the overall incidence of adverse events was 19.8% and events potentially related to Gd–BOPTA administration were reported in 15.1% of adult patients. Headache, injection site reaction, nausea, abnormal taste, and flushing were the most common adverse events, with a reported frequency of between 1.0 and 2.6%. Serious adverse events potentially related to Gd–BOPTA were reported in five (0.2%) patients. An apparent tendency towards a greater incidence of both total and study agent related events was noted in patients younger than 65 years and in studies conducted in the US compared to Europe.

A study comparing gadobenate dimeglumine and gadopentetate dimeglumine for MR imaging of liver tumors reported an incidence of adverse events of 4.7% (6/128) for gadobenate vs. 1.6% (2/127) for gadopentetate, but the difference was not significant

(KUWATSURU et al. 2001). Results of controlled studies were available in 410 patients and revealed no differences between Gd–BOPTA and Gd–DTPA or placebo in the incidence and type of adverse events. For the controlled liver study and for patients with renal impairment, end-stage renal disease or hepatic impairment, the incidence of adverse events following Gd–BOPTA administration was similar to that following placebo administration. There were no clinically important changes in vital signs, clinical laboratory data, or ECG findings. The most frequently reported adverse event among the hematology parameters was hypochromic anemia (0.6%). In the pediatric population ($n = 110$ subjects), the incidence of adverse events was 12.7%; one event was classified as severe but not related to the study agent, and two events were classified as serious (one report of worsening of vomiting that was considered to be possibly related, and one report of hypoxia that was considered to be not related). In a review evaluating the safety and tolerability of gadobenate dimeglumine relative to that of gadopentetate dimeglumine in 924 subjects (including 174 pediatric subjects) enrolled in 10 clinical trials, Shellock et al. showed that the safety profile of gadobenate dimeglumine was similar to gadopentetate dimeglumine in patients and volunteers (SHELLOCK et al. 2006). No case of nephrogenic systemic fibrosis (NSF) that could be related to the administration of gadobenate dimeglumine has been reported. Gadobenate dimeglumine has a very high conditional stability constant and no excess chelate. It is as yet not known whether biliary excretion conveys a decreased risk for developing NSF. Because of the increased relaxivity of gadobenate dimeglumine, it may be possible to inject a half dose (0.05 mmol kg^{-1}) without losing efficacious contrast enhancement. This possible advantage should be evaluated by further research (LIN and BROWN 2007).

Safety and efficacy of gadobenate dimeglumine have not been established in patients under 18 and gadobenate dimeglumine is not approved in patients less than 18 years old. The package insert indicates that patients should be observed during the 15 min following injection as the majority of severe adverse events occurs within 15 min after injection.

25.2.2
Gadoxetic Acid

Gadoxetic acid disodium (Gd–EOB–DTPA, Primovist®, Schering AG, Berlin, Germany) is a para-magnetic hepatobiliary contrast medium with hepatocellular uptake via the anionic-transporter protein and a molecular weight of 726 Da. In human plasma, it has a higher T1-relaxivity compared to Gd–DTPA (R1 8.2 mM^{-1} s^{-1}) because of a greater degree of protein binding (~10%). At body temperature, the aqueous formulation of 0.25 mol l^{-1} has an osmolality of 890 mOsmol kg^{-1} water, a viscosity of 1.22 mPa, and a thermodynamic stability constant of 10^{20}. Biodistribution studies revealed dose-dependent renal (40.9% ± 2.35%) and biliary (57.0% ± 2.49%) excretion without signs for metabolism and an enterohepatic recirculation of approximately 2.1% ± 0.56% (SCHUHMANN-GIAMPIERI et al. 1992; WIENMANN et al. 1992; HAMM et al. 1995).

Like other gadolinium agents, gadoxetic acid disodium behaves as a conventional extracellular contrast agent in the first minutes following administration and can be administered as a fast intravenous bolus. The liver-specific, delayed phase starts earlier than Gd–BOPTA and delayed imaging can be started as early as 15–20 min after administration, giving it a logistic advantage over the other liver-specific media (GIOVAGNONI and PACI 1996; REIMER et al. 2004). Since it is given as a bolus, dynamic imaging is possible. The uptake of Gd–EOB–DTPA by the hepatocytes allows imaging to be performed in parenchymal phases as well. Therefore, twofold lesion information is obtained: lesion vascularity during the dynamic phase and lesion cell composition during the late phase of imaging (HALAVAARA et al. 2006). The excretion by the biliary system is significantly greater than Gd–BOPTA (2–4%), making contrast-enhanced MR cholangiography also feasible (BOLLOW et al. 1997).

A recent preclinical safety evaluation study of gadoxetic acid disodium concluded that it was well tolerated with high safety margins between the single diagnostic dose and the doses showing adverse effects in animal studies (DOHR et al. 2007). No indications of reproductive or developmental toxicity, potential contact allergenic, and genotoxic effects were observed. No organ toxicity was observed.

For gadoxetic acid disodium, only premarketing safety data in humans are available from registration clinical trials. In phase I trials with tested doses between 0.01 and 0.1 mmol kg^{-1} body weight, no serious side effects or changes in laboratory values were seen in 44 healthy volunteers (HAMM et al. 1995). The phase II trials were conducted in two parts. As a result of these trials, 0.025 mmol kg^{-1} body weight (or 7 ml for a 70 kg adult) was considered to be the optimum dose for clinical use. While no adverse events in any patient were reported in 33 patients in the first part (Reimer et al. 1996), in the second part eight minor adverse events were reported in six of 171 patients. No adverse effects were graded as serious. Also, there were no significant changes in vital parameters or laboratory values (Stern et al. 2000). In the phase III multicenter trial reported by Huppertz et al. in 2004, 162 patients received Gd–EOB–DTPA and showed improved liver lesion detection. A total of 21 adverse events was recorded in 11 patients (6.8%). Of these, 13 were definitely, possibly, or probably related to the contrast medium, and most frequent symptoms included nausea, headache, altered taste, vasodilatation, and injection site pain (Bollow et al. 1997; Huppertz et al. 2004). In a review summarizing the safety data on Gd–EOB–DTPA from phase II and phase III clinical studies conducted in Europe, Japan, and USA (Breuer et al. 2003), a total of 120 (8.5%) of the 1,404 patients experienced one or more adverse effects, which in 3.4% of the patients were considered by the investigator to be definitely, possibly, or probably related to the drug. None of the eight serious adverse events that occurred in five patients were considered to be drug related. The excellent clinical tolerance of Gd–EOB–DTPA was confirmed by the results of the phase III study conducted by Bluemke et al. (2005), which enrolled 172 adult patients who had liver lesions and were scheduled to undergo liver surgery. They received 25 µmol kg^{-1} (0.1 ml kg^{-1}) Gd–EOB–DTPA as an intravenous bolus injection at a rate of 2 ml s^{-1}. Fifteen events in 10 patients were classified as definitely, probably, or possibly contrast material-related and were all mild or moderate in intensity. The authors concluded that compared with precontrast imaging, postcontrast MR imaging with Gd–EOB–DTPA demonstrated improved sensitivity for lesion detection in two of three blinded readers, with no substantial adverse events (Bluemke et al. 2005). No case of NSF has been reported that could be related to the administration of Gd–EOB–DTPA. However, the number of patients with reduced renal function who have received this contrast agent is not known.

Interactions of Gd–EOB–DTPA with commercially available drugs were only tested in animal models. In a rat model, only rifampicin significantly decreased hepatic enhancement, while prednisolone, doxorubicin, cisplatin, and propanolol led to a slight increase in enhancement (Kato et al. 2002).

25.3
MR Angiography Blood Pool Agent Gadofosveset Trisodium

Gadofosveset (MS-325, Vasovist®, EPIX Pharmaceuticals, Cambridge, Mass, USA and Bayer Schering Pharma AG, Berlin, Germany) is the first intravascular contrast agent approved in the European Union for magnetic resonance angiography (MRA) of vessels in the abdomen, pelvis, and lower extremity in adults. It is a newly developed gadolinium-based blood-pool contrast agent that noncovalently binds to albumin in the blood. This reversible binding to albumin enhances the paramagnetic effectiveness of gadolinium and allows the administration of lower contrast agent doses compared with the doses needed for conventional MR angiography (Nikolaou et al. 2006). Gadofosveset is 2–3 times more stable than Gd–DTPA at pH 7.4 and is 10–100 times more kinetically inert (Caravan et al. 2001). In addition, the albumin-binding characteristic extends the vascular life-time of the agent and thus allows longer vascular imaging time, potentially higher spatial resolution, and larger anatomic coverage. T½ of the agent is about 18 h in patients with normal renal function or 12 times longer than that of the traditional extracellular gadolinium-based contrast agents. The recommended dose is only 1/3–1/4 of the standard dose recommended for the extracellular agents. Hepatic uptake accounts for 9% of the injected dose of gadofosveset with 91% excreted by the kidney. This contrast agent has been reported to provide significant improvement in effectiveness (increase in accuracy, sensitivity, and specificity) over unenhanced MRA for the assessment of aortoiliac occlusive disease (Goyen et al. 2005; Rapp et al. 2005) and arterial disease of the foot (Bosch et al. 2008).

Results of previous dose-range studies have shown that 0.03 mmol kg^{-1} was the most clinically appropriate dose for MR angiography of aortoiliac occlusive disease (Perreault et al. 2003). Steger-Hartmann et al. investigated the toxicity of this compound (Steger-Hartmann et al. 2006), including studies of acute, repeated-dose, reproductive, and developmental toxicity as well as local tolerance, immunotoxicity, and mutagenic potential. They concluded that Vasovist® was well tolerated with reasonable safety margins between the single diagnostic dose of 0.03 mmol kg^{-1} in humans and the doses resulting in adverse effects in animal studies. In 2006, Shamsi et al. published a summary of safety of gadofosveset at 0.03 mmol kg^{-1} body weight dose in phase II and phase II clinical trials. No severe adverse events were reported in the phase II trial. Overall safety data were pooled from eight studies that included subjects with known or suspected vascular disease who were administered 0.03 mmol kg^{-1} gadofosveset (767 subjects) or placebo (49 subjects). Pooled data revealed no clinically significant trends in adverse events, laboratory assays, vital signs, oxygen saturation, physical examination, and electrocardiography. Contrast agent related adverse events were reported by 176 (22.9%) patients receiving gadofosveset and by 16 (32.7%) patients receiving placebo (SHAMSI et al. 2006). The most common adverse events were nonspecific and as follows: feeling hot, nausea, headache, burning sensation, feeling cold, paresthesia, vasodilatation, and dry mouth (BOSCH et al. 2008; RAPP et al. 2005). Most of the treatment-related adverse events occurred within 5 min after gadofosveset administration, and most of them resolved spontaneously within 15 min (BOSCH et al. 2008). It is not known how many patients with end-stage renal failure have been examined with gadofosveset and as yet no cases of NSF following its administration have been reported.

Other possible applications of blood-pool agents are now being considered. They include assessment of venous thromboembolism, coronary artery disease, sinus venous thrombosis, perfusion MR studies, and monitoring of inflammatory changes.

25.4
Conclusions

Organ-specific contrast agents were developed later than conventional extracellular gadolinium chelates and fewer data exist about their safety. They belong to different classes of agent and therefore exhibit different physicochemical properties, modes of action, and metabolic pathways. In each category, at least one agent has been approved for clinical use to improve lesion detection and characterization on MR examinations. Despite the inherent toxicity of the Gd ion and the relatively newness of Gd-based organ-specific contrast agents, these contrast agents are simple to use and appear in general to be safe and well tolerated. Guidelines on the safety aspects are

presented in Chap. 29. The European Regulatory Authorities classify all three agents as having "intermediate risk of NSF" (STENVER 2008).

References

Bellin MF, Zaim S, Auberton E et al (1994) Liver metastases: safety and efficacy of detection with superparamagnetic iron oxide in MR imaging. Radiology 193:657–663

Bellin MF, Vasile M, Morel-Precetti S (2003) Currently used non-specific extracellular MR contrast media. Eur Radiol 13:2688–2698

Bluemke AD, Sahani D, Amendola M et al (2005) Efficacy and safety of MR imaging with liver specific contrast agent: US multicenter phase III study. Radiology 237:89–98

Bollow M, Taupitz M, Hamm B et al (1997) Gadolinium-ethoxybenzyl-DTPA as a hepatobiliary contrast agent for use in MR cholangiography: results of an in vivo phase-I clinical evaluation. Eur Radiol 7:126–132

Bosch E, Kreitner KF, Peirano MF et al (2008) Safety and efficacy of gadofosveset-enhanced MR angiography for evaluation of pedal arterial disease: multicenter comparative phase 3 study. Am J Roentgenol 190:179–186

Breuer J, Balzer T, Shamsi K et al (2003) Clinical experience from phase II and phase III studies for Gd-EOB-DTPA: a new liver specific MR contrast agent. Eur Radiol 13 (Suppl 2):S109

Caravan P, Comuzzi C, Crooks W et al (2001) Thermodynamic stability and kinetic inertness of MS-325, a new blood pool agent for magnetic resonance imaging. Inorg Chem 40:2170–2176

Caudana R, Morana G, Pirovano GP et al (1996) Focal malignant hepatic lesions: MR imaging enhanced with gadolinium benzyloxypropionictetra-acetate (BOPTA) – preliminary results of phase II clinical application. Radiology 199:513–520

Cavagna FM, Maggioni F, Castelli PM et al (1997) Gadolinium chelates with weak binding to serum proteins: a new class of high-efficiency, general purpose contrast agents for magnetic resonance imaging. Invest Radiol 32:780–796

Dohr O, Hofmeister R, Treher M, Schweinfurth H (2007) Preclinical safety evaluation of Gd-EOB-DTPA (Primovist). Invest Radiol 42:830–841

Giovagnoni A, Paci E (1996) Liver III: Gadolinium-based hepatobiliary contrast agents (Gd-EOB-DTPA and Gd-BOPTA/Dimeg). Magn Reson Imaging Clin North Am 4:61–72

Goyen M, Edelman M, Perreault P et al (2005) MR angiography of aortoiliac occlusive disease: a phase III study of the safety and effectiveness of the blood-pool contrast agent MS-325. Radiology 236:825–833

Grazioli L, Morana G, Caudana R et al (2000) Hepatocellular carcinoma: correlation between gadobenate dimeglumine-enhanced MRI and pathological findings. Invest Radiol 35:25–34

Halavaara J, Breuer J, Ayuso C et al (2006) Liver tumor characterization: comparison between liver-specific Gd-EOB-DTPA –enhanced MRI and biphasic CT: a multicenter trial. J Comput Assist Tomogr 30:345–354

Hamm B, Staks T, Mühler A et al (1995) Phase I clinical evaluation of Gd-EOB-DTPA as a hepatobiliary MR contrast agent: safety, pharmacokinetics, and MR imaging. Radiology 195:785–792

Hamm B, Kirchin M, Pirovano G et al (1999) Clinical utility and safety of MultiHance in magnetic resonance imaging of liver cancer: results of multicenter studies in Europe and the USA. J Comput Assist Tomogr 23(Suppl 1): S53–S60

Huppertz A, Balzer T, Blakeborough A et al for the European EOB Study Group (2004) Improved detection of focal liver lesions at MR imaging: multicenter comparison of gadoxetic acid-enhanced MR images with intraoperative findings. Radiology 230:266–275

Kato N, Yokawa T, Tamura A et al (2002) Gadolinium-ethoxybenzyl-diethylenetriamine-pentaacetic acid interaction with clinical drugs in rats. Invest Radiol 37:680–684

Kirchin MA, Runge VM (2003) Contrast agents for magnetic resonance imaging: safety update. Top Magn Reson Imaging 14:426–435

Kirchin MA, Pirovano G, Spinazzi A (1998) Gadobenate dimeglumine (Gd-BOPTA): an overview. Invest Radiol 33:798–809

Kirchin MA, Pirovano G, Venetianer C et al (2001) Safety assessment of gadobenate dimeglumine (MultiHance): extended clinical experience from phase I studies to post-marketing surveillance. J Magn Reson Imaging 14:281–294

Kuwatsuru R, Kadoya M, Ohtomo K et al (2001) Comparison of gadobenate dimeglumine with gadopentetate dimeglumine for magnetic resonance imaging of liver tumors. Invest Radiol 36:632–641

Lin SP and Brown JJ (2007) MR contrast agents: physical and pharmacologic basics. J Magn Reson Imaging 25:884–899

Manfredi R, Maresca G, Baron RL et al (1998) Gadobenate dimeglumine (BOPTA)-enhanced MR imaging: patterns of enhancement in normal liver and cirrhosis. J Magn Reson Imaging 8:862–867

Manfredi R, Maresca G, Baron RL et al (1999) Delayed MR imaging of hepatocellular carcinoma enhanced by gadobenate dimeglumine (Gd-BOPTA). J Magn Reson Imaging 9:704–710

Nikolaou K, Kramer H, Grosse D et al (2006) High-spatial-resolution multistation MR angiography with parallel imaging and blood pool agent: initial experience. Radiology 241:861–872

Perreault P, Edelman MA, Baum RA et al (2003) MR angiography with gadofosveset trisodium for peripheral vascular disease phase II trial. Radiology 229:811–820

Peterstein J, Spinazzi A, Giovagnoni A et al (2000) Evaluation of the efficacy of gadobenate dimeglumine in magnetic resonance imaging of focal liver lesions: a multicenter phase III clinical study. Radiology 215:727–736

Rapp JH, Wolff SD, Quinn JA et al (2005) Aortoiliac occlusive disease in patients with known or suspected peripheral vascular disease: safety and efficacy of gadofosveset-enhanced MR angiography- Multicenter comparative phase III study. Radiology 236:71–78

Reimer P, Rummeny EJ, Shamsi K et al (1996) Phase II clinical evaluation of Gd-EOB-DTPA: dose, safety aspects, and pulse sequence. Radiology 199:177–183

Reimer P, Schneider G, Schima W (2004) Hepatobiliary contrast agents for contrast-enhanced MRI of the liver: properties, clinical development and applications. Eur Radiol 14:559–578

Rosati G, Pirovano G, Spinazzi A (1994) Interim results of phase II clinical testing of gadobenate dimeglumine. Invest Radiol 29:S183–S185

Schuhmann-Giampieri G, Schmitt-Willich H, Press WR et al (1992) Preclinical evaluation of Gd-EOB-DTPA as a contrast agent in MR imaging of the hepatobiliary system. Radiology 183:59–64

Shamsi K, Yucel EK, Chamberlin P (2006) A summary of safety of gadofosveset (MS-325) at 0.03 mmol/kg body weight dose: phase II and phase III clinical trials data. Invest Radiol 41:822–830

Shellock FG, Parker JR, Pirovano G et al (2006) Safety characteristics of gadobenate dimeglumine: clinical experience from intra- and interindividual comparison studies with gadopentetate dimeglumine. J Magn Reson Imaging 24: 1378–1385

Spinazzi A, Lorusso V, Pirovano G et al (1999) Safety, tolerance, biodistribution and MR imaging enhancement of the liver with Gd-BOPTA: results of clinical pharmacologic and pilot imaging studies in non-patient and patient volunteers. Acad Radiol 6:282–291

Steger-Hartmann T, Graham PB, Müller S, Schweinfurth H (2006) Preclinical safety assessment of Vasovist (gadofosveset trisodium), a new paramagnetic resonance imaging contrast agent for angiography. Invest Radiol 41:449–459

Stenver DI (2008) Pharmacovigilance: What to do if you see an adverse reaction and the consequences. Eur J Radiol 66:184–186

Stern W, Schick F, Kopp AF et al (2000) Dynamic MR imaging of liver metastases with Gd-EOB-DTPA. Acta Radiol 41: 255–262

Vogl TJ, Stupavsky A, Pegios W et al (1997) Hepatocellular carcinoma: evaluation with dynamic and static gadobenate dimeglumine-enhanced MR imaging and histopathologic correlation. Radiology 205:721–728

Weinmann HJ, Schuhmann-Gampieri G, Schmitt-Willich H et al (1992) A new lipophilic gadolinium chelate as a tissue-specific contrast medium for MRI. Magn Reson Med 22: 233–237

Non-Gadolinium-Based Contrast Agents

Marie-France Bellin

CONTENTS

26.1
Introduction

A variety of organ-specific contrast agents designed to overcome the limitations of nonspecific tissue uptake by conventional extracellular gadolinium chelates have been developed for contrast-enhanced MR imaging. (Bellin et al. 2003). Commercially available contrast agents are mainly targeted at the liver (Gandhi et al. 2006), and also at MR angiography (Table 26.1). Lymph node-specific contrast agents are still awaiting approval. Liver-specific non-Gd-based agents include superparamagnetic iron oxide particles and manganese-based preparations (manganese chelate (mangafodipir trisodium) and free manganese for oral intake).

Marie-France Bellin
Université Paris –Sud 11, AP-HP, Service de Radiologie,
Hôpital Paul Brousse, 12–14 avenue Paul Vaillant Couturier,
94804 Villejuif Cedex, France

An oral agent containing manganese is still awaiting approval. The superparamagnetic iron oxide particles accumulate in the reticuloendothelial cells and are mainly T2-agents, which produce a decrease in signal intensity, while the gadolinium and manganese-based products accumulate in the hepatocytes and are mainly T1 agents, which produce an increase in signal intensity. Ultrasmall superparamagnetic iron oxide particles have the potential to improve noninvasive lymph node assessment and to characterize vulnerable atherosclerotic plaques. One USPIO agent (Supravist®) has recently been approved for MR angiography. The literature about tolerance and safety of non-Gd-based organ-specific agents is limited and the incidence of adverse events has not been studied in randomized clinical trials. Nonetheless, non-Gd-based organ-specific MR contrast agents appear to be safe and well tolerated in clinical use. The rate of adverse events seems to be higher with liver-specific contrast agents than with extracellular gadolinium chelates (Bellin et al. 1994, 2003; Reimer 2004a; Kirchin and Runge 2003). In addition, the mode of administration of superparamagnetic iron oxide particles, either infusion or intravenous bolus administration, may be a factor influencing their tolerance (Blume et al. 1994; Kehagias et al. 2001; Kopp et al. 1997; Reimer and Balzer 2003). The manganese-based agents may be tolerated differently when they are given orally or intravenously.

26.2
Superparamagnetic Iron Oxides (SPIOS)

26.2.1
Agents

Superparamagnetic iron oxide particles are one of an increasing number of MR contrast agents that target

Table 26.1. Overview of the various organ specific non-gadolinium-based MR contrast agents

Organ specific MR agents	Target cell	Main effect on signal intensity		Generic names (trade names)	Main route of elimination
		T1	T2		
Superparamagnetic iron oxides	Reticuloendothelial cells (Kupffer cells of the liver)	↑a	↓	Ferumoxides (Endorem®, Feridex®)	Metabolized
Superparamagnetic iron oxides	Reticuloendothelial cells (Kupffer cells of the liver)	↑a	↓	Ferucarbotran (Resovist®/ Cliavist®)	Metabolized
Ultrasmall superpara-magnetic iron oxides	Blood pool agent MR angiography	↑	↓a	Ferucarbotran (Supravist®)	Metabolized
Manganese based contrast agents	Hepatocytes	↑	↓a	Mangafodipir trisodium (Teslascan®)	Biliary+++ and renal (15% in 24 h)

a Slight effect

specific cellular processes. They are composed of a magnetic iron oxide core covered by a dextran or carboxydextran coat. The coat prevents uncontrollable aggregation and sedimentation of the particles in aqueous solutions, achieves high biological tolerance, and prevents toxic side effects. SPIO particles can be manufactured with different particle sizes and surface coatings. The core size ranges from 2 nm to less than 10 nm, and the hydrodynamic diameter ranges from 20 to 150 nm. Large SPIO particles, called superparamagnetic iron oxides (SPIOs), with a diameter ranging from 50 to 150 nm, are used for MR imaging of the liver and spleen and mainly produce a signal decrease or T2-shortening. They include the following commercially available contrast agents: ferumoxides (AMI-25, Endorem® in Europe, Laboratoire Guerbet, Aulnay-sous-Bois, France, Feridex®, in the USA, Berlex Laboratories, Wayne, NJ, USA) and ferucarbotran (SHU-555A, Resovist®/Cliavist®, Bayer Schering Pharma AG, Berlin, Germany). Smaller particles (<30 nm), called ultrasmall superparamagnetic iron oxides (USPIOs), have a different organ distribution. The future development of SPIO and USPIO particles with a modified coat may include molecular imaging, such as receptor-directed imaging, stem cell labeling, and labeling of gene constructs for localization in gene therapy (SCHÄFER et al. 2007; TAUPITZ et al. 2006).

Superparamagnetic iron oxides (SPIO) are extremely effective T_2 relaxation agents, which pro-

duce a long-range disturbance in magnetic field homogeneity and thus reduce the T_2 relaxation time, producing signal loss on T_2 and T_2^*-weighted images (BELLIN et al. 1994; BLUEMKE et al. 2003; ROS et al. 1995). The strong T_2 effect (susceptibility effect) is particularly apparent when SPIO particles are distributed inhomogeneously after uptake by Kupffer cells. After intravenous injection, SPIO particles are specifically taken up within minutes by the reticuloendothelial system (RES), mostly in the liver (approximately 80% of the injected dose) and spleen (5–10% of the injected dose) (WANG et al. 2001). In the liver they are taken up by normal RES Kupffer cells and decrease the signal intensity of the normal liver parenchyma on T_2 and T_2^*-weighted images. Since most liver lesions (including metastases and the vast majority of hepatocellular carcinomas) do not have an intact RES, they retain their signal intensity, so that the contrast between normal and abnormal liver tissue is increased. Some uptake of SPIO particles has been observed in focal nodular hyperplasia (PRECETTI-MOREL et al. 1999) and very rare cases of well differentiated hepatocellular adenomas and carcinomas. SPIO particles also have a T_1 effect, which is substantially less than their T_2 effect and can be used for lesion characterization when the agent is given as a bolus injection and for the characterization of hemangiomas (MONTET et al. 2004).

Two different preparations are available: ferumoxides and ferucarbotran. The commercial preparation of ferumoxides sold in the USA contains 11.2 mg of iron ml^{-1}, whereas in Europe the concentration of the agent is 22.4 mg of iron ml^{-1}. The approved dose is 0.8 mg of iron kg^{-1} body weight for ferumoxides and for ferucarbotran 0.56 mg iron kg^{-1} body weight.

The overall size of the particles, the coating of the iron core, and the electrical charge of the surfaces influence their pharmacodynamic and clinical properties. In principle, smaller particles circulate longer in the blood space and may accumulate in the macrophages of the lymph nodes, liver, and spleen while larger particles have a shorter half life and target the liver more specifically (STARK et al. 1988), being preferentially entrapped by Kupffer cells, which line the hepatic sinusoids. Ferumoxides have a mean diameter of 160 nm, a blood half life of 8 min, and a high T_2 relaxivity of 0.95×10^{-5} l mol^{-1} s^{-1} at 0.47 T, while ferucarbotran has a smaller mean diameter of 60 nm, a blood half life similar to that of ferumoxides, and a 1.9×10^{-5} l mol^{-1} s^{-1} T_2 relaxivity. The package inserts indicate that these agents are approved for adult patients and liver imaging. Safety and efficacy studies in patients under 18-years-old have not been carried out. The recommended dose for ferumoxides is 15 µmol Fe kg^{-1} (i.e., 0.075 ml kg^{-1}) and 10 µmol Fe kg^{-1} for ferucarbotran for T_2-weighted imaging at retention phase. Dosage remains the same in subjects with liver or renal insufficiency.

For ferumoxides, the dose of contrast agent should be diluted in 100 ml of 5% isotonic glucose solution and slowly infused intravenously for a period of at least 30 min. The imaging window is large: 0.5–6 h after administration for T_2- to T_2^*-weighted imaging (BELLIN et al. 1994). Because of the smaller size of the particles of ferucarbotran and since this agent can be injected as a bolus, it has stronger T_1 relaxivity properties and can also be used for T_1-weighted imaging and MR angiography following a bolus injection. A study published in 2003 (BLUEMKE et al. 2003) showed that direct undiluted injection of ferumoxides administered at 2 ml min^{-1} had safety and effectiveness profiles similar to those of slow infusion. Ferucarbotran is approved for bolus injection at a dose of 10 µmol Fe kg^{-1}.

SPIO particles are metabolized into a soluble, non-superparamagnetic form of iron. Dextrans follow the metabolism cycle while iron is incorporated into the body iron pool (e.g., ferritin, hemosiderin, and hemoglobin) within a few days. Iron is progressively cleared from the liver (half life, 3 days) and spleen (half life, 4 days). The total additional iron load per single dose does not exceed 2% of the total iron content of the human body (Ros et al. 1995; STARK et al. 1988).

26.2.2
Safety of Ferumoxides

In the original clinical trial performed with ferumoxides at a dose of 40 µmol Fe kg^{-1} (STARK et al. 1988), two adverse reactions were seen in two of the 15 patients, including one rash and one case of transient hypotension. Subsequent trials were performed with new formulations (a sodium citrate solvent was replaced by a mannitol solution), lower doses, and slower injection rates. In a phase II clinical trial that included 30 adult patients with liver metastases (BELLIN et al. 1994), no adverse events were seen and there were no significant changes in heart rate, blood pressure, or urine analyses. There were significant changes in the following parameters: protein level, serum iron, transferrin and ferritin levels, and transferrin saturation coefficient.

The largest series evaluating safety was a phase III clinical trial of 208 patients conducted in the US (Ros et al. 1995). The patients received 213 doses of 10 µmol Fe kg^{-1} given as a slow IV infusion. Eight percent experienced adverse reactions classified as possibly or probably related to drug administration. No serious adverse reactions to ferumoxides were reported. The intensity of adverse events reported was mild-to-moderate except for severe back pain in two patients and severe flushing in one. Back pain and flushing were reported in 4 and 2% of the patients, respectively, and were the most frequently reported adverse events. The exact mechanism of back pain is unknown but has been associated with a variety of colloids, emulsions, and other particulate agents. The package insert indicates that in the event of lumbar pain, chest pain, hypotension, or dyspnea, the infusion must be stopped and the patient kept under medical surveillance until the symptoms disappear. The administration of ferumoxides can be then continued under medical supervision by reducing the infusion rate and extending the infusion over at least 60 min. In Ros et al.'s (1995) series, none of the changes in clinical laboratory, vital signs, and electrocardiographic findings were reported to be clinically significant. Ferumoxides are contraindicated in patients with known allergy or hypersensitivity to dextran or to any of the other components and should be used with caution in patients with hemosiderosis or hemochromatosis.

26.2.3
Safety of Ferucarbotran (SPIO) SHU-555A

Three main papers have addressed the safety of ferucarbotran in clinical trials (KEHAGIAS et al. 2001; KOPP et al. 1997; REIMER and BALZER 2003). The phase II clinical trial (KEHAGIAS et al. 2001) included 36 patients who received a bolus injection of ferucarbotran at a dose of 4, 8, or 16 μmol Fe kg^{-1} BW. No drug related adverse event occurred and there were no significant changes in heart rate following bolus administration of ferucarbotran. Serum iron and ferritin levels were increased at all doses. The serum iron level reached a maximum 24 h after injection. A statistically significant but transient decrease in the serum level of factor XI was observed with the highest dose level. The series of KOPP et al. (1997) included 19 patients as part of a phase III clinical trial, and only one patient experienced moderate adverse events that were probably related to the injection of ferucarbotran. The adverse events was a diffuse erythematous rash associated with a feeling of pressure in the thorax, which lasted for 30 min. Changes in vital signs and laboratory tests were minimal and did not affect the patient's clinical condition. In their review, REIMER and BALZER (2003) summarized the safety data obtained during the whole clinical development of ferucarbotran. One hundred sixty-two adverse reactions were documented in 1,053 patients, of which 75 were classified as possibly, probably, or definitely related to the injection of ferucarbotran. In all, 73 of 75 adverse events occurred within the first 3 h and were of mild intensity, and one anaphylactoid reaction was observed. The frequency of adverse events was within the range of other approved MR contrast agents; no significant cardiovascular changes were observed. These authors concluded that ferucarbotran was a safe contrast agent.

26.3
Ultrasmall Superparamagnetic Iron Oxides (USPIOs)

There are two contrast agents containing ultrasmall superparamagnetic iron oxides. The first is ferucarbotran (SHU-555C, Supravist®, Bayer Schering Pharma AG, Berlin, Germany), which is used for MR angiography of the trunk, peripheral vessels, and coronary arteries. The second, which is still awaiting approval, is ferumoxtran (AMI-227, Sinerem, Laboratoire Guerbet, Aulnay-sous-Bois, France, or Combidex in the USA, Advanced Magnetics, Cambridge, Mass, USA). Ferumoxtran has the potential to detect and characterize lymph node metastases (MR lymphography) and to characterize vulnerable atherosclerotic plaques. In experimental studies, USPIOs have also been used to assess perfusion parameters in tumors and in tissues like the myocardium.

26.3.1
Ferucarbotran (USPIO) SHU-555c

SHU-555C (preliminary trade name Supravist®, Bayer Schering Pharma AG, Berlin, Germany) is a positive enhancer blood pool agent that can be administered as an IV bolus up to doses of 80 μmol kg^{-1}. The mean core particle size is 3–5 nm and the mean hydrodynamic diameter is about 20 nm in an aqueous environment. It has been proposed that this agent is suitable for first-pass and steady-state angiography (TOMBACH et al. 2004). In a phase I dose-finding study of MR assessment of myocardial perfusion and MR angiography of the chest in healthy volunteers, Reimer et al. (REIMER et al. 2004b) showed a dose-dependent increase in signal intensity enhancement during both the first pass and equilibrium phases. In this study, SHU-555C was injected intravenously at four doses (5, 10, 20, and 40 μmol iron [Fe] per kg of body weight) and was well tolerated; no cardiovascular reactions occurred. In an experimental study published in 2003, WACKER et al. showed that one intravenous injection of SHU-555C produced long, continuous intravenous signal intensity enhancement for MR angiography and allowed MR imaging-guided intravascular interventions to be undertaken in an open MR imaging system. More recently, phase III trials in patients with peripheral arterial disease and renal vascular disease have been completed, but results have not yet been published (BREMERICH et al. 2007).

26.3.2
Ferumoxtran AMI-227

Ferumoxtran (AMI-227, Sinerem, Laboratoire Guerbet, Aulnay-sous-Bois, France, or Combidex in the USA, Advanced Magnetics, Cambridge, Mass,

USA) is being developed for MR lymphography to improve the detection of node metastases. It is still in the experimental stage.

In ferumoxtran, USPIO particles are composed of iron oxide crystals coated with polymers to avoid uncontrolled aggregation of the magnetic crystals. USPIO salt solutions are prepared by coprecipitation of magnetite in the presence of a coating material. Electron microscopy shows that they contain an electron-dense crystal core consisting of multiple crystal aggregates covered with low-molecular-weight Dextran. The preparation method determines the number of crystals per particle, the size of each individual iron oxide crystal, and the dispersion of the crystal within the carrier particle. Overall particle size depends on the core size and its surface coating. With fe rumoxtran the mean particle size is 20 nm. The T1 and T2 relaxivities are, respectively, 2.3×10^4 and $5.3 \times 10^4 \mathrm{mol^{-1}\ s^{-1}}$ (20 MHz, 39°C) in 0.5% agar.

In normally functioning lymphatic tissue, USPIO particles are taken up by macrophages and cause a decrease in signal intensity (SI) on T_2 and T_2*-weighted images by their magnetic susceptibility effect and T_2-shortening effects. Metastatic nodes, in which macrophages are replaced by tumor cells, do not exhibit USPIO uptake and their signal intensity remains unchanged on postcontrast images. In 1990, WEISSLEDER et al. identified two mechanisms for USPIO uptake: direct transcapillary passage of the particles from the vascular bed into the medullary sinuses and extravasation throughout the body followed by a subsequent uptake by the macrophages which line the peripheral sinuses of the nodes. In addition, because of increased vascular permeability in cancer tissue, minimal leakage of USPIO particles into the extracellular space of metastases has been described. This produces a low local concentration of USPIO particles and a consequent positive enhancement, known as the "T_1 effect" of USPIO particles. The iron oxides are biodegraded in phagolysosomes within macrophages. The iron oxide core is incorporated into the plasma iron pool and is subsequently incorporated into hemoglobin.

Clinical tolerance of ferumoxtran is generally excellent (BELLIN et al. 1998; HARISINGHANI et al. 2003) and the total rate of adverse events does not exceed 2%. Most adverse events are minor. They include lumbar pain, rash, a transient decrease in blood pressure, arrhythmia, etc. The mechanism of postinjection lumbar pain is unknown, but lumbar pain is observed with other particulate agents. It usu-

ally disappears when the injection is stopped or its speed is reduced. Seventy-five percent of adverse events disappear without treatment. USPIOs do not significantly modify laboratory parameters, except for serum iron and ferritin levels.

26.4
Manganese-Based Contrast Agents

Mangafodipir trisodium (Teslascan®, GE Healthcare, USA) is a manganese chelate, which has been developed as a MR paramagnetic contrast agent for the hepatobiliary system. It comprises a manganese ion (Mn^{2+}) bound to a large linear ligand (fodipir; DPDP), which reduces the intravenous acute toxicity of free Mn^{2+} (ELIZONDO et al. 1991; FEDERLE et al. 2000). The metal chelate has a net electric charge of −3 (resulting from the +2 charge of the manganese ion and the −5 charge of DPDP), which is counterbalanced by the presence in the solution of three sodium ions, each having a charge of +1. In Europe, this agent is available in one preparation for 10–15-min infusion with a concentration of $0.01 \mathrm{mol\ l^{-1}}$. It was removed from the US market in 2003, because of problems (e.g. impurities) during production. Manganese is a paramagnetic ion, which causes increased signal intensity on T_1-weighted images, but it has also a minor T_2 effect causing reduction in the signal intensity.

An initial study (LIM et al. 1991) in healthy male volunteers showed that liver enhancement begins early, within 1–2 min of injection, with steady-state enhancement reached in 5–10 min. Liver enhancement persists for several hours allowing greater flexibility of scanning protocols and patient scheduling when compared to Gd chelates. The degree of liver enhancement depends on the physiological status of the liver parenchyma.

The Mn^{2+} ion has five unpaired electrons and is a powerful T_1 relaxation contrast agent that produces positive enhancement of normal hepatic tissue (increased signal intensity). The approved dose is $5\,\mu\mathrm{mol\ kg^{-1}}$ ($0.1\,\mathrm{ml\ kg^{-1}}$), with the injection given over 1 min. Manganese (as manganese chloride ($MnCl_2$)) can also be administrated orally (THOMSEN et al. 2004a, b). The manganese is absorbed in the gut and reaches the liver via the portal system and so circulation of free manganese is largely avoided. Between 0.8 and 1.6 g manganese chloride dissolved in 400 ml of fluid is given per patient (THOMSEN et al. 2004a, 2007).

Following intravenous injection, the manganese ion accumulates in the liver, bile, pancreas, kidneys, and cardiac muscle (GALLEZ et al. 1996; HUSTVEDT et al. 1997). Biliary excretion is first visible at 5 min after injection. Complete delineation of the biliary tree may require more than 15 min. Following oral intake, manganese accumulates only in the liver and bile (THOMSEN et al. 2004a). Cirrhosis may cause heterogeneous enhancement, while fibrosis may account for decreased enhancement. A meta-analysis comparing safety and efficacy of mangafodipir trisodium in patients with liver lesions and cirrhosis showed that a significantly higher number of lesions was found on the postcontrast images than on precontrast images, both in the cirrhotic (n = 137 patients) and non-cirrhotic patients (n = 480 patients) (MARTI-BONMATI et al. 2003). This increase was not influenced by the presence of liver cirrhosis. Lesion characterization was significantly improved in cirrhotic patients after administration of mangafodipir trisodium but not in non-cirrhotic patients. The number and severity of adverse events did not differ significantly between the two groups of patients. They were recorded in 6.7% of patients in the cirrhotic group and 7.0% in the non-cirrhotic group. Most adverse events were mild or moderate, with only one patient in each group having a severe adverse event. With the oral agent a few patients expressed some discomfort associated with drinking 400 ml of fluid, but no adverse reactions were reported (THOMSEN et al. 2007).

Mangafodipir trisodium has been shown to be a safe contrast agent at the approved dose of 5 µmol kg⁻¹ (0.1 ml kg⁻¹), as a slow infusion of 2–3 ml min⁻¹ (TORRES et al. 1997) or with higher injection rates (MARTI-BONMATI et al. 2001). The first large series evaluating mangafodipir trisodium was a phase II trial, which included 141 patients, of which 38 (27%) exhibited minor side effects (RUMMENY et al. 1991). Flushing and warmth were reported in 21/141 patients (14%), and nausea in 3 (2.1%). In 1993, AICHER et al. reported side effects in six of 20 (30%) patients, including flushing, warmth, and/or metallic taste. The results of a small European phase III trial that included 82 patients reported mild or moderate adverse events in 17% while 4% experienced infusion related discomfort (WANG et al. 1997).

The rate of adverse events observed in a large European phase III clinical trial was 7% in 624 patients (TORRES et al. 1997). The largest study of efficacy and safety is a multicenter phase III clinical trial of 404 adult patients in 18 institutions in the US (FEDERLE et al. 2000; WANG et al. 1997). The study design included

an initial contrast-enhanced CT examination followed by unenhanced MRI, injection of Mn-DPDP (5 µmol kg⁻¹ IV), and enhanced MRI at 15 min post-injection. Mangafodipir-enhanced MRI provided additional diagnostic information in 48% of the patients and altered patient management in 6%. Twenty-three percent of the patients reported at least one adverse event, and 146 adverse events in all were reported (WANG et al. 1997). The most frequent adverse reactions associated with the administration of mangafodipir trisodium are nausea, headache, and pruritus (FEDERLE et al. 2000; TORRES et al. 1997). Sensations of heat and flushing are most common with high injection rates and are probably related to peripheral vasodilatation (FEDERLE et al. 2000; TORRES et al. 1997). Transient decrease in alkaline phosphatase levels have also been reported with the use of mangafodipir trisodium.

The exact mechanism of these adverse events is unknown but may be due, at last in part, to in vivo dechelation of the contrast agent, with rapid incorporation of the manganese ion into hepatocytes. The dechelation of mangafodipir trisodium may induce flushing, as well as uptake by the intestinal mucosa and pancreas (BLUME et al. 1994; MAYO-SMITH et al. 1998; WANG et al. 1997). After dechelation, the manganese ions bind to human serum proteins. Cardiovascular effects may be seen because of increased circulating concentrations of manganese. Mn^{2+} given intravenously interferes with myocardial processing of Ca^{2+} and can act as a Ca^{2+} blocker affecting cardiac contractility and muscle physiology. Manganese also uncouples myocardial as well as smooth muscle excitation and contraction, leading to further decrease in cardiac contractility and hypotension. In the brain it may also interfere with the electrochemical potential of cell membranes. Approximately 15% of the manganese ion contained in the initial injection is eliminated in the urine by 24 h and 59% in the feces by 5 days (data from package insert). Mangafodipir trisodium should not be administered to pregnant women and whether it is safe for lactating women to breastfeed after receiving it is unknown (REIMER et al. 2004).

26.5
Conclusions

Because of improvements in contrast agent design, a large number of contrast agents are now available for MR imaging, among which the organ specific agents provide specific advantages in terms of sensitivity of lesion detection and characterization. They have unique features that include greater relaxivity when compared to extracellular Gd chelates, and both T2- and T1-shortening properties in the case of ferucarbotran. Although mangafodipir, SPIOs, and USPIOs are all known to dissociate or be metabolized in vivo, organ-specific contrast agents appear in general to be safe and well tolerated. No studies comparing the safety of the organ-specific iron oxides and the gadolinium-based agents have been published, so as yet it is not known whether the incidence of adverse reactions differs between them. Comparative clinical trials between the different agents should be undertaken. Guidelines on the safety aspects are presented in Chap. 29.

References

Aicher KP, Laniado M, Kopp AF et al (1993) Mn-DPDP-enhanced MR imaging of malignant liver lesions: efficacy and safety in 20 patients. J Magn Reson Imaging 3:731–737

Bellin MF, Zaim S, Auberton E et al (1994) Liver metastases: safety and efficacy of detection with superparamagnetic iron oxide in MR imaging. Radiology 193:657–663

Bellin MF, Roy C, Kinkel K et al (1998) Lymph node metastases: safety and effectiveness of MR imaging with ultrasmall superparamagnetic iron oxide particles. Initial clinical experience. Radiology 207:799–808

Bellin MF, Vasile M, Morel-Precetti S (2003) Currently used non-specific extracellular MR contrast media. Eur Radiol 13:2688–2698

Bluemke DA, Weber TM, Rubin D et al (2003) Hepatic MR imaging with ferumoxides: multicenter study of safety and effectiveness of direct injection protocol. Radiology 228:457–464

Bremerich J, Bilecen D, Reimer P (2007) MR angiography with blood pool contrast agents. Eur Radiol 17:3017–3024

Blume J, Palmie S, Aue B et al (1994) Pancreatic contrast enhancement with Mn-bis pyridoxal ethylene diamine diacetic acid and the influence of a hormonal stimulation of the pancreas in pigs. Acad Radiol 1:253–260

Elizondo G, Fretz CJ, Stark DD et al (1991) Preclinical evaluation of Mn-DPDP: new paramagnetic hepatobiliary contrast agent for MR imaging. Radiology 178:73–78

Federle M, Chezmar J, Rubin DL et al (2000) Efficacy and safety of mangafodipir trisodium (MnDPDP) Injection for hepatic MRI in adults: results of the US multicenter phase III clinical trials. Efficacy of early imaging. J Magn Reson Imaging 12:689–701

Gallez B, Bacic G, Swartz HM (1996) Evidence for the dissociation of the hepatobiliary MRI contrast agent Mn-DPDP. Magn Reson Med 35:14–19

Gandhi SN, Brown MA, Wong JG (2006) MR contrast agents for liver imaging: what, when, how. RadioGraphics 26:1621–1636

Harisinghani MG, Barentsz J, Hahn PF et al (2003) Noninvasive detection of clinically occult lymph-node metastases in prostate cancer. N Engl J Med 348:2491–2499

Hustvedt SO, Grant D, Southon TE et al (1997) Plasma pharmacokinetics, tissue distribution and excretion of MnDPDP in the rat and dog after intravenous administration. Acta Radiol 38:690–699

Kehagias DT, Gouliamos AD, Smyrniotis V et al (2001) Diagnostic efficacy and safety of MRI of the liver with superparamagnetic iron oxide particles (SHU 555 A). J Magn Reson Imaging 14:595–601

Kirchin MA, Runge VM (2003) Contrast agents for magnetic resonance imaging: safety update. Top Magn Reson Imaging 14:426–435

Kopp AF, Laniado M, Dammann F et al (1997) MR imaging of the liver with Resovist: safety, efficacy, and pharmacodynamic properties. Radiology 204:749–756

Lim KO, Stark DD, Leese PT et al (1991) Hepatobiliary MR imaging: first human experience with MnDPDP. Radiology 178:79–82

Manfredi R, Maresca G, Baron RL et al (1999) Delayed MR imaging of hepatocellular carcinoma enhanced by gadobenate dimeglumine (Gd-BOPTA). J Magn Reson Imaging 9:704–710

Marti-Bonmati L, Torregrosa A, Miguel A et al (2001) Safety and efficacy of a bolus administration of mangafodipir trisodium in MR studies. Poster presented in ninth scientific meeting ISMRM and 14th annual meeting ESMRMB, Glasgow. Proc ISMRM 2036

Marti-Bonmati L, Fog AF, Op de Beeck B et al (2003) Safety and efficacy of mangafodipir trisodium in patients with liver lesions and cirrhosis. Eur Radiol 13:1685–1692

Mayo-Smith WW, Schima W, Saini S et al (1998) Pancreatic enhancement and pulse sequence analysis using low-dose mangafodipir trisodium. Am J Roentgenol 170:649–652

Montet X, Lazeyras F, Howarth N et al (2004) Specificity of SPIO particles for characterization of liver hemangiomas using MRI. Abdom Imaging 29:60–70

Precetti-Morel S, Bellin MF, Ghebontni L et al (1999) Focal nodular hyperplasia of the liver on ferumoxides-enhanced MR imaging: features on conventional spin-echo, fast spin-echo and gradient-echo pulse sequences. Eur Radiol 9:1535–1542

Reimer P, Balzer T (2003) Ferucarbotran (Resovist), a new clinically approved RES-specific contrast agent for contrast-enhanced MRI of the liver: properties, clinical development, and applications. Eur Radiol 13:1266–1276

Reimer P, Schneider G, Schima W (2004a) Hepatobiliary contrast agents for contrast-enhanced MRI of the liver: properties, clinical development, and applications. Eur Radiol 14:559–578

Reimer P, Bremer C, Allkemper T (2004b) Myocardial perfusion and MR angiography of chest with SHU 555 C: results of placebo-controlled clinical phase I study. Radiology 231:474–481

Ros PR, Freeny PC, Harms SE et al (1995) Hepatic MR imaging with ferumoxides: a multicenter clinical trial of the safety and efficacy in the detection of focal hepatic lesions. Radiology 196:481–488

Rummeny E, Ehrenheim C, Gehl HB et al (1991) Manganese-DPDP as a hepatobiliary contrast agent in the magnetic resonance imaging of liver tumors. Results of clinical phase

II trials in Germany including 141 patients. Invest Radiol 26(Suppl 1):S142–S145 Discussion S150–S155

Schäfer R, Kehlbach R, Wiskirchen J et al (2007). Transferrin receptor upregulation: in vitro labeling of rat mesenchymal stem cells with superparamagnetic iron oxide. Radiology 224:514–523

Stark DD, Weissleder R, Elizondo G et al (1988) Superparamagnetic iron oxide: clinical application as a contrast agent for MR imaging of the liver. Radiology 168:297–301

Taupitz M, Schimtz S, Hamm B (2006) Superparamagnetic iron oxide particles: current state and future development. RöFo 175:752–765

Tombach B, Reimer P, Bremer C et al (2004) First-pass and equilibrium-MRA of the aortoiliac region with a superparamagnetic iron oxide blood pool MR contrast agent (SH U 555 C): results of a human pilot study. NMR Biomed 17:500–506

Thomsen HS, Loegager V, Noergaard H et al (2004a) Oral manganese for liver imaging at three different field strengths. Acad Radiol 11:630–636

Thomsen HS, Svendsen O, Klastrup S (2004b) Increased manganese concentration in the liver after oral intake. Acad Radiol 11:38–44

Thomsen HS, Barentsz JO, Burcharth F et al (2007) Initial clinical experience with oral manganese (CMC-001) for liver imaging. Eur Radiol 17:273–278

Torres CG, Lundby B, Sterud AT et al (1997) MnDPDP for MR imaging of the liver. Results from the European phase III studies. Acta Radiol 38:631–637

Wacker FK, Reither K, Ebert W et al (2003) MR image-guided endovascular procedures with the ultrasmall superparamagnetic iron oxide SH U 555 C as an intravascular contrast agent: study in pigs. Radiology 226:459–464

Wang C, Ahlstrom H, Ekholm S et al (1997) Diagnostic efficacy of MnDPDP in MR imaging of the liver. A phase III multicenter study. Acta Radiol 38:643–649

Wang Y X J, Hussain SM, Krestin GP (2001) Superparamagnetic iron oxide contrast agents: physicochemical characteristics and applications in MR imaging. Eur Radiol 11:2319–2331

Weissleder R, Elizondo G, Wittenberg J et al (1990) Ultrasmall superparamagnetic iron oxide: characterization of a new class of contrast agents for MR imaging. Radiology 175:489–493

Ultrasonographic Contrast Media

Safety of Ultrasonographic Agents

Raymond Oyen

CONTENTS

27.1

Introduction

Microbubble contrast agents for ultrasound have gained increasing interest in recent years (QUAIA 2007). It is generally considered that ultrasound contrast agents approved for clinical use are well tolerated and serious adverse reactions are rarely observed. In this chapter, the evidence supporting this impression is reviewed.

Raymond Oyen
Department of Radiology, Katholieke Universiteit Leuven, Herestraat 49, 3000 Leuven, Belgium

27.2

General Considerations on the Acoustic Properties of Microbubble-Based Ultrasound Contrast Media

Ultrasound contrast media for intravenous injections are usually gas-filled microbubbles with a mean diameter less than that of a red blood cell (i.e., 2–$6\,\mu m$). They are composed of a shell of biocompatible materials, including proteins, lipids, or biopolymers containing a filling gas. The contrast agents can be described according to the concentration of particles, size of particles or microbubbles, volume of gas, kind of gas, kind of shell, additives, etc. The microbubble shell may be stiff (e.g., denatured albumin) or flexible (phospolipids) and has a thickness from 10 to 200 nm. High molecular weight and low-solubility filling gases (perfluorocarbon or sulfur hexafluoride) produce a raised vapor concentration inside the microbubble relative to surrounding blood and increase the microbubble stability in the peripheral circulation. There are only a few products approved for clinical use, and they are all based on microbubbles (Table 27.1).

Microbubbles have a pure intravascular distribution even though some agents have a postvascular hepato- and/or spleno-specific phase from 2 to 5 min after i.v. injection. This phenomenon is probably determined by the adherence of the microbubbles to the hepatic sinusoids or by the selective uptake by the phagocytic cells of the reticuloendothelial system (HARVEY et al. 2001). From 10 to 15 min after injection, the microbubble gas content is exhaled via the lungs, while the components of the shell are metabolized or filtered by the kidney and eliminated by the liver (MOREL et al. 2000).

Table 27.1. Ultrasound contrast agents available for clinical use. Generic names are given in parenthesis

Product name	Clinical nature
Imavist® (AF0150)	Perfluorohexane and nitrogen gas in stabilized microbubbles
SonoVue® (BR1)	Sulphur hexafluoride gas in polymer with phospholipids
Definity™ (DMP 115)	Fluorocarbon gas in liposomes
Albunex™	Air-filled protein shell
Optison™ (FS069)	Octafluropropane-filled albumin microspheres
Echovist®	Galactose-based gas bubbles
Levovist® (SHU 508A)	Galactose-based, palmitic acid stabilized air-bubbles

The effect of ultrasound contrast media is mainly produced by increased backscattering intensity as compared to that from blood, other fluids, and most tissues (JAKOBSEN 1996). The spectral Doppler intensity is also increased, with a brighter spectral waveform displayed and a stronger sound heard. When color Doppler technique is used, ultrasound contrast media enhance the frequency or the power intensity and give rise to stronger color encodings. The effect of ultrasound contrast media is most efficient when various contrast-specific nonlinear techniques are used. Typically, the microbubbles oscillate as a response to the external sound field during scanning, both in a linear and in a nonlinear way. This is the basis for nonlinear techniques such as second harmonic imaging (BURNS 1996), pulse or phase inversion, or pulse cancellation, which improve the detection of microbubbles specifically (BURNS et al. 2000). The effect on microbubble behavior is dependent on the acoustic pressure created by the ultrasound probe. Usually, with increasing wave pressure, the effect on imaging may come from reflection, then asymmetrical vibration, and finally disruption of microbubbles, in that order (CORREAS et al. 2001). These changes in microbubble behavior may induce the unwanted effects described later in this paper. Therefore, the effect of insonation on microbubble behavior is dependent on the level of the mechanical index (MI), as well as the properties of the contrast agent and the imaging mode chosen.

27.3
Experimental Findings on Microbubble-Based Ultrasound Contrast Media

The cavitation phenomenon refers to formation, growth, and collapse by implosion of microbubbles. The "cavitation threshold" is the point where the amount of energy being introduced into the fluid initiates cavitation. The implosion causes large changes in pressure and temperature in the close vicinity. This cavitation phenomenon has caused some concern in relation to the safety of ultrasound contrast agents.

In vitro studies have shown that ultrasound contrast agents may cause hemolysis, platelet aggregation, and endothelial damage (MILLER and GIES 1998; POLIACHIK et al. 1999; CARSTENSEN et al. 1993; EVERBACH et al. 1998). The amount of hemolysis seems to correlate with the amount of microbubbles present, the acoustic pressure exerted on the blood, and varies with the type of ultrasound contrast medium. Cavitation is considered the cause of most of these effects.

In vivo studies of pigs and dogs with pulmonary hypertension have shown that pulmonary function can be affected by high doses of ultrasound contrast media (WALDAY et al. 1994; OSTENSEN et al. 1992; YAMAYA et al. 2002). The interaction between ultrasound contrast media and pulsed ultrasound waves seems to cause no pulmonary damage (RAEMAN et al. 1997).

Animal studies showed no significant influence of ultrasound contrast media on left ventricular (LV) function or myocardial blood flow (MAIN et al. 1997; MEZA et al. 1996). However, CHEN et al. (2002) reported an increase in troponin T (a marker of myocardial ischemia) when a high mechanical index for bubble destruction was transmitted. This was not associated with LV dysfunction or histopathological evidence of myocardial damage. Furthermore, in one study on rats, several types of arrhythmias were observed when ultrasound contrast media and ultrasound were combined (ZACHARY et al. 2002).

Disruption of the blood brain barrier may occur in rats after intravenous injection of ultrasound contrast media (MYCHASKIW et al. 2000). However, left ventricular injection of air-filled contrast agents in rats did not damage the brain or its microvasculature (HAGGAG et al. 1998). The combination of ultrasound exposure and ultrasound contrast media may damage the endothelial cells and venules and capillaries of rat mesentery (KOBAYASHI et al. 2002, 2003; RASMUSSEN et al. 2003). Amplification of the Doppler echo alters the measurements during both high and low flow, so that the flow rate cannot be recorded very precisely (LIEPSCH et al. 2004).

27.4
Clinical Safety of Ultrasound Contrast Media

The side effects observed in animal studies have not been observed in clinical practice despite extensive investigation (NANDA and CARSTENSEN 1997; MOREL et al. 2000; MYRENG et al. 1999; ROBBIN et al. 1998; BORGES et al. 2002). The microbubbles are so small that obstruction or trapping in the capillaries does not seem to be a problem. Adverse reactions caused by cavitation have not been shown in humans. The galactose content of some agents, and human protein content of others have been considered to be potential causes of adverse reactions, but clinical investigations have shown no major problems so far.

The most common general adverse events reported are the same as those seen with other types of contrast media, that is, headache, warm sensation, and flushing. More unusual events are nausea and vomiting, dizziness, chills and fever, altered taste, dyspnoea, chest pain, etc. (0%–5%) (CORREAS et al. 2001; MYRENG et al. 1999; BOKOR et al. 2001; CLAUDON et al. 2000; ROTT 1999; TER HAAR 2002; GOLDBERG 1997; COHEN et al. 1998; KAPS et al. 1999; FRITSCH and SCHLIEF 1995). Similar findings were, however, observed in placebo groups. Such adverse reactions are rare, usually transient, mild, and the same with many agents (CORREAS et al. 2001). Allergy-like reactions occur rarely; general flush with erythema and papules has been reported (CORREAS et al. 2001). Three anaphylactic reactions have been reported, two in women aged 59 and 70 years, and one in a man of 70 years (DE GROOT et al. 2004). In a large retrospective analysis of the safety of SonoVue, the overall reporting rate of serious adverse events was 0.0086% (PISCAGLIA et al. 2006). Asymptomatic premature ventricular contractions have been observed during triggered imaging with ultrasound contrast medium (VAN DER WOUW et al. 2000). Based on the large clinical experience accu-

mulated in several clinical trials, it can be concluded that the overall risk of serious adverse reactions during contrast-enhanced echocardiography is small, if not negligible (HAYAT and SENIOR 2005).

It has been recommended that therapeutic ultrasound and lithotripsy should be avoided in the day following the use of ultrasound contrast agents (BRAYMAN and MILLER 1997; DALECKI et al. 1997; DELIUS 1994). Decisions about the use of contrast materials in the maternal circulation depend on the clinical condition of the mother (ROTT 1999; ECMUS 2004).

The European Medicine Agency (EMEA) recently took precautionary measures (DE GROOT et al. 2004) to limit the use of ultrasonographic contrast agent sulphur hexafluoride in patients with cardiac disease (including acute coronary syndrome, unstable angina, recent acute myocardial infarction, recent coronary artery intervention, acute or class III/IV chronic heart failure, or severe rhythm disorders). Throughout Europe a number of serious reactions have been reported with probable secondary cardiovascular problems including severe hypotension, bradycardia, anaphylactic shock. In addition to this, there have been three reports of a fatal outcome soon after administration of this agent. All of these patients were, however, at risk of serious cardiac complications because of underlying cardiac problems (DE GROOT et al. 2004). (Table 27.2)

27.5
Recommendation on the Use of Ultrasound Contrast Media

The European Committee for Medical Ultrasound Safety (ECMUS) recommends that ultrasound contrast media only be used if there is a good clinical indication, and the risk/benefit ratio must be carefully assessed (ECMUS 2004). In addition this Committee emphasized that high values of Mechanical Index should be used only when essential for a particular clinical study (ECMUS 2003). It is important to acknowledge that ultrasound contrast media are fairly new products and it may take several years of accurate surveillance to document possible adverse reactions to them. It is also not clear whether there are important differences in the safety among the products currently available.

Table 27.2. Frequency of adverse events during intravenous administration of Levovist®, Optison®, and SonoVue®

Adverse event reported 0.5%–5%	Adverse event reported less than 1%
Body as a whole Headache Hypersensitivity at injection site	**Body as a whole** Abdominal pain Weakness Pain Back Pain Chest Pain Fatigue
Cardiovascular system Hypertension	**Cardiovascular system** Atrial fibrillation Palpitation Tachycardia
Digestive system Nausea	**Digestive system** Anorexia Diarrhea Dyspepsia
Nervous system Dizziness Dry mouth Vasodilatation	**Nervous system** Paresthesia
Special senses Abnormal smell or taste	**Musculoskeletal system** Leg cramps
	Respiratory system Dyspnoea
	Skin and appendages Sweating Rash Pruritus

27.6
Conclusion

In vitro and animal studies have shown adverse effects of ultrasound contrast media related to the properties of the particles and the interaction between microbubble destruction and ultrasound beam energy. However, clinical studies have not shown such adverse events and indicate that ultrasound contrast media are generally safe. Most adverse events seen clinically are nonspecific and probably unrelated to the constituents of the various products. Any rare adverse events should be treated symptomatically.

The use of ultrasound contrast media should always be clinically justified. It is important that the exposure time to ultrasound and the acoustic output shown be kept to lowest level consistent with obtaining diagnostic information. Guidelines on the safety of ultrasound contrast media can be found in Chap. 29.

References

Bokor D, Chambers JB, Rees PJ, Mant TGK, Luzzani F, Spinazzi A (2001) Clinical safety of SonoVue, a new contrast agent for ultrasound imaging, in healthy volunteers and in patients with chronic obstructive pulmonary disease. Invest Radiol 36:104–109

Borges AC, Walde T, Reibis RK, Grohmann A, Ziebig R, Rutsch W et al (2002) Does contrast echocardiography with Optison induce myocardial necrosis in humans? J Am Soc Echocardiogr 15:1080–1086.

Brayman AA, Miller MW (1997) Acoustic cavitation nuclei survive the apparent ultrasonic destruction of Albunex® microspheres. Ultrasound Med Biol 23:793–796

Burns PN (1996) Harmonic imaging with ultrasound contrast agents (1996) Clin Radiol 51:S50–S55

Burns PN, Wilson SR, Simpson DH (2000) Pulse inversion imaging of liver blood flow: improved method for characterizing focal masses with microbubble contrast. Invest Radiol 35:58–71

Carstensen EL, Kelly P, Church CC, Brayman AA, Child SZ, Raeman CH, Schery L (1993) Lysis of erythrocytes by exposure to CW ultrasound. Ultrasound Med Biol 19:147–165

Chen S, Kroll MH, Shohet RV, Frenkel P, Mayer SA, Grayburn PA (2002) Bioeffects of myocardial contrast microbubble destruction by echocardiography. Echocardiography 19:495–500

Claudon M, Pouin PF, Baxter G, Ohban T, Maniez Devos D (2000) Renal arteries in patients at risk of renal arterial stenosis: multicenter evaluation of the echo-enhancer SH U 508A at color and spectral Doppler US. Levovist Renal Artery Stenosis Study Group. Radiology 214:739–746

Cohen JL, Cheirif J, Segar DS, Gillam LD, Gottdiener JS, Hausnerova E (1998) Improved left ventricular endocardial border delineation and opacification with Optison (FS069), a new echocardiographic contrast agent. Results of a phase III Multicenter Trial. J Am Coll Cardiol 32:746–752

Correas J-M, Bridal L, Lesavre A, Méjean A, Claudon M, Hélénon O (2001) Ultrasound contrast agents: properties, principles of action, tolerance, and artifacts. Eur Radiol 11:1316–1328

Dalecki D, Raeman CH, Child SZ, Penney DP, Carstensen EL. (1997) Remnants of Albunex® nucleate acoustic cavitation. Ultrasound Med Biol 23:1405–1412

De Groot MC, van Zwieten-Boot BJ, van Grootheest AC (2004) Severe adverse reactions after the use of sulphur hexafluoride (SonoVue) as an ultrasonographic contrast agent. Ned Tijdschr Geneesk 48:1887–1888

Delius M (1994) Medical applications and bioeffects of extracorporeal shock waves. Shock Waves 4:55–72

ECMUS Safety Committee tutorial paper (1999) Safety of ultrasonic contrast agents. www.efsumb.org/tutpap11.htm, Accessed on 14 December 2004

European Committee of Medical Ultrasound Safety (ECMUS) (2003) Clinical safety statement for digital ultrasound. www.efsumb.org/safstat2003.htm

Everbach EC, Makin IR, Francis CW, Meltzer RS (1998) Effect of acoustic cavitation on platelets in the presence of an echo-contrast agent. Ultrasound Med Biol 24:129–136

Fritsch T, Schlief R (1995) Levovist®. Drugs of the Future 20:1224–1227

Goldberg BB (1997) Ultrasound contrast agents. Martin Dunitz Ltd, London, UK

Haggag KJ, Russell D, Walday P, Skiphamn A, Torvik A (1998) Air-filled ultrasound contrast agents do not damage the cerebral microvasculature or brain tissue in rats. Invest Radiol 33:129–135

Harvey CJ, Blomley MJK, Eckersley RJ, Cosgrove DO (2001) Developments in ultrasound contrast media. Eur Radiol 11:675–689

Hayat SA, Senior R (2005) Safety: the heart of the matter. Eur J Echocardiogr 6(4):235–237

Jakobsen J (1996) Echo-enhancing agents in the renal tract. Clin Radiol 51:S40–S43

Kaps M, Seidel G, Bokor D, Modrau B, Algermissen C (1999) Safety and ultrasound enhancing potentials of a new sulphur hexafluoride-containing agent in the cerebral circulation. J Neuroimaging 9:150–154

Kobayashi N, Yasu T, Yamada S, Kudo N, Kuroki M, Kawakami M et al (2002) Endothelial cell injury in venule and capillary induced by contrast ultrasonography. Ultrasound Med Biol 28:949–956

Kobayashi N, Yasu T, Yamada S, Kudo N, Kuroki M, Miyatake K et al (2003) Influence of contrast ultrasonography with perflutren lipid microspheres on microvessel injury. Circ J 67:630–636

Liepsch D, Schmid T, McLean J, Weigand C (2004) Do contrast agents affect ultrasound flow measurements? Technol Health Care 12(6):411–423

Main ML, Escobar JF, Hall SA, Grayburn PA (1997) Safety and efficacy of QW7437, a new fluorocarbon-based echo cardiographic contrast agent. J Am Soc Echocardiogr 10:798–804

Meza M, Greener Y, Hunt R, Perry B, Revall S, Barbee W et al (1996) Myocardial contrast echocardiography: reliable, safe, and efficacious myocardial perfusion assessment after intravenous injections of a new echocardiographic contrast agent. Am Heart J 132:871–881

Miller DL, Gies RA (1998) Enhancement of ultrasonically-induced hemolysis by perfluorocarbon-based compared to air-based echo-contrast agents. Ultrasound Med Biol 24:285–292

Morel DR, Schwieger I, Hohn L, Terrettaz J, Llull JB, Cornioley YA et al (2000) Human pharmacokinetics and safety evaluation of SonoVue, a new contrast agent for ultrasound imaging. Invest Radiol 35:80–85

Mychaskiw G II, Badr AE, Tibbs R, Clower BR, Zhang JH (2000) Optison (FS069) disrupts the blood-brain barrier in rats. Anesth Analg 91:798–803

Myreng Y, Molstad P, Ytre-Arne K, Aas M, Stoksflod L, Nossen J et al (1999) Safety of the transpulmonary ultrasound contrast agent NC100100: a clinical and hemodynamic evaluation in patients with suspected or proven coronary artery disease. Heart 82:333–335

Nanda NC, Carstensen EL (1997) Echo-enhancing agents: safety. In: Nanda NC, Schlief R, Goldberg BB (eds) Advances in Echo imaging using contrast enhancement. Kluwer, Dordrecht, pp 115–131

Ostensen J, Hede R, Myreng Y, Ege T, Holtz E (1992) Intravenous injection of Albunex microspheres causes thromboxane mediated pulmonary hypertension in pigs, but not in monkeys or rabbits. Acta Physiol Scand 144:307–315

Piscaglia F, Bolondi L, Italian Society for Ultrasound in Medicine and Biology (SIUMB) Study group on ultrasound contrast agents (2006) The safety of Sonovue in abdominal applications: retrospective analysis of 23188 investigations. Ultrasound Med Biol 32(9):1369–1375

Poliachik SL, Chandler WL, Mourad PD, Bailey MR, Bloch S, Cleveland RO et al. (1999) Effect of high-intensity focused ultrasound on whole blood with and without microbubble contrast agent. Ultrasound Med Biol 25:991–998

Quaia E (2007) Microbubble ultrasound contrast agents: an update. Eur Radiol 17:1995–2008

Raeman CH, Dalecki D, Child SZ, Meltzer RS, Carstensen EL (1997) Albunex does not increase the sensitivity of the lung to pulsed ultrasound. Echocardiography 14:553–558

Rasmussen H, Dirven HA, Grant D, Johnsen H, Midtvedt T (2003) Etiology of cecal and hepatic lesions in mice after administration of gas-carrier contrast agents used in ultrasound imaging. Toxicol Appl Pharmacol 188:176–184

Robbin ML, Eisenfeld AJ (For the EchoGen Contrast Ultrasound Study Group) (1998) Perflenapent emulsion: a US contrast agent for diagnostic radiology – multicenter, double-blind comparison with a placebo. Radiology 207:717–722

Rott HD (1999) Safety of ultrasonic contrast agents. European Committee for Medical Ultrasound Safety. Eur J Ultrasound 9:195–197

ter Haar GR (2002) Ultrasonic contrast agents: safety considerations reviewed. Eur J Radiol 41:217–221

Van Der Wouw PA, Brauns AC, Bailey SE, Powers JE, Wilde AA (2000) Premature ventricular contractions during triggered imaging with ultrasound contrast. J Am Soc Echocardiogr 13:288–294

Walday P, Tolleshaug H, Gjoen T, Kindberg GM, Berg T, Skotland T, Holtz E (1994) Biodistributions of air-filled albumin microspheres in rats and pigs. Biochem J 299:437–443

Yamaya Y, Niizeki K, Kim J, Entin PL, Wagner H, Wagner PD (2002). Effects of Optison on pulmonary gas exchange and hemodynamics. Ultrasound Med Biol 28:1005–1013

Zachary JF, Hartleben SA, Frizzell LA, O'Brien WD Jr (2002) Arrhythmias in rat hearts exposed to pulsed ultrasound after intravenous injection of a contrast agent. J Ultrasound Med 21:1347–1356

Barium Preparations

Barium Preparations: Safety Issues

28

Sameh K. Morcos

28.1
Introduction

The use of barium sulphate to image the gastrointestinal tract (GIT) was first proposed in 1910 by Bechem and Gunther. Since those early days barium sulphate preparations have improved markedly and now they are used routinely in radiology departments worldwide. Adverse effects directly related to the oral or rectal administration of barium preparations will be discussed in this chapter (Table 28.1). Technique related complications of barium examinations are beyond the scope of this account.

28.2
Barium Sulphate

All barium preparations are based on barium sulphate, which is a heavy insoluble material produced from barite. Pure barium sulphate suspension is not suitable for imaging the GIT as it flocculates easily and produces very poor mucosal coating. Therefore, additives (e.g., pectin, sorbitol, agar-agar, carboxy-

Sameh K. Morcos
Department of Diagnostic Imaging, Northern General Hospital NHS Trust, Sheffield S5 7AU, UK

methyl-cellulose) are used in the commercial barium preparations to enhance the mucosal coating properties of the suspension, prevent flocculation, and improve the taste for oral use (Almen and Aspelin 1995). More than 90 different additives have been described in the literature. However, the manufacturers of the barium suspensions very often keep the exact type and proportions of additives in each barium preparation secret for commercial reasons.

28.3
Adverse Effects of Barium Sulphate Preparations

Barium sulphate is insoluble in water and theoretically nontoxic (Morcos 2000). The particles of barium sulphate suspension remain in the intestinal lumen and are not absorbed. Barium ions are toxic, but the extremely small amounts of barium ions that are present in the suspension and available for intestinal absorption are regarded as being of no practical importance (Almen and Aspelin 1995).

Oral or rectal administration of barium sulphate is usually safe but constipation and abdominal pain may occur after barium meals or enemas (Smith et al. 1988). An overview of the adverse effects of barium preparations is given in Table 28.1. The main risk is that barium may remain in the colon for 6 weeks or longer in elderly patients or patients with partial colonic obstruction. Prolonged stasis of barium may occur following a barium enema into the distal loop of a colostomy (Morcos 2000). Baroliths (barium feco-liths) are rare complications of barium contrast examinations and usually seen in diverticula of the colon. Baroliths are often asymptomatic but may be associated with abdominal pain, appendicitis, bowel obstruction, or perforation. They may even have to be removed surgically (Smith et al. 1988; Morcos and

Table 28.1. Adverse effects of barium preparations

Adverse effect	Result
Retention of barium in colon	Abdominal discomfort
	Constipation
Formation of barolith	Bowel obstruction
	Appendicitis
Aggravation of toxic dilatation of the colon	Colonic perforation may be precipitated
Leakage of barium into peritoneal cavity	Peritonitis
	Peritoneal adhesions and bowel obstruction
Extraperitoneal leakage of barium	Granulomatous inflammatory reaction
	Fibrosis
Aspiration of barium into bronchial tree	Respiratory failure
	Chemical pneumonia
Intravasation of barium suspension	Barium pulmonary emboli
	Disseminated intravascular coagulation
	Septicaemia
	Hypotension
Allergic reactions to barium preparations	Severe anaphylactic reactions may develop to the additives of the barium preparations
	Bronchospasm
	Angioedema
	Urticaria

BROWN 2001). Baroliths of the small bowel are rare. A case of small bowel obstruction secondary to barolith which developed at the site of narrowing of a loop of ileum secondary to a carcinoid tumour has been reported (REGAN et al. 1999). Interference with the flow of barium at this segment precipitated the development of the barolith.

Toxic dilatation of the colon may be aggravated by barium enema (MORCOS 2000; WILLIAMS and HARNED 1991).

Barium sulphate even when sterile can cause marked peritoneal irritation with considerable fluid loss into the peritoneal cavity (MORCOS 2000). Perforation into the peritoneal cavity following barium enema occurs rarely. Those at risk are children, debilitated adults, or patients in whom the colon is already weakened by inflammatory, malignant, or parasitic disease. The perforation may be triggered by manipulations involved in giving the barium enema or result from hydrostatic pressure (MORCOS

2000). Perforation of the colon by barium enema may result in death (MORCOS 2000). The incidence of perforation is approximately one in 6,000 examinations. The mixture of barium and faeces produces severe peritonitis and dense adhesions. The mortality has been reported to be 58% with conservative treatment, and still as high as 47% with surgical intervention (ZHEUTLIN et al. 1952). Early surgery is indicated and large volumes of intravenous fluids improve the prognosis. Patients who recover may develop fibrogranulomatous reactions and adhesions, which can lead to bowel obstruction or ureteric occlusion (MORCOS 2000). Perforation of the duodenum and barium leakage into the peritoneal cavity may also occur rarely in patients with duodenal ulcer (MORCOS 2000).

Extraperitoneal perforation and leakage of barium into the retroperitoneum or mediastinum may cause few immediate symptoms, but delayed endotoxic shock can develop 12 h later and is frequently fatal.

Inflammatory reaction leading to formation of barium granulomata and fibrosis may occur. Painful masses, rectal strictures, and ulcers have been described following extraperitoneal leakage (MORCOS 2000).

Intravenous barium intravasation after enema examination has also been reported and may be associated with mortality of up to 55%. Barium emboli in the lungs, disseminated intravascular coagulation, septicaemia, and severe hypotension have been documented following barium intravasation. Most cases have been attributed to trauma from the tip of the enema tube or retention balloon, mucosal inflammation, or misplacement of the tube in the vagina. The amount and speed of intravasation of the barium, as well as the site of the intravasation and the general health of the patient determine the outcome of this complication (MORCOS 2000; WILLIAMS and HARNED 1991).

Disseminated intravascular coagulation, septicaemia, and severe hypotension have also been documented following venous intravasation of Gastrografin (a high osmolar water soluble contrast medium preparation containing sodium and meglumine diatrizoate used for imaging of the GIT and suitable only for oral or rectal administration) (GLAUSER et al. 1999).

Low osmolar water soluble contrast media should be used in preference to Gastrografin or barium preparations in patients with suspected compromise of bowel wall integrity. Barium leaking into a sigmoid abscess during a barium enema examination and intravasating into the portal venous system has been reported (WHEATLEY and ECKHAUSER 1991).

Accidental administration of a barium enema into the vagina instead of the rectum may occur and can be very hazardous: in a number of these patients there has been rupture of the vagina with fatal venous intravasation of barium (MORCOS 2000).

Aspiration of barium sulphate preparation into the lungs during barium meal examination can cause significant respiratory embarrassment particularly in patients with poor respiratory function and general condition. If thick barium paste is inhaled, it occludes small bronchi and may cause fatal asphyxiation. Aspiration of barium may also cause fatal pneumonia (MORCOS and BROWN 2001; TAMM and KORTSIK 1999; LAREAU and BERTA 1976; GRAY et al. 1980). Persistent alveolar deposition of barium sulphate on the chest radiograph, which only decreases slightly compared to the initial X-ray, will be observed (TAMM and KORTSIK 1999). It has been recommended that bronchoscopy should be performed early following barium aspiration to extract barium from the bronchial tree, and prophylactic antibiotic therapy is important to prevent lung infection (TAMM and KORTSIK 1999). Water-soluble low osmolar contrast media, which are better tolerated, should be used instead of barium preparations if there is a possibility of aspiration during an upper GIT examination (GINAI et al. 1994).

Hypersensitivity reactions to products used during barium meal examinations are extremely rare (MORCOS 2000). Barium sulphate is generally regarded as an inert and insoluble compound that is neither absorbed nor metabolized and is eliminated unchanged from the body. However, some studies have demonstrated that very small amounts of barium ions can be absorbed from the GIT. Isolated cases of barium encephalopathy have been attributed to absorption of barium following the use of barium sulphate (MORCOS 2000). Plasma and urine barium levels can be elevated after oral barium sulphate administration. In addition, many additives are present in commercial barium products and are essentially the same as the additives used in food products. Some of these agents are capable of inducing an immune response. A patient with a history of a severe reaction to barium agents should not receive barium products again (MORCOS and BROWN 1999; SEYMOUR and KESACK 1997; STRINGER et al. 1993).

Reactions to other constituents of barium sulphate enemas are now being recognized with increasing frequency and could be as common as one in 1,000 (MORCOS 2000). They vary from urticarial rashes to severe anaphylactic collapse, and can be particularly severe in patients with asthma (MORCOS 2000). Hypersensitivity to the latex balloon catheter used in double contrast barium enemas appears to be a common mechanism (OWNBY et al. 1991), but hypersensitivity to glucagon, to the preservative methylparaben, or to other additives seems to be responsible in some cases (MORCOS 2000).

A fatal case of poisoning resulted from the use of barium sulfide that had been mistaken for barium sulphate has been reported (MORCOS 2000). A guideline on the safe use of barium preparations can be found in the Chap. 29.

References

Almen T, Aspelin P (1995) Contrast media in diagnostic radiology. In: Pettersson H (ed) The NICER centennial book 1995. A global textbook of radiology, Chap 7. NICER Institute, Lund, p 131

Bechem C, Gunther H (1910) Barium sulphate as a shadow-forming contrast medium in radiological investigations. Z Rontgenk Radiumfortschr 12:369–376

Ginai AZ, Ten Kate FJW, Ten Berg RGM, Hoornstra K (1994) Experimental evaluation of various available contrast agents for use in the upper gastrointestinal tract in case of suspected leakage. Effects on lungs. Br J Radiol 57:895–901

Glauser T, Savioz D, Grossholz M et al (1999) Venous intravasation of Gastrografin: a serious but underestimated complication. Eur J Surg 165:274–277

Gray C, Sivaloganathan S, Simkins KC (1980) Aspiration of high-density barium contrast medium causing acute pulmonary inflammation – report of two fatal cases in elderly women with disordered swallowing. Clin Radiol 40:397

Lareau DG, Berta JW (1976) Fatal aspiration of thick barium. Radiology 120:317

Morcos SK (2000) Radiological contrast media. In: Dukes MNG, Aronson JKS (eds) Side effects of drugs, 14th edn, Chap 46.1. Elsevier, Amsterdam, pp 1603–1605

Morcos SK, Brown P (1999) Radiological contrast agents. In: Aronson JK (ed) Side effects of drugs, annual 24, Chap 46. Elsevier, Amsterdam, p 503

Morcos SK, Brown P (2001) Radiological contrast agents. In: Aronson JK (ed) Side effects of drugs, annual 24, Chap 46. Elsevier, Amsterdam, pp 524–525

Ownby DR, Tomlanovich M, Sammons N et al (1991) Anaphylaxis associated with latex allergy during barium enema examinations. AJR Am J Roentgenol 156:903–908

Regan JK, O'Neil HK, Aizenstein RI (1999) Small bowel carcinoid presenting as a barolith. Clin Imaging 23:22–25

Seymour PC, Kesack CD (1997) Anaphylactic shock during a routine upper gastrointestinal series. AJR Am J Roentgenol 168:957–958

Smith HJ, Jones K, Hunter TB (1988) What happens to patients after upper and lower gastrointestinal studies? Invest Radiol 23:822

Stringer DA, Hassal E, Ferguson AC et al (1993) Hypersensitivity reaction to single contrast barium meal studies in children. Paediatr Radiol 23:587–588

Tamm I, Kortsik C (1999) Severe barium sulfate aspiration into the lung: clinical presentation, prognosis and therapy. Respiration 66:81–84

Wheatley MJ, Eckhauser FE (1991) Portal venous barium intravasation complicating barium enema examination. Surgery 109:788–791

Williams SM, Harned RK (1991) Recognition and prevention of barium enema complications. Curr Probl Diagn Radiol 20:123–151

Zheutlin N, Lasser EC, Rigler LG (1952) Clinical studies on the effect of barium in the peritoneal cavity following rupture of the colon. Surgery 32:967

Appendix

ESUR Guidelines on Contrast Media

ACADEMIC MEMBERS* OF THE CONTRAST MEDIA SAFETY COMMITTEE

29.1

Introduction

Since 1996, the Contrast Media Safety Committee has reviewed all safety aspects of contrast media to produce a comprehensive set of simple, practical guidelines. The evidence on which the guidelines are based has been summarized in the preceding chapters. The most recent version of the guidelines (version 7.0) is presented in this chapter.

29.2

Non-Renal Adverse Reactions

29.2.1
Acute Adverse Reactions

Definition: An adverse reaction that occurs within 1 h of contrast medium injection.

---

*Academic members of the Contrast Medium Safety Committee during preparation of the Guidelines:
Henrik S. Thomsen, Sameh K. Morcos, Torsten Almén, Peter Aspelin, Per Liss, Marie-France Bellin, Raymond Oyen, Gertraud Heinz-Peer, Jarl Å. Jakobsen, Fulvio Stacul, Judith A. W. Webb, and Aart van der Molen

Classification	
Mild	Nausea, mild vomiting, urticaria, itching
Moderate	Severe vomiting, marked urticaria, bronchospasm, facial/laryngeal edema, vasovagal attack
Severe	Hypotensive shock, respiratory arrest, cardiac arrest, convulsion

29.2.1.1
Acute Adverse Reactions to Iodinated Contrast Media

Risk factors for acute reactions	
Patient related	Patient with a history of • Previous moderate or severe acute reaction (see classification above) to an iodinated agent • Asthma • Allergy requiring medical treatment
Contrast medium related	• High osmolality ionic contrast media
To reduce the risk of an acute reaction	
For all patients	• Use a nonionic contrast medium • Keep the patient in the Radiology Department for 30 min after contrast medium injection • Have the drugs and equipment for resuscitation readily available (see Sect. 29.2.1.3)
For patients at increased risk of reaction (see risk factors above)	• Consider an *alternative test* not requiring an iodinated contrast agent • Use a *different iodinated agent* for previous reactors to contrast medium • Consider the use of *premedication*. Clinical evidence of the effectiveness of premedication is limited. If used, a suitable premedication regime is prednisolone 30 mg (or methylprednisolone 32 mg) orally given 12 and 2 h before contrast medium
Extravascular administration of iodinated contrast media	When absorption or leakage into the circulation is possible, take the same precautions as for intravascular administration.

29.2.1.2
Acute Adverse Reactions to Gadolinium Contrast Media (Non-organ Specific)

Note: The risk of an acute reaction to a gadolinium contrast agent is significantly lower than the risk with an iodinated contrast agent.

Risk factors for acute reactions	
Patient related	Patients with a history of • Previous acute reaction to gadolinium contrast agent • Asthma • Allergy requiring medical treatment
Contrast medium related	The risk of reaction is not related to the osmolality of the contrast agent: the low doses used make the osmolar load very small
To reduce the risk of an acute reaction	
For all patients	• Keep the patient in the Radiology Department for 30 min after contrast medium injection • Have the drugs and equipment for resuscitation readily available (see Sect. 29.2.1.3)
For patients at increased risk of reaction (see risk factors above)	• Consider an *alternative test* not requiring a gadolinium agent • Use a *different gadolinium agent* for previous reactors to contrast medium • Consider the use of *premedication*. There is no clinical evidence of the effectiveness of premedication. If used, a suitable premedication regime is prednisolone 30 mg (or methylprednisolone 32 mg) orally given 12 and 2 h before contrast medium

29.2.1.3
Management of Acute Adverse Reactions

First line emergency drugs and instruments that should be in the examination room.

Oxygen
Adrenaline 1:1,000
Antihistamine H1 – suitable for injection
Atropine
β2-agonist metered dose inhaler
I.V. Fluids – normal saline or Ringers solution
Anti-convulsive drugs (diazepam)
Sphygmomanometer
One-way mouth "breather" apparatus

Simple guidelines for first line treatment of acute reactions to contrast media

Nausea/Vomiting

Transient: Supportive treatment

Severe, protracted: Appropriate antiemetic drugs should be considered.

Urticaria

Scattered, transient: Supportive treatment including observation.

Scattered, protracted: Appropriate H1-antihistamine intramuscularly or intravenously should be considered. Drowsiness and/or hypotension may occur.

Profound: Consider adrenaline 1:1,000, 0.1–0.3 ml (0.1–0.3 mg) intramuscularly in adults, 50% of adult dose to children between 6 and 12 years old and 25% of adult dose to children below 6 years old. Repeat as needed.

Bronchospasm

1. Oxygen by mask ($6–10\,l\,min^{-1}$)
2. β-2-agonist metered dose inhaler (2–3 deep inhalations)
3. Adrenaline
   Normal blood pressure
   Intramuscular: 1:1,000, 0.1–0.3 ml (0.1–0.3 mg) [use smaller dose in a patient with coronary artery disease or elderly patient]
   In pediatric patients: $0.01\,mg\,kg^{-1}$ up to 0.3 mg max.
   Decreased blood pressure
   Intramuscular: 1:1,000, 0.5 ml (0.5 mg),
   In pediatric patients:
      6–12 years: 0.3 ml (0.3 mg) intramuscularly
      <6 years: 0.15 ml (0.15 mg) intramuscularly

Laryngeal edema

1. Oxygen by mask ($6–10\,l\,min^{-1}$)
2. Intramuscular adrenaline (1:1,000), 0.5 ml (0.5 mg) for adults, repeat as needed.
   In pediatric patients:
      6–12 years: 0.3 ml (0.3 mg) intramuscularly
      <6 years: 0.15 ml (0.15 mg) intramuscularly

Hypotension
Isolated hypotension

1. Elevate patient's legs
2. Oxygen by mask (6–10 l min^{-1})
3. Intravenous fluid: rapidly, normal saline, or lactated Ringer's solution
4. If unresponsive: adrenaline: 1:1,000, 0.5 ml (0.5 mg) intramuscularly, repeat as needed
     In pediatric patients:
          6–12 years: 0.3 ml (0.3 mg) intramuscularly
          <6 years: 0.15 ml (0.15 mg) intramuscularly

Vagal reaction (hypotension and bradycardia)

1. Elevate patient's legs
2. Oxygen by mask (6–10 l min^{-1})
3. Atropine 0.6–1.0 mg intravenously, repeat if necessary after 3–5 min, to 3 mg total (0.04 mg kg^{-1}) in adults. In pediatric patients give 0.02 mg kg^{-1} intravenously (max 0.6 mg per dose) repeat if necessary to 2 mg total.
4. Intravenous fluids: rapidly, normal saline, or lactated Ringer's solution

29.2.1.4
Generalized anaphylactoid reaction

1. Call for resuscitation team
2. Suction airway as needed
3. Elevate patient's legs if hypotensive
4. Oxygen by mask (6–10 l min^{-1})
5. Intramuscular adrenaline (1:1,000), 0.5 ml (0.5 mg) in adults. Repeat as needed.
     In pediatric patients:
          6–12 years: 0.3 ml (0.3 mg) intramuscularly
          <6 years: 0.15 ml (0.15 mg) intramuscularly
6. Intravenous fluids (e.g., normal saline, lactated Ringer's)
7. H1-blocker, for example, diphenhydramine 25–50 mg intravenously

29.2.2
Late Adverse Reactions

Definition: An adverse reaction which occurs 1 hour to 1 week after contrast medium injection.

Type of reaction	
Iodinated contrast media	• A variety of late symptoms (e.g., nausea, vomiting, headache, musculoskeletal pain, fever) have been described following contrast medium, but many are not related to contrast medium. • *Skin reactions* of similar type to other drug eruptions are true late adverse reactions. They are usually mild to moderate and self limiting.
Gadolinium contrast media	Nephrogenic systemic fibrosis usually presents after 1 week but may occur earlier (see Sect. 29.2.3)
Skin reactions following iodinated contrast medium administration	
Risk factors	• Previous contrast medium reaction • Interleukin-2 treatment

Prophylaxis	Generally not recommended
	Patients who have had a previous serious late adverse reaction can be given steroid prophylaxis (see Sect. 29.2.1.1)
Management	Symptomatic and similar to the management of other drug induced skin reactions
Recommendation	Tell patients who have had a previous contrast reaction or who are on interleukin-2 treatment that a late skin reaction is possible and that they should contact a doctor if they have a problem.

29.2.3
Very Late Adverse Reactions

Definition: An adverse reaction that usually occurs more than 1 week after contrast medium injection.

Type of reaction	
Iodinated contrast media	Thyrotoxicosis
Gadolinium contrast media	Nephrogenic systemic fibrosis
Thyrotoxicosis	
At risk	• Patients with untreated Graves' disease
	• Patients with multinodular goiter and thyroid autonomy, especially if they are elderly and/or live in area of dietary iodine deficiency
Not at risk	Patients with normal thyroid function
Recommendations	• *Iodinated contrast media should not be given to patients with manifest hyperthyroidism.*
	• Prophylaxis is generally not necessary.
	• In selected high-risk patients, prophylactic treatment may be given by an endocrinologist; this is more relevant in areas of dietary iodine deficiency.
	• Patients at risk should be closely monitored by endocrinologists after iodinated contrast medium injection.
	• Intravenous cholangiographic contrast media should not be given to patients at risk.

Nephrogenic systemic fibrosis

The link between nephrogenic systemic fibrosis (NSF) and gadolinium-based contrast agents was recognized only in 2006. Information about NSF continues to be collected and it may be necessary to review these guidelines as new information becomes available.

Clinical features of NSF	**Onset:** From the day of exposure for up to 2–3 months, sometimes up to years after exposure.
	Initially
	• Pain
	• Pruritus
	• Swelling
	• Erythema
	• Usually starts in the legs
	Later
	• Thickened skin and subcutaneous tissues – "woody" texture and brawny plaques
	• Fibrosis of internal organs, e.g., muscle, diaphragm, heart, liver, lungs
	Result
	• Contractures
	• Cachexia
	• Death, in a proportion of patients

Patients	
At higher risk	• Patients with CKD 4 and 5 (GFR <30 ml min^{-1}) • Patients on dialysis • Patients with reduced renal function who have had or are awaiting liver transplantation
At lower risk	• Patients with CKD 3 (GFR 30–59 ml min^{-1}) • Children under 1 year, because of their immature renal function
Not at risk of NSF	Patients with normal renal function

Contrast agents: Classification and Recommendations	

Highest risk of NSF
• *Contrast agents*
	Gadodiamide (Omniscan®)
	    Ligand: Nonionic linear chelate (DTPA-BMA)
	    Incidence of NSF: 3–7% in at-risk subjects
	
	Gadopentetate dimeglumine (Magnevist®)
	    Ligand: Ionic linear chelate (DTPA)
	    Incidence of NSF: Estimated to be 0.1–1% in at-risk subjects
	
	Gadoversetamide (Optimark®)
	    Ligand: Nonionic linear chelate (DTPA-BMEA)
	    Incidence of NSF: Unknown.

• *Recommendations*	These agents are CONTRAINDICATED in
	    • patients with CKD 4 and 5 (GFR <30 ml min^{-1}), including those on dialysis
	    • patients with reduced renal function who have had or are awaiting liver transplantation
	
	These agents should be used with CAUTION in
	    • patients with CKD 3 (GFR 30–60 ml min^{-1})
	    • children less than 1 year old
	
	Serum creatinine (eGFR) measurement before administration: **Mandatory**

Intermediate risk of NSF
• *Contrast agents*
	Gadobenate dimeglumine (Multihance®)
	    Ligand: Ionic linear chelate (BOPTA)
	    Incidence of NSF: No unconfounded* cases have been reported.
	    Special feature: Similar diagnostic results can be achieved with lower doses because of its 2–3% protein binding.
	
	Gadofosveset trisodium (Vasovist®)
	    Ligand: Ionic linear chelate (DTPA-DPCP)
	    Incidence of NSF: No unconfounded* cases reported, but experience is limited
	    Special feature: It is a blood pool agent with affinity to albumin. Diagnostic results can be achieved with 50% lower doses than extracellular Gd-CM. Biological half-life is 12 times longer than for extracellular agents (18 h compared to 1½ h, respectively).
	
	Gadoxetate disodium (Primovist®)
	    Ligand: Ionic linear chelate *(EOB-DTPA)*
	    Incidence of NSF: No unconfounded* cases have been reported but experience is limited.
	    Special feature: Organ specific gadolinium contrast agent with 10% protein binding and 50% excretion by hepatocytes. Diagnostic results can be achieved with lower doses than extracellular Gd-CM.

• *Recommendation*	Serum creatinine (eGFR) measurement before administration: **Not mandatory**

Lowest risk of NSF
• *Contrast agents*
	Gadobutrol (Gadovist®)
	    Ligand: Nonionic cyclic chelate (BT-DO3A)
	    Incidence of NSF: No unconfounded* cases have been reported.

	Gadoterate meglumine (Dotarem®)
	    Ligand: Ionic cyclic chelate (DOTA)
	
	    Incidence of NSF: No unconfounded* cases have been reported.
	
	Gadoteridol (Prohance®)
	    Ligand: Nonionic cyclic chelate (HP-DO3A)
	
	    Incidence of NSF: No unconfounded* cases have been reported.

• *Recommendation*	Serum creatinine (eGFR) measurement before administration: **Not mandatory**
Confounded cases	If two different Gd-CM had been injected, it is impossible to determine with certainty which agent triggered the development of NSF and the situation is described as "confounded." However the agent which is most likely responsible is the one which has triggered NSF in other unconfounded situations.
Recommendation for all patients	In all patients use the smallest amount of contrast medium necessary for a diagnostic result. Never deny a patient a clinically well-indicated enhanced MRI examination. Always use an agent that leaves the smallest amount of gadolinium in the body.

29.3

Renal Adverse Reactions

Definition: Contrast medium nephrotoxicity is a condition in which an impairment in renal function *(an increase in serum creatinine by more than 25% or 44 μmol l⁻¹ (0.5 mg dl⁻¹))* occurs within 3 days following the intravascular administration of a contrast medium (CM) in the absence of an alternative etiology.

29.3.1
Renal Adverse Reactions to Iodinated Contrast Media

Risk factors for contrast medium induced nephropathy	
Patient related	• eGFR less than 60 ml min⁻¹ 1.73 m⁻² (or raised serum creatinine) particularly if secondary to diabetic nephropathy • Dehydration • Congestive heart failure • Gout • Age over 70 • Concurrent administration of nephrotoxic drugs, e.g., non-steroid anti-inflammatory drugs.
Contrast medium related	• High osmolality contrast media • Large doses of contrast medium
Risk of iodinated contrast media in patients taking metformin	
Lactic acidosis	Metformin is excreted unchanged in the urine. In the presence of renal failure, either pre-existing or induced by iodinated contrast medium, metformin may accumulate in sufficient amounts to cause lactic acidosis
Note	Metformin does not cause renal failure

29.3.1.1
Time of Referral

Elective Examination

(1) Identify patients with eGFR less than 60 ml min^{-1} 1.73 m^{-2} (or raised serum creatinine)	

• Patients with known eGFR less than 60 ml min^{-1} 1.73 m^{-2} (or raised serum creatinine)
• Diabetic patients taking metformin
• Patients who will receive intra-arterial contrast medium
• Patients who have a history suggesting the possibility of reduced GFR:
   ○ Renal disease
   ○ Renal surgery
   ○ Proteinuria
   ○ Diabetes mellitus
   ○ Hypertension
   ○ Gout
   ○ Recent nephrotoxic drugs
	Measure eGFR (or serum creatinine) within 7 days of contrast medium administration

(2) Identify diabetic patients taking metformin	
	Depending on eGFR/ serum creatinine level, metformin will have to be stopped either before or at the time of contrast medium administration (see 29.3.1.2)

Emergency Examination

(1)   Identify patients with eGFR less than 60 ml min^{-1} 1.73 m^{-2} (or raised serum creatinine) if possible.

(2)   Identify diabetic patients taking metformin
- Measure eGFR (or serum creatinine) if the procedure can be deferred until the result is available without harm to the patient
- In extreme emergency, if eGFR (or serum creatinine) measurement cannot be obtained, follow the protocol for patients with eGFR less than 60 ml min^{-1} 1.73 m^{-2} (or raised serum creatinine) as closely as clinical circumstances permit.

29.3.1.2
Before the Examination

Elective examination	
Patients *with eGFR less than 60 ml min^{-1} 1.73 m^{-2} (or raised serum creatinine)* and those *at increased risk of nephrotoxicity* (see risk factors above)	• Consider an alternative imaging method not using iodinated contrast media • Stop nephrotoxic drugs, mannitol, and loop diuretics at least 24 h before contrast medium administration • Start hydration. A suitable intravenous regime is 1 ml kg^{-1} b.w. per hour of normal saline for at least 6 h before and after the procedure. In hot climates the volume should be increased.
Diabetic patients taking metformin	• If *eGFR is greater than 60 ml min^{-1} 1.73 m^{-2}* the patient can continue to take metformin • If *eGFR is between 30 and 60 ml min^{-1} 1.73 m^{-2} (or serum creatinine is raised)* stop metformin 48 h before contrast medium administration and remain off metformin for 48 h after contrast medium. Only restart metformin if serum creatinine is unchanged 48 h after contrast medium. • If *eGFR is less than 30 ml min^{-1} 1.73 m^{-2}*, metformin is not approved in most countries and iodinated contrast medium should be avoided if possible.

Emergency examination	
Patients at increased risk of nephrotoxicity	• Consider an alternative imaging method not using iodinated contrast media. • Start intravenous hydration as early possible before contrast medium administration (See elective examination, above).

Diabetic patients taking metformin	• If *eGFR is greater than 60 ml min^{-1} 1.73 m^{-2} (or serum creatinine is normal)*, follow instructions for elective patients.
	• If *eGFR is between 30 and 60 ml min^{-1} 1.73 m^{-2} (or serum creatinine is raised) or unknown*, weigh the risks and benefits of contrast medium administration and consider an alternative imaging method. If contrast medium is deemed essential take the following precautions:
	  ° Metformin therapy should be stopped.
	  ° The patient should be hydrated (e.g., at least 1 ml h^{-1} kg^{-1} b.w. of intravenous normal saline up to 6 h after contrast medium administration – In hot climates more fluid should be given).
	  ° Monitor renal function (eGFR/serum creatinine), serum lactic acid and pH of blood.
	  ° Look for symptoms of lactic acidosis (vomiting, somnolence, nausea, epigastric pain, anorexia, hyperpnea, lethargy, diarrhea, and thirst). Blood test results indicative of lactic acidosis: pH ≤ 7.25 with plasma lactate ≥5 mmol l^{-1}.

29.3.1.3
Time of Examination

In patients at increased risk of contrast medium induced nephropathy	• Use low or iso-osmolar contrast media • Use the lowest dose of contrast medium consistent with a diagnostic result
In patients with no increased risk of contrast medium induced nephropathy	• Use the lowest dose of contrast medium consistent with a diagnostic result

29.3.1.4
After the Examination

In patients with eGFR less than 60 ml min^{-1} 1.173 m^{-2} (or raised serum creatinine)	Continue hydration for at least 6 h
In diabetic patients taking metformin who have eGFR less than 60 ml min^{-1} 1.173 m^{-2}	Measure eGFR (or serum creatinine) at 48 h after contrast medium administration. If it has not worsened, metformin can be restarted. Metformin is not approved in most countries in patients with abnormal renal function.

Note: No **pharmacological manipulation** (with renal vasodilators, receptor antagonists of endogenous vasoactive mediators, or cytoprotective drugs) has yet been shown to offer consistent protection against contrast medium induced nephropathy.

29.3.2
Renal Adverse Reactions to Gadolinium Contrast Media (Non-organ Specific)

MR Examinations

• The risk of nephrotoxicity is very low when gadolinium contrast media are used in approved doses.

Radiographic Examinations

• Gadolinium contrast media should not be used for radiographic examinations in patients with renal impairment.
• Gadolinium contrast media are more nephrotoxic than iodinated contrast media in equivalent X-ray attenuating doses.

29.3.3
Dialysis and Contrast Medium Administration

All contrast media, iodinated and gadolinium, can be removed by hemodialysis or peritoneal dialysis. However, there is no evidence that hemodialysis protects patients with impaired renal function from contrast medium induced nephropathy or nephrogenic systemic fibrosis. To avoid the risk of NSF please refer to Sect. 29.2.3.

Patients on dialysis who receive iodinated or gadolinium contrast medium	
Hemodialysis	• Avoid osmotic and fluid overload • Correlation of time of the contrast medium injection with the hemodialysis session is unnecessary. • Extra hemodialyis session to remove contrast medium is unnecessary.
Continuous ambulatory peritoneal dialysis	• Hemodialyis to remove the contrast medium is unnecessary

29.4
Miscellaneous

29.4.1
Contrast Medium Extravasation

Type of injuries	• Most injuries are minor • Severe injuries include skin ulceration, soft tissue necrosis, and compartment syndrome
Risk factors	
Technique related	• Use of a power injector. • Less optimal injection sites including lower limb and small distal veins • Large volume of contrast medium • High osmolar contrast media
Patient related	• Inability to communicate • Fragile or damaged veins • Arterial insufficiency • Compromised lymphatic and/or venous drainage • Obesity
To reduce the risk	• Intravenous technique should always be meticulous using an appropriate sized plastic cannula placed in a suitable vein to handle the flow rate used during the injection • Test injection with normal saline • Use nonionic iodinated contrast medium

Treatment	• Conservative management is adequate in most cases
	  ○ limb elevation
	  ○ apply ice packs
	  ○ careful monitoring
	• If a serious injury is suspected, seek the advice of a surgeon

29.4.2
Pulmonary Effects of Iodinated Contrast Media

Pulmonary adverse effects	• Bronchospasm • Increased pulmonary vascular resistance • Pulmonary edema
Patients at high risk	• History of asthma • History of pulmonary hypertension • Incipient cardiac failure
To reduce the risk of pulmonary adverse effects	• Use low or iso-osmolar contrast media • Avoid large doses of contrast media

29.4.3
Effects of Iodinated Contrast Media on Blood and Endothelium

The clinically important adverse effect of iodinated contrast media on blood and endothelium is thrombosis. It is recognized that

- All contrast media have anticoagulant properties, especially ionic agents
- High osmolar ionic contrast media may induce thrombosis due to endothelial damage, particularly in phlebographic procedures
- Drugs and interventional devices that decrease the risk of thromboembolic complications during interventional procedures minimize the importance of the effects of contrast media

Guidelines

- Meticulous angiographic technique is mandatory and is the most important factor in reducing thromboembolic complications.
- Low- or isoosmolar contrast media should be used for diagnostic and interventional angiographic procedures including phlebography.

29.4.4
Contrast Media and Catecholamine Producing Tumors
(Pheochromocytoma and Paraganglioma)

Preparation

Tumor localization when catecholamine-producing tumor detected biochemically
(a) Before intravenous contrast medium (iodinated or gadolinium): α- and β-adrenergic blockade with orally administered drugs under the supervision of the referring physician is advised. Further α-blockade with intravenous phenoxybenzamine is not necessary.
(b) Before intra-arterial iodinated contrast medium: α- and β-adrenergic blockade with orally administered drugs and α-blockade with intravenous phenoxybenzamine under the supervision of the referring physician are recommended
Characterization of incidentally detected adrenal mass
No special preparation

Type of contrast medium that should be used

Iodinated: nonionic agent
Gadolinium: any agent, ionic or nonionic

29.4.5
Pregnancy and Lactation

	Iodinated agents	Gadolinium agents
Pregnancy	(a) In exceptional circumstances, when radiographic examination is essential, iodinated contrast media may be given to the pregnant female. (b) Following administration of iodinated agents to the mother during pregnancy, thyroid function should be checked in the neonate during the first week.	(a) When there is a very strong indication for enhanced MR, the smallest possible dose of the most stable gadolinium contrast agent (macrocyclic agents) may be given to the pregnant female. (b) Following administration of gadolinium agents to the mother during pregnancy, no neonatal tests are necessary.
Lactation	Breast feeding may be continued normally when iodinated agents are given to the mother.	Breast feeding should be avoided for 24 h after contrast medium.
Pregnant or lactating mother with renal impairment	See renal adverse reactions (29.3). No additional precautions are necessary for the fetus or neonate.	Do not administer gadolinium-based contrast agents

29.4.6
Interaction with Other Drugs and Clinical Tests

General recommendation	
	Be aware of the patient's drug history Keep a proper record of the contrast medium injection (time, dose, name) Do not mix contrast media with other drugs in tubes and syringes
Drugs needing special attention	
Metformin	Refer to Sect. 29.3

Nephrotoxic drugs
    Cyclosporine
    Cisplatin
    Aminoglycosides
    Non-steroid anti-inflammatory drugs
	Refer to Sect. 29.3

β-blocker	β-blockers may impair the response to treatment of bronchospasm induced by contrast medium
Interleukin-2	Refer Sect. 29.2.2

Biochemical assays	
Recommendation	Do not perform nonemergency biochemical analysis of blood and urine collected within 24 h of contrast medium injection.

Isotope studies and/or treatment	
Thyroid	Patients undergoing therapy with radioactive iodine should not have received iodinated contrast media for at least two months before treatment Isotope imaging of the thyroid should be avoided for two months after iodinated contrast medium injection
Bone, red blood cell labeling	Avoid iodinated contrast medium injection for at least 24 h before the isotope study

29.4.7
Safety of Ultrasound Contrast Media

Statement	• Ultrasound contrast media are generally safe
Contraindication	• Severe heart disease (e.g., New York class III/IV)
Type and severity of reactions	• The majority of reactions are minor (e.g., headache, nausea, sensation of heat, altered taste) and self-resolving
	• Allergy-like reactions occur rarely
To reduce the risk	• Check for intolerance to any of the components of the contrast agent
	• Use the lowest level of acoustic output and shortest scanning time to allow a diagnostic examination
Treatment	• If a serious event occurs – see 29.2.1.3

29.4.8
Safety of Liver Specific MR Contrast Media

Types of adverse reactions	Similar to reactions observed with other types of contrast media such as nausea, vomiting, urticaria, rash, generalized anaphylactoid reactions. Back pain may also occur with superparamagnetic iron oxides. Serious life threatening reactions are rare
Patients <18 years old	Safety has not yet been established

Contraindications	Iron oxides
	    Known allergy or hypersensitivity to parenteral iron or dextran
	
	Manganese based contrast media
	  • Known allergy to the preparation
	  • Pregnancy
	  • Lactation
	  • Severe liver impairment
	
	Gadolinium based contrast media
	    Known allergy to the preparation

Cautions	Iron oxides
	    In patients with hemosiderosis or hemochromatosis: iron-overload may be aggravated
	
	Manganese-based contrast media
	    Liver impairment and heart failure
	
	Gadolinium-based contrast media
	  • Agent with high hepatocyte uptake: liver and renal failure
	  • Agent with low hepatocyte uptake: renal failure
	  • Hepato-renal syndrome – see also Sect. 29.2.3

29.4.9
Safety of Barium Contrast Media

		Recommended action
Contraindications	Integrity of gut wall compromised	Use iodinated water-soluble contrast media
		In neonates and patients at risk of leakage into mediastinum and/or lungs use low- or isoosmolar contrast media
	Previous allergic reactions to barium products	Use iodinated water-soluble contrast media and be prepared to treat a reaction

Cautions	Bowel strictures	Use only small amounts
	Extensive colitis	Avoid barium enemas
Complications	Reduced bowel motility	Encourage fluid intake
	Venous intravasation	• Early identification and careful observation • Antibiotics and intravenous fluids • Emergency treatment may be needed
	Aspiration	• Bronchoscopic removal for large amounts • Chest physiotherapy • Antibiotics

29.5

Questionnaires to be Completed by Clinicians Referring Patients for Examinations Using Iodinated or Gadolinium Contrast Media

Questionnaire for iodine-based contrast media administration to be completed by the referring clinician

1. History of moderate or severe reaction to an iodinated contrast medium   ☐ Yes ☐ No
2. History of allergy requiring treatment   ☐ Yes ☐ No
3. History of asthma   ☐ Yes ☐ No
4. Hyperthyroidism   ☐ Yes ☐ No
5. Heart Failure   ☐ Yes ☐ No
6. Diabetes Mellitus   ☐ Yes ☐ No
7. History of renal disease   ☐ Yes ☐ No
8. Previous renal surgery   ☐ Yes ☐ No
9. History of proteinuria   ☐ Yes ☐ No
10. Hypertension   ☐ Yes ☐ No
11. Gout   ☐ Yes ☐ No
12. Most recent measurement of eGFR or serum creatinine   • Value...........................
       • Date ....
13. Is the patient currently taking any of the following drugs
    • Metformin   ☐ Yes ☐ No
    • Interleukin 2   ☐ Yes ☐ No
    • NSAIDs   ☐ Yes ☐ No
    • Aminoglycosides   ☐ Yes ☐ No
    • β-blockers   ☐ Yes ☐ No

Completed by _____ Date _____

Questionnaire for gadolinium contrast media administration to be completed by the referring clinician

1. History of moderate or severe reaction to a MRI contrast medium   ☐ Yes ☐ No
2. History of allergy requiring treatment   ☐ Yes ☐ No
3. History of asthma   ☐ Yes ☐ No
4. Has the patient end-stage renal failure (eGFR < 30 ml/min/1.73m^2) or is the patient on dialysis ?   ☐ Yes ☐ No
5. Has the patient reduced renal function (eGFR between 30 and 60 ml/min/1.73 m^2)   ☐ Yes ☐ No
6. History of hemosiderosis or hemochromatosis   ☐ Yes ☐ No
7. Previous reaction to dextran   ☐ Yes ☐ No

Completed by _____ Date _____

Aspelin P, Stacul F, Thomsen HS, Morcos SK, Molen AJvd, Members of Contrast Media Safety Committee of European Society of Urogenital Radiology (ESUR) (2006) Iodinated contrast media and blood interactions. Eur Radiol 16:1041–1049

Bellin M-F, Jakobsen JÅ, Tomassin I, Thomsen HS, Morcos SK, Members of the Contrast Media Safety Committee of the European Society of Urogenital Radiology (2002) Contrast medium extravasation injury: guidelines for prevention and management. Eur Radiol 12:2807–2812

Bellin M-F, Webb JAW, Molen AJvd, Thomsen HS, Morcos SK, Members of Contrast Media Safety Committee of European Society of Urogenital Radiology (ESUR) (2005) Safety of MR liver specific contrast media. Eur Radiol 15:1607–1614

ESUR Contrast Media Safety Committee (Thomsen HS) (2007) ESUR guideline: gadolinium-based contrast media and nephrogenic systemic fibrosis. Eur Radiol 17:2692–2696

Jakobsen JÅ, Oyen R, Thomsen HS, Morcos SK, Members of Contrast Media Safety Committee of European Society of Urogenital Radiology (ESUR) (2005) Safety of ultrasound contrast agents. Eur Radiol 15:941–945

Molen AJvd, Thomsen HS, Morcos SK, Members of Contrast Media Safety Committee of European Society of Urogenital Radiology (ESUR) (2004) Effect of iodinated contrast media on thyroid function in adults. Eur Radiol 14:902–906

Morcos SK, Bellin M-F, Thomsen HS, Almén T, Aspelin P, Heinz-Peer G, Jakobsen JÅ, Liss P, Oyen R, Stacul F, Van der Molen AJ, Webb JAW (2008) Reducing the risk of iodine-based and MRI contrast media administration: recommendation for a questionnaire at the time of booking. Eur J Radiol 66:225–229

Morcos SK, Thomsen HS, Exley CM, Members of Contrast Media Safety Committee of European Society of Urogenital Radiology (ESUR) (2005) Contrast media: interaction with other drugs and clinical tests. Eur Radiol 15:1463–1468

Morcos SK, Thomsen HS, Webb JAW, Members of Contrast Media Safety Committee of the European Society of Urogenital Radiology (ESUR) (1999) Contrast media induced nephrotoxicity: a consensus report. Eur Radiol 9:1602–1613

Morcos SK, Thomsen HS, Webb JAW, Members of Contrast Media Safety Committee of the European Society of Urogenital Radiology (ESUR) (2001) Prevention of generalized reactions to contrast media: a consensus report and guidelines. Eur Radiol 11:1720–1728

Morcos SK, Thomsen HS, Webb JAW, Members of the Contrast Media Safety Committee of European Society of Urogenital Radiology (2002) Dialysis and contrast media. Eur Radiol 12:3026–3030

Thomsen HS (ed.) (2006) Contrast media. Safety issues and ESUR guidelines, 1st ed. Heidelberg, Springer

Thomsen HS, Almén T, Morcos SK, Members of Contrast Media Safety Committee of European Society of Urogenital Radiology (2002) Gadolinium-containing contrast media for radiographic examinations: a position paper. Eur Radiol 12:2600–2605

Thomsen HS, Morcos SK, Members of Contrast Media Safety Committee of the European Society of Urogenital Radiology (ESUR) (1999) Contrast media and metformin. Guidelines to diminish the risk of lactic acidosis in non-insulin dependent diabetics after administration of contrast media. Eur Radiol 9:738–740

Thomsen HS, Morcos SK, Members of Contrast Media Safety Committee of European Society of Urogenital Radiology (ESUR) (2004) Management of acute adverse reactions to contrast media. Eur Radiol 14:476–481

Thomsen HS, Morcos SK, Members of Contrast Media Safety Committee of European Society of Urogenital Radiology (ESUR) (2005) In which patients should serum-creatinine be measured before contrast medium administration? Eur Radiol 15:749–754

Webb JAW, Stacul F, Thomsen HS, Morcos SK, Members of the Contrast Media Safety Committee of the European Society of Urogenital Radiology (ESUR) (2003) Late adverse reactions to intravascular iodinated contrast media. Eur Radiol 13:181–184

Webb JAW, Thomsen HS, Morcos SK, Members of Contrast Media Safety Committee of European Society of Urogenital Radiology (ESUR) (2005) The use of iodinated and gadolinium contrast media during pregnancy and lactation. Eur Radiol 15:1234–1240

Members of the Contrast Media Safety Committee (Spring 2008)

Henrik S. Thomsen (DK) **Chairman**, Sameh K. Morcos (UK) **Secretary**, Torsten Almén (SE), Peter Aspelin (SE), Per Liss (SE), Marie-France Bellin (FR), Raymond Oyen (BE), Edwin T. den Braber (DE) *Covidien*, Gertraud Heinz-Peer (AT), Jean-Marc Idée (FR) *Guerbet*, Andrea Löwe (DE) *Bayer-Schering-Pharma*, Jarl Å. Jakobsen (NO), Alberto Spinazzi (IT) *Bracco*, Fulvio Stacul (IT), Judith A. W. Webb (UK), Aart van der Molen (NL)

Subject Index

List of Contributors

Peter Aspelin, MD
Department of Radiology
Karolinska University Hospital
SE-14186 Stockholm
Sweden

Email: peter.aspelin@ki.se

Marie-France Bellin, MD
Professor, Department of Radiology
University Paris-Sud 11
Paul Brousse Hospital
AP-HP, 12-14 Av. Paul Vaillant Couturier
FR-94804 Villejuif Cedex,
France

Email: marie-france.bellin@pbr.ap-hop-paris.fr

Giuseppe Biondi-Zoccai, MD
Meta-Analysis and Evidence Based Medicine Training
in Cardiology (METCARDIO)
Via Aurelia Levante 5
IT-18104 Ospedaletti
Italy

Email: gbiondizoccai@gmail.com

Gertraud Heinz-Peer, MD
Department of Radiology
Medical University of Vienna, AKH
Waehringer Gurtel 18-20
AT-1090 Vienna
Austria

Email: gertraud.heinz@meduniwien.ac.at

Jarl Å. Jakobsen, MD
Professor, Department of Diagnostic Radiology
Rikshospitalet
NO-0027 Oslo
Norway

Email: jarl.jakobsen@rikshospitalet.no

Marzia Lotrionte, MD
Cardiology and Cardiac Rehabilitation Unit
Catholic University
Largo A. Gemelli 8
IT-00136 Rome
Italy

Sameh K. Morcos, FRCS, FFRRCSI, FRCR
Department of Diagnostic Imaging
Northern General Hospital
Sheffield Teaching Hospitals NHS Trust
Herries Road
Sheffield S5 7AU
UK

Email: sameh.morcos@sth.nhs.uk

Raymond Oyen, MD, PHD
Adjunct Clinic Head
Department of Radiology
Catholic University of Leuven
Herestraat 49
BE-3000 Leuven
Belgium

Email: raymond.oyen@uzleuven.be

June M. Raine, MD
Medicines Control and Healthcare Products Agency
Market Towers
1 Nine Elms Lane
London, SW8 5NQ
UK

Email: June.Raine@mhra.gsi.gov.uk

Fulvio Stacul
S.C. Radiologia
Ospedale Maggiore
Piazza Ospitale 1
IT-34134 Trieste
Italy

Email: fulvio.stacul@aots.sanita.fvg.it

Doris I. Stenver, MD, MPA
Chief Medical Officer, Danish Medicines Agency
Member of the CHMP Pharmacovigilance Working Party
Danish Medicines Agency
Axel Heides Gade 1
DK-2300 Copenhagen S
Denmark

Email: dis@dkma.dk

Henrik S. Thomsen, MD
Professor of Radiology
Chairman, Department of Diagnostic Radiology 542E
Copenhagen University Hospital, Herlev
Faculty of Health Sciences
University of Copenhagen
Herlev Ringvej 75
DK-2730 Herlev
Denmark

Email: hentho01@heh.regionh.dk

Aart J. van der Molen, MD
Department of Radiology – C2-S
Leiden University Medical Center
P.O. Box 9600
NL-2300 RC Leiden
The Netherlands

Email: Aart.vdmolen@planet.nl and molen@lumc.nl

Judith A.W. Webb, MD, FRCP, FRCR
Consultant (retired)
Department of Diagnostic Radiology
St Bartholomews Hospital
West Smithfield
London EC1A 7BE
UK

Email: jawwebb@btopenworld.com

MEDICAL RADIOLOGY Diagnostic Imaging and Radiation Oncology

Titles in the series already published

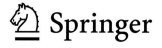

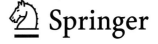 Springer

Printing and Binding: Stürtz GmbH, Würzburg